Label-Free Technologies For Drug Discovery

T0375239

Label-Free Technologies
For Drug Discovery

Editors

Matthew Cooper
Institute for Molecular Bioscience,
University of Queensland, Australia

Lorenz M. Mayr
Biology Unit, Protease Platform, Novartis Pharma AG,
Basel, Switzerland

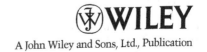

A John Wiley and Sons, Ltd., Publication

This edition first published 2011
© 2011 John Wiley & Sons, Ltd

Registered office
John Wiley & Sons Ltd, The Atrium, Southern Gate, Chichester, West Sussex, PO19 8SQ,
United Kingdom

For details of our global editorial offices, for customer services and for information about how to
apply for permission to reuse the copyright material in this book please see our website at
www.wiley.com.

Library of Congress Cataloging-in-Publication Data

Label-free technologies for drug discovery / editors, Matthew Cooper, Lorenz M. Mayr.
   p. ; cm.
   Includes bibliographical references and index.
   ISBN 978-0-470-74683-7 (cloth)
   1. Drug development.   I. Cooper, M. A. (Matthew A.)   II. Mayr, M. Lorenz.
   [DNLM: 1. Drug Discovery   2. Biosensing Techniques.   3. Drug Design. QV 744]
   RM301.25.L33   2011
   615'.19–dc22
                                     2010042191

A catalogue record for this book is available from the British Library.

Print ISBN: 9780470746837
ePDF ISBN: 9780470979136
oBook ISBN: 9780470979129
ePub ISBN: 9781119990277

Typeset in 10.5/13pt Sabon by Aptara Inc., New Delhi, India.

Contents

Preface

In the 1980s, surface plasmon resonance (SPR) and related techniques exploiting evanescent waves were first applied to the interrogation of biological and chemical interactions. These techniques allowed us to study the interaction between immobilized receptors and analytes in real time and without labelling of the analyte; leading to the term 'label-free'. While initially intended as a method of determining affinities, the use of a microfluidic delivery system to the sensor interface allowed kinetics (on and off rates of binding) to be measured. This, in turn, allowed new questions on compound action to be addressed and new compound optimization strategies to be explored. Today it is generally accepted that observed binding rates and binding levels can be interpreted to provide information on the specificity, kinetics and affinity of a drug–receptor interaction that relate to compound mode of action. This builds on the most often quoted maxim used in selecting bioactive compounds; *'Corpora non agunt nisi fixate'*: a drug will not work unless it is bound (Paul Ehrlich; 1854–1915). This now axiomatic statement guided Ehrlich through many scientific discoveries covering haematology, immunology, bacteriology and early chemotherapy. In the drug discovery process, we are now having to consider not just equilibrium-based, static descriptors of drug–receptor interactions (e.g. IC_{50} and EC_{50}), but also descriptors of the *dynamic* nature of drug action. For example, similarly structured molecules can bind to a target with similar affinity. However, only one may have a slow enough off rate to effectively block action of an endogenous ligand; only one may bind in an orientation suitable for a catalytic reaction; only one may induce a conformational change in the receptor. At the extreme, two similarly structured molecules may bind with similar affinity, but one may initiate the receptor response (an agonist), whereas the other may block the response (an antagonist). Optimal binding mechanisms can thus define the therapeutic index and the utility of a drug. Label-free techniques can hence help us understand and optimize these parameters, particularly with respect to predictive pharmacodynamics, competition/interaction with endogenous ligands, binding to side effect profiling targets and metabolic enzyme, and many other attributes that lead to differentiation of a drug candidate from competitor compounds.

Since the development of the first commercial label-free biosensors in the late 1980s, their use in research and development has been described in over 5000 scientific publications covering most disciplines found in the pharmaceutical and diagnostic industries. Traditional solution-based thermodynamic techniques, such as isothermal titration calorimetry (ITC), have evolved from cumbersome, labour-intensive techniques to automated systems with much lower requirements for reagents and reduced (200 µl) sample volume. Nonfluorescent (white light) high content cell-based assays have been developed together with automated microscope systems combining rapid auto-focusing, automated stage movement and dedicated analysis software capable of batch processing large numbers of images from 96 and 384 well plates. Mass spectrometry combined with high throughput size exclusion and solid phase extraction methods now allows quantification of free and bound species in minutes. Mass spectrometry is thus now a powerful label-free technique that has transitioned from an analytical quality control tool to a mainstream compound profiling and screening platform. In a similar manner, nuclear magnetic resonance (NMR) has evolved from a method to confirm compound structure to a powerful screening tool for identifying low molecular weight drug 'fragment' binders, and even elucidate the specific target binding site of a fragment or lead compound. This approach was pioneered by scientists at Abbott Laboratories, who identified hits from changes in NMR chemical shifts (^{15}N-^{1}H HSQC) and Vertex, who relied on detecting changes in the NMR relaxation properties of the fragments themselves when bound to a protein target.

Finally, in the last five years, the advent of 384- and 1536-well screening systems based on resonant waveguide patterned microtitre plates and electrical impedance 96- and 384-plates has led to an explosion in the application of label-free to GPCR screening. This is highly significant for drug discovery, as at least 800 distinctive human G-protein coupled receptors (GPCRs) are known, with ~350 being estimated to be useful drug targets. Although only ~7% of GPCRs are currently targeted by drugs, this accounts for ~35% of blockbuster pharmaceuticals. Here label-free can really challenge current screening paradigms. It has emerged that different ligands (agonists or antagonists) that bind to the same GPCR, even the same subtype, can display profoundly different biological properties (ligand directed signalling) arising through different regulation of intracellular pathways (e.g. IP3 flux, ERK 1/2 phosphorylation, cAMP activation, Ca^{2+} release, β-arrestins, etc.). GPCR-mediated pathways, initially thought to be independent, are now known to cross-communicate with other activation paths. For instance, GPCR stimulation can lead to activation of 'traditional' tyrosine kinase pathway components such as Raf, MEK and ERK.

Drug candidate screening paradigms typically involve selection of a transfected cell line, over-expressing the target GPCR. This cell line is then used with one, or a variety, of downstream markers of receptor activation, such as Ca^{2+}, cAMP, inositol phosphate and diacylglyercol flux. Standard assay development can be summarized as: (i) compound selection and synthesis, (ii) cell line selection and (iii) downstream reporter assay selection, all of which lead to a data set predicated by cell line and assay format chosen in the first instance. Although this standard approach has become well-accepted for compound screening and pharmacological characterization, it is *fundamentally limited in scope* in profiling target-related response outcomes. An 'agonist' or 'antagonist' may only be so in the specific screen used; a response in a transfected or transduced cell line may not be the same as that found in the disease relevant endogenous cell. In contrast, label-free screening, which can be carried out using parental cell lines, is thought to be indicative of ligand binding induced changes in cell morphology and holistic behaviour. The readout is noninvasive, temporal, cumulative and most importantly, *signalling pathway independent*. Kinetic responses or 'fingerprints' elicited by a compound are mechanistically informative, and profiles for particular G-protein coupling can be determined. Hence, the combination of label-free, pathway independent receptor and whole cell profiling with standard reporter and pathway dependent screening should provide new insight into compound mode of action, in addition to identifying new hits that could be missed by traditional assays.

Label-free continues to grow from a niche technology with a user base comprised of early adopters, towards a mainstream, easy to use (but sometimes not easy to understand) technology. We hope the reader finds this compendium of chapters describing label-free technologies and case studies both useful and thought provoking.

Matt Cooper and Lorenz M. Mayr
Brisbane, Australia and Basel, Switzerland, July 2010

List of Contributors

Yama A. Abassi
ACEA Biosciences Inc., 6779 Mesa Ridge Rd, San Diego, CA 92121, USA

J. Bradley
Pfizer Global Research and Development, Sandwich, Kent CT13 9NJ, UK

Tsafrir Bravman
Bio-Rad Laboratories, Inc., Gutwirth Park, Technion, Haifa 32000, Israel

Vered Bronner
Bio-Rad Laboratories, Inc., Gutwirth Park, Technion, Haifa 32000, Israel

Jason Brown
Neurosciences Centre of Excellence in Drug Discovery, GlaxoSmith-Kline, New Frontiers Science Park, Harlow, CM19 5AW, UK

Richard Brown
GE Healthcare, MicroCal Products Group, 22 Industrial Drive East, Northampton, MA, USA

Xun Chen
FAST (Facility for Automation & Screening Technologies), Merck Research Laboratories, Rahway, NJ, USA

Yen-Wen Chen
Molecular Devices, Inc., 1311 Orleans Drive, Sunnyvale, CA 94089, USA

Mike Chin
Novartis Institutes for Biomedical Research, 4560 Horton Street, Emeryville, CA 94608, USA

Bernard K. Choi
FAST (Facility for Automation & Screening Technologies), Merck Research Laboratories, Rahway, NJ, USA

Steven S. Choi
Micro and Nanotechnology Laboratory, Department of Electrical and Computer Engineering, University of Illinois at Urbana-Champaign, 1406 West Green Street, Urbana, IL 61801 USA

Chun-Wa Chung
GlaxoSmithKline, New Frontiers Science Park, Stevenage, Essex CM19 5AW, UK

Brian T. Cunningham
Micro and Nanotechnology Laboratory, Department of Electrical and Computer Engineering, University of Illinois at Urbana-Champaign, 1406 West Green Street, Urbana, IL 61801 USA

Mike Doyle
Novartis Institutes for Biomedical Research, 4560 Horton Street, Emeryville, CA 94608, USA

Claude Dufresne
FAST (Facility for Automation & Screening Technologies), Merck Research Laboratories, Rahway, NJ, USA

J. Gary Eden
Laboratory for Optical Physics and Engineering, Department of Electrical and Computer Engineering University of Illinois at Urbana-Champaign, 1406 West Green Street, Urbana, IL 61801 USA

E. Fairman
Pfizer Global Research and Development, Sandwich, Kent CT13 9NJ, UK

Paul Feucht
Novartis Institutes for Biomedical Research, 4560 Horton Street, Emeryville, CA 94608, USA

Ernesto Freire
Department of Biology, Johns Hopkins University, Baltimore, MD 21218, USA

Debra L. Gallant
Molecular Devices, Inc., 1311 Orleans Drive, Sunnyvale, CA 94089, USA

E. Gbekor
Pfizer Global Research and Development, Sandwich, Kent CT13 9NJ, UK

Chun Ge
Micro and Nanotechnology Laboratory, Department of Electrical and Computer Engineering, University of Illinois at Urbana-Champaign, 1406 West Green Street, Urbana, IL 61801 USA

Neil S. Geoghagen
FAST (Facility for Automation & Screening Technologies), Merck Research Laboratories, Rahway, NJ, USA

Robert Graves
GE Healthcare Life Sciences, 800 Centennial Avenue, Piscataway, New Jersey 08855-1327, USA

P. Hayter
Pfizer Global Research and Development, Sandwich, Kent CT13 9NJ, UK

Tom G. Holt
Facility for Automation & Screening Technologies (FAST), Merck Research Laboratories, Rahway, NJ, USA

Walter Huber
F.Hoffmann-La RocheAG, Pharma Research Basel, Grenzacherstrasse, 4070 Basel, Switzerland

Kristian K. Jensen
FAST (Facility for Automation & Screening Technologies), Merck Research Laboratories, Rahway, NJ, USA

Jeffrey C. Jerman
Molecular Discovery Research, 1–3 Burtonhole Lane, London NW7 1AD, UK

Maxine Jonas
BioTrove, Inc., Woburn, MA, USA

William A. LaMarr
BioTrove, Inc., Woburn, MA, USA

Lukas Leder
Novartis Institutes for Biomedical Research, Lichtstrasse 35, CH-4056, Basel, Switzerland

Melanie Leveridge
GlaxoSmithKline, New Frontiers Science Park, Stevenage, Essex CM19 5AW, UK

Meng Lu
Micro and Nanotechnology Laboratory, Department of Electrical and Computer Engineering, University of Illinois at Urbana-Champaign, 1406 West Green Street, Urbana, IL 61801 USA

Ming-Juan Luo
FAST (Facility for Automation & Screening Technologies), Merck Research Laboratories, Rahway, NJ, USA

Qi Luo
FAST (Facility for Automation & Screening Technologies), Merck Research Laboratories, Rahway, NJ, USA

Lorraine Malkowitz
FAST (Facility for Automation & Screening Technologies), Merck Research Laboratories, Rahway, NJ, USA

Eric Martin
Novartis Institutes for Biomedical Research, 4560 Horton Street, Emeryville, CA 94608, USA

Julio Martin
GlaxoSmithKline, Centro de Investigacion Basica, Parque Tecnologico de Madrid, 28760 Tres Cantos, Spain

Ryan P. McGuinness
Molecular Devices, Inc., 1311 Orleans Drive, Sunnyvale, CA 94089, USA

Marco Meyerhofer
Novartis Institutes for Biomedical Research, Lichtstrasse 35, CH-4056, Basel, Switzerland

David G. Myszka
Center for Biomolecular Interaction Analysis, University of Utah, Salt Lake City, UT 84132, USA

Oded Nahshol
Bio-Rad Laboratories, Inc., Gutwirth Park, Technion, Haifa 32000, Israel

Thomas Neumann
Graffinity Pharmaceuticals GmbH, INF 518, 69120 Heidelberg, Germany

Ronan O'Brien
GE Healthcare, MicroCal Products Group, 22 Industrial Drive East, Northampton, MA, USA

Johannes Ottl
Novartis Institute for BioMedical Research, Centre for Proteomic Chemistry, Forum 1, Novartis Campus, CH-4056, Basel, Switzerland

Can C. Ozbal
BioTrove, Inc., Woburn, MA, USA

John M. Proctor
Molecular Devices, Inc., 1311 Orleans Drive, Sunnyvale, CA 94089, USA

S. Ramsey
Pfizer Global Research and Development, Sandwich, Kent CT13 9NJ, UK

Rebecca L. Rich
Center for Biomolecular Interaction Analysis, University of Utah, Salt Lake City, UT 84132, USA

Magalie Rocheville
Molecular Discovery Research, GlaxoSmithKline, New Frontiers Science Park, Harlow, CM19 5AW, UK

Renate Sekul
Graffinity Pharmaceuticals GmbH, INF 518, 69120 Heidelberg, Germany

Kevin Shoemaker
Novartis Institutes for Biomedical Research, 4560 Horton Street, Emeryville, CA 94608, USA

Alexander Sieler
Roche Diagnostics GmbH, BP-C1 Nonnenwald 2, 82377 Penzberg, Germany

F. Stuhmeier
Pfizer Global Research and Development, Sandwich, Kent CT13 9NJ, UK

David C. Swinney
iRND3, Institute for Rare and Neglected Diseases Drug Discovery, 1514 Ridge Road, Belmont, CA 94002, USA

Blisseth Sy
Novartis Institutes for Biomedical Research, 4560 Horton Street, Emeryville, CA 94608, USA

H. Roger Tang
Molecular Devices, Inc., 1311 Orleans Drive, Sunnyvale, CA 94089, USA

Georg C. Terstappen
Faculty of Pharmacy, University of Siena, Via Fiorentina 1, 53100 Siena, Italy

Trisha A. Tutana
Molecular Devices, Inc., 1311 Orleans Drive, Sunnyvale, CA 94089, USA

Clark J. Wagner
Laboratory for Optical Physics and Engineering, Department of Electrical and Computer Engineering, University of Illinois at Urbana-Champaign, 1406 West Green Street, Urbana, IL 61801 USA

John Wang
Novartis Institutes for Biomedical Research, 4560 Horton Street, Emeryville, CA 94608, USA

Jun Wang
FAST (Facility for Automation & Screening Technologies), Merck Research Laboratories, Rahway, NJ, USA

Xiaobo Wang
ACEA Biosciences Inc., 6779 Mesa Ridge Rd, San Diego, CA 92121, USA

Bob Warne
Novartis Institutes for Biomedical Research, 4560 Horton Street, Emeryville, CA 94608, USA

Charles Wartchow
FortéBio, Inc., 1360 Willow Road, Suite 201, Menlo Park, CA 94025-1516, USA

Trevor Wattam
GlaxoSmithKline, New Frontiers Science Park, Stevenage, Essex CM19 5AW, UK

Manfred Watzele
Roche Diagnostics GmbH, BP-C1 Nonnenwald 2, 82377 Penzberg, Germany

Glyn Williams
Astex Therapeutics Ltd, 436 Cambridge Science Park, Milton Road, Cambridge CB4 0QA, UK

Donna L. Wilson
Molecular Devices, Inc., 1311 Orleans Drive, Sunnyvale, CA 94089, USA

Yusheng Xiong
FAST (Facility for Automation & Screening Technologies), Merck Research Laboratories, Rahway, NJ, USA

Xiao Xu
ACEA Biosciences Inc., 6779 Mesa Ridge Rd, San Diego, CA 92121, USA

Kelly Yan
Novartis Institutes for Biomedical Research, 4560 Horton Street, Emeryville, CA 94608, USA

Danfeng Yao
FortéBio, Inc., 1360 Willow Road, Suite 201, Menlo Park, CA 94025-1516, USA

Jiamin Yu
Novartis Institutes for Biomedical Research, 4560 Horton Street, Emeryville, CA 94608, USA

Isabel Zaror
Novartis Institutes for Biomedical Research, 4560 Horton Street, Emeryville, CA 94608, USA

1

The Revolution of Real-Time, Label-Free Biosensor Applications

Rebecca L. Rich and David G. Myszka
Center for Biomolecular Interaction Analysis, University of Utah, Salt Lake City, UT, USA

1.1 INTRODUCTION

Initially, we had planned to discuss the revolution of real-time, label-free biosensor applications. This revolution has been monumental. In the early days, biosensors were used as immunosensors to characterize antibody/antigen interactions. It didn't take long for researchers to

Label-Free Technologies for Drug Discovery Edited by Matthew Cooper and Lorenz M. Mayr
© 2011 John Wiley & Sons, Ltd

exploit the technology's capabilities to examine other biological systems, including receptors, nucleic acids, and lipids. Once people recognized that low intensity signals were reliable, the biosensor quickly became a tool for characterizing small molecules and even membrane-associated systems.

Upon reflection, we realized a greater development was in users' understanding of how to apply biosensor technology. How we design experiments and analyse data today is different than in years past. Improvements in data processing and global fitting have eliminated much, but not all, of the confusion biosensor users experience when interpreting binding responses. With these advances it is now easier to recognize well performed experiments. So a better title for this discussion may be "Evolution in Our Understanding of Biosensor Analysis".

When we look at how people use biosensors today, we realize that many users still don't know what they are doing with the technology and the problems are not because of the biosensor (it's a poor craftsman that blames his tools). Instead, far too often, users don't employ basics tenets of the scientific method. They don't include controls, test replicates, or even show data when presenting results. As a result, they end up publishing experimental artifacts or misinterpreting the interaction. Unfortunately, poor quality analysis gives all biosensor technology a bad name. In fact, based on the published data, we wonder if a better title for this chapter might be "Why are Biosensor Users Such Poor Scientists?"

Before we examine why most biosensor users aren't good scientists, let's have a short review of where the technology came from. In 1990, a Swedish company called Pharmacia released Biacore, the first commercially viable biosensor. As depicted in Figure 1.1a, the system was operated by a 486 Hz personal computer (PC for short) – boy, does that bring back memories. To put things into perspective, Figures 1.1b–1.1f pictorially depict other significant advances that occurred in 1990. You might not remember it but the World Wide Web (Figure 1.1b) was launched then and changed forever how we gather information and communicate. The Super Nintendo Entertainment System (Figure 1.1c) revolutionized home video gaming, making it possible to play sports without going outside. Researchers who had been using Perrier water as a solvent in their chromatography systems (presumably because of its high level of purity) found some bottles were actually contaminated with benzene (Figure 1.1d). In one of the biggest upsets in boxing history, James Buster Douglas knocked out Mike Tyson (Figure 1.1e). And Pons and Fleischmann discovered cold fusion (Figure 1.1f); thanks to them we now have an

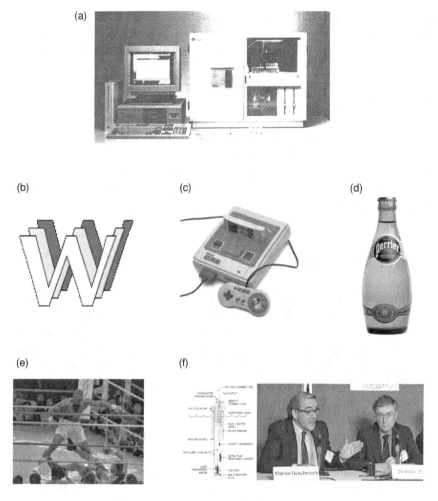

Figure 1.1 Memorable events in 1990. (a) The first commercial optical biosensor, Biacore, was released by Pharmacia. Advent of (b) the World Wide Web and (c) Nintendo's SuperNES gaming console; (d) the Perrier scandal; (e) the Douglas/Tyson boxing match; and (f) Pons and Fleischmann's announcement of cold fusion.

endless supply of cheap, clean energy but of course the cost of Perrier has skyrocketed.

Since the release of the first biosensor, we have seen an explosion in the number and variety of commercial biosensors. Today there are around twenty different instrument manufacturers and about forty different platforms available. These numbers fluctuate as established companies offer new products, old companies falter, and new companies acquire old companies' products (the circle of biosensors cannot be broken). This diversity in instrumentation is a godsend for bench-top scientists because it means there is a system available to meet each user's sensitivity, throughput, and cost requirements.

While it is true that today's biosensors often employ a variety of detection methods (e.g., surface plasmon resonance, reflectometric interference, evansescent wave, acoustic wave, and dual polarization interferometry to name a few), we think people are too often distracted by a particular platform's detection method. It is not necessary to understand the physics of how a detector works to use it properly. It is far more important to understand how to set up a biosensor experiment and analyse the data properly.

1.2 SPR PESSIMISTS

Unfortunately, there is still significant skepticism in the general scientific community about the validity of biosensor data. Most people can be classified into one of the three categories (Figure 1.2). There are the naysayers who say biosensors don't work (Figure 1.2a), users who think they are experts (Figure 1.2b), and scientists who really love the technology and will do what it takes to get reliable biosensor data (Figure 1.2c).

Let's start with the first group. The naysayers often declare the biosensor has insurmountable problems with instrument drift, nonspecific binding, mass transport, and avidity effects. (Actually, these effects can be minimized and/or accounted for if an experiment is performed properly.) But their fundamental claim is that immobilizing one binding partner on a surface produces artificial binding constants. Sure, taking something

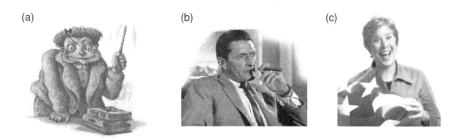

(a)   (b)   (c)

Figure 1.2 Opinions of biosensor technology. (a) "Biosensors don't work." (b) "I'm an expert. I've been using biosensors for years and am not going to change how I do an experiment." (c) "I think biosensors are great and I'm eager to learn about the latest developments."

(a)   (b)   (c)

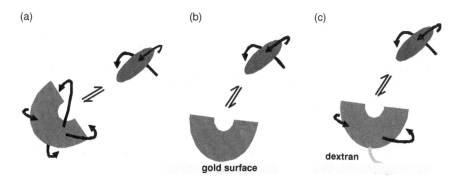

gold surface   dextran

Figure 1.3 Rotational freedom in solution (a) and when the target is immobilized on a flat surface (b) or tethered to a dextran matrix (c).

in solution, as shown in Figure 1.3a, and putting it on a surface could change its entropic properties; perhaps then it cannot freely rotate and would be accessible in only two dimensions (Figure 1.3b) rather than three dimensional space by an approaching binding partner. But, for the vast majority of binding studies the immobilized partner is not actually stuck directly on the flat surface. It is suspended in a dextran layer (Figure 1.3c), which provides a solution-like environment. Maybe the problem with understanding this concept is the word "immobilize". When the ligand is linked to the dextran-coated surface, the binding partner is not immobile. Instead, it is tethered: it is still free to rotate and is accessible in three dimensions for binding.

Relying on its experience using dextran in column chromatography resins, Pharmacia recognized the advantages of using this surface matrix. The dextran layer provides a hydrophilic environment and reduces nonspecific binding. Often the dextran layer is illustrated as a homogeneous forest of seaweed but in reality it is more like cotton candy, whose height depends on buffer conditions, for example, salt concentration. Not only does the dextran layer permit target mobility, but it also introduces a "pre-concentration effect" (1), which allows targets to be readily immobilized, um,... we mean tethered. Coupling a protein on a planar carboxyl surface, for example, requires a higher protein concentration, but with the dextran's capacity to pre-concentrate material through charge effects, a protein could be extracted from a solution of comparably lower concentration and still immobilized at high surface densities. Of course, high densities may not always be optimal (read on).

Coating the sensor surface with dextran was a brilliant decision by Pharmacia when it was developing the biosensor for commercial release. It turned out that the dextran layer is one of the primary reasons its technology has been so successful. Several manufacturers have produced novel biosensor detection systems but have stumbled in surface chemistry development. Pharmacia's (later Biacore, now GE Healthcare) longevity in the biosensor field is due to its proprietary dextran surfaces. As patents on the use of dextran surfaces begin to expire in 2010, we should see other manufacturers quickly adopt this surface chemistry.

Naysayers often claim that solution- and sensor-determined binding parameters do not match up. To counter this charge, we demonstrated that rate constants and affinities determined using the two approaches do in fact agree when the experiments are done properly. In one study, we determined the kinetics of a small molecule binding to an enzyme using both Biacore technology and a stopped-flow fluorescence instrument (2). The rate constants obtained from the two experiments correlated well. We expanded this investigation to include other biosensor platforms and a panel of compounds that display different affinities for the enzyme and compared results with those obtained from calorimetry measurements (3–8).

A few years ago we began a series of benchmark studies to show that other users can get reliable data from biosensors (2, 3, 7–10). In each study, a panel of participants tested the same interaction. For example, in one study, twenty-two different biosensor users determined the affinities of four compound/target interactions at six temperatures. From these numbers we calculated interaction enthalpies and entropies and compared these values with thermodynamic parameters determined using calorimetry (8). Once again, results from the two approaches matched and the coefficient of variation in the biosensor-determined rate constants was about 10%.

In another benchmark study, we examined a high-affinity antibody/antigen system (9) to demonstrate that even systems with slow off rates could be interpreted reliably. Others have also compared the binding constants for mAb/antigen interactions obtained from Biacore and Kinexa (11), again demonstrating the kinetics and affinity matched between methods.

Recently, we expanded these comparisons to include even more biologically relevant assays. In collaboration with Anthony Giannetti, we compared the biosensor-determined K_Ds of about a hundred kinase inhibitors to the IC_{50}'s measured in biochemical and cellular analyses (Figure 1.4) (12). In both panels the data points lie along a diagonal, which indicates excellent correlation between the biosensor and other methods.

These (and other) comparative studies we have overseen span the range of biosensor variables: testing both small and large analytes

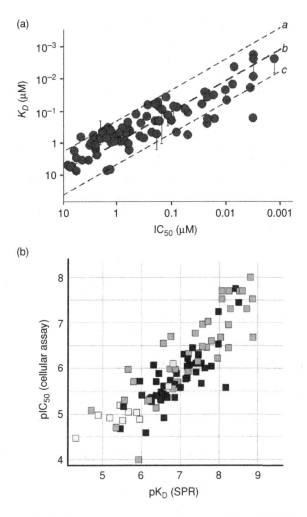

Figure 1.4 Correlation between parameters determined for ~100 kinase inhibitors using biosensor vs. biochemical (top panel) and cellular (bottom panel) assays. In the top panel the heavy dashed line (b) corresponds to $K_D = IC_{50}$. The shorter dashed lines (a and c) correspond to $K_D = 1/5 \times IC_{50}$ and $K_D = 5 \times IC_{50}$, respectively. Error bars not visible are smaller than the symbols used. (Top panel reproduced from (12) with permission from Elsevier © 2008.)

having affinities that differ by more than 100 000-fold, including users (more than 200 to date) of widely different skill levels, and evaluating instruments from the highly automated, high throughput platforms to the manual bench-top models. Across this array of variables, the parameters determined using the biosensor compare well with kinetics, affinities, thermodynamics, and even activity data measured using solution-based biophysical, biochemical, and cellular assays.

Of course, the key to getting the parameters to agree is to do both of the experiments properly. We find the biggest problem is that most users do not take the time to do the biosensor experiment right. And it's not just new users. We often see in the literature data from more seasoned users who are not setting up the experiment properly. They have the attitude "I've been doing this for years so I know what I'm doing" (Figure1.2b). They have stagnated, not realizing the application of the technology has evolved well past what they consider to be state-of-the-art.

In general we find that many biosensor users have absolutely dreadful technique. We can defend this statement because we read the literature – every single article containing commercial biosensor results that has been published – and for the past decade we have written an annual review of the year's literature (13–22). Most often the problems arise from poor experimental design and execution, as well as inadequate or inappropriate data analysis. It is common to read a paper that suffers from one (or more) of these problems, which renders the authors' conclusions suspect.

1.3 SETTING UP EXPERIMENTS

Bad data often start with bad reagents. The number-one issue to worry about in any biosensor experiment is the quality of the reagents. Unfortunately, the problem is that this is often out of the biosensor user's control. For example, sometimes we are asked to analyse two proteins that were prepared by someone else or simply purchased from a vendor, so we don't have any information about their activities. Remember that what the biosensor is measuring is the activity of the reagents. Unlike mass spectrometry measurements, in which the results are independent of whether the sample is active or inactive, we need two properly folded, conformationally homogeneous, active binding partners for a successful biosensor experiment. There is no way to get meaningful biosensor data from inactive proteins. And the argument that a protein appears as a single band on a SDS-PAGE gel is not good enough. We don't care about purity. We care about ACTIVITY!

But what is the cutoff for being a bad or good reagent? Would we do an experiment if only 50% of each sample was active? Maybe. But if we collect binding data and we see aggregation, complexity, or nonspecific binding in the data set then we really need to consider how the quality of the reagents is affecting the responses. The issue is not that the technology requires ultra-high-quality reagents. Rather, expectations have to be adjusted based on the quality of reagents. For example, if someone wants to study small molecules binding to an enzyme and they tell us their enzyme preparation can be crystallized, we feel a little more confident that we will be able to get good quality data for that interaction, since the protein has been shown to be well behaved. If, instead, someone brings us protein that has precipitated at the bottom of a centrifuge tube and they cannot see any enzymatic activity but want us to do a binding assay on the sample, we may still do the experiment but we already know to proceed with caution. If we do not see binding or if we see very complex binding we think "Aha! The unusual responses may relate to the quality of the reagents." All too often in the literature we see people over-interpret complex binding responses as something meaningful. The latest fad in interpreting complex binding responses is what we call the "Look everyone, I've got a conformational change" syndrome (more about this later).

Now, assuming your reagents are good, you can move on to starting the biosensor experiment. But stay alert. There are a number of potential pitfalls in each of the steps needed to get good biosensor data. Firstly, consider ligand immobilization. When the biosensor was first released everyone immobilized ligands via amine coupling because it is fast and easy. While this method works great for a number of systems, it does have limitations. For example, the drop in pH and salt concentration required for effective preconcentration may inactivate some ligands. So, a number of alternative chemistries and capturing methods have been developed over the years. Unfortunately, what we most often see users do (and what is presented in the literature) is only one approach: they immobilized the target using amine coupling and got some data, so they stopped optimizing the assay conditions. But if you only do it one way, you are not considering if/how immobilization may affect binding. How do you know you are getting native activity of your ligand without trying other methods?

The opportunity to use several immobilization approaches is one example of how the technology and its applications have evolved over time. With any new system, we recommend trying multiple methods of immobilization. In our laboratory, we set up a preliminary experiment in which we prepare surfaces of the same target immobilized by amine coupling, minimal biotinylation and, if possible, capture via a suitable tag; we then test them side by side for analyte binding.

Another issue with amine coupling is that it is random, which can cause trouble. Amine coupling can produce a heterogeneous ligand population. If you use random coupling, the ligand on the surface may not all be equally accessible for binding. If, instead, the ligand is captured or otherwise homogenously tethered to the surface, the population should be equally accessible for binding. Remember, we are talking about being chemically, not physically, similarly oriented. A big misconception people have is that oriented immobilization leads to a uniform physical presentation of the molecules on the surface, like all the binding sites are facing up. But, in fact, the dextran layer is flexible and mobile, so an oriented population of immobilized ligand is not all necessarily pointed in the same direction; it is all tethered to the dextran via the same functional group. This beauty of the dextran layer brings to mind an ancient haiku:

> *Ligands hung in fluid breeze*
> *Some face up, some may face down*
> *Now bind damn it, bind.*

The next step is to consider how much target to immobilize. As the technology evolved we showed that for kinetic studies it is important to use lower density surfaces (23,24). In the old days (and you still see this sometimes) people measured very large responses but the binding was mechanistically very complex because they introduced effects like crowding, aggregation, and/or mass transport. We found that as you lowered the surface density the binding responses became simpler and could be described by a single exponential.

We often are asked: "How low in surface density should you go?" The answer is, let the sensor be your guide. Immobilize your ligand at a density that produces low analyte binding signals and run something we call "replicates". Replication is the art of taking the same sample and analyzing it more than one time to determine how reproducible a response is.

It is indeed shocking just how few examples there are in the biosensor literature of doing replicate experiments, even the simple test of injecting the same analyte twice over the same chip. This is even more disappointing given that most commercially available biosensors are fully automated, so you could set up the assay to run ten times while you go to lunch or leave for the day. When you come back to the laboratory, you have an answer about how reproducible your data set is.

Figure 1.5a shows the data obtained from a simple reproducibility test in which analyte was injected across the same surface three times. The triplicate responses overlay, indicating the binding was reproducible

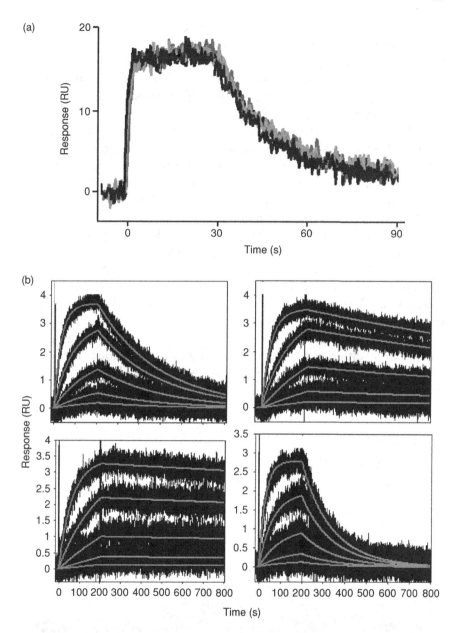

Figure 1.5   Reproducible responses obtained from low density surfaces. (a) Overlay of the responses obtained for an analyte tested three times. (b) Light gray lines depict the fit of a 1:1 interaction model; black lines are the responses (triplicates overlaid) from each analyte concentration.

and therefore reliable, even at this low response level. Figure 1.5b shows the full analyses of antigen binding to four low density antibody surfaces. In each panel, every antigen concentration was tested three times. The responses are so reproducible you cannot see that there are three individual curves overlaid. While the responses in Figure 1.5 are only a few RU (resonance units) in intensity, they are easily discernable above background and the overlay of the replicates, as well as their fit to a 1:1 interaction model, demonstrate these data are reliable.

Keep in mind that there is a lot of information in replicate data sets, even if the responses are not exactly reproducible. First of all, we do not believe any response until we see it at least twice. Then, if the responses overlay, we know the binding partners are stable and the regeneration condition is working. If the replicate responses decrease over time, one (or both) of the partners may be losing activity during the experiment. Working with unstable reagents is still possible in some experiments, but again we would need to adjust our expectations of the quality of data we could obtain. Knowing the reproducibility of a binding event is a critical first step to evaluating an interaction.

How many replicates do you really need? The data set in Figure 1.6 consists of 80 different analyte concentrations measured four times each. Admittedly, this is an extreme example – you don't need to do this many replicates of such a narrow dilution series to prove a mechanism or define

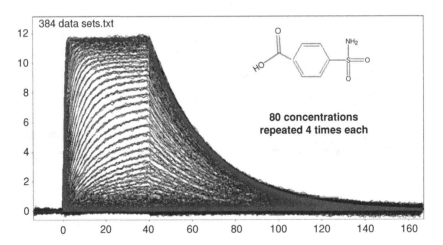

Figure 1.6 Overlaid responses obtained for eighty concentrations of a small molecule (shown in the inset) binding to an immobilized target. Each analyte concentration was tested four times. The light gray lines depict the fit of the responses (black lines) to a 1:1 interaction model.

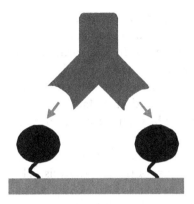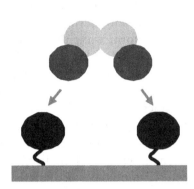

Figure 1.7 Poor experimental design: testing bivalent analytes (left: antibody; right, GST-tagged protein) in solution binding to immobilized binding partners introduces avidity.

the binding constants. We ran this experiment years ago because at the time naysayers were claiming that nothing measured using the biosensor ever fits a simple interaction model. But Figure 1.6 contains over 600 000 data points, spanning more than a 1000-fold concentration range, all fit simultaneously to a 1:1 interaction model, which proves that some data sets can all be fit by a simple interaction model if you know what you are doing.

The key to getting data to fit a simple model is to get good quality data. The problem is that too many experiments are poorly designed. One classic problem is testing a bivalent system in solution (for example, antibodies or GST-tagged proteins) against a monomeric partner immobilized on the surface (Figure 1.7). With this set-up you will get avidity effects. People who design an experiment this way either don't understand avidity or choose to ignore it, but as a consequence they end up reporting an artificially tight affinity for the interaction. Unfortunately, this is just one example of scientific carelessness. There are a number of other experimental factors to consider and we have tackled them in a number of publications (25–27). The bottom line is: if you set up the experiment incorrectly in the beginning you cannot expect to get good data out.

1.4 DATA PROCESSING AND ANALYSIS

The next big issue is proper data processing, which can account for systematic noise, instrument drift, and even nonspecific binding. Over the years there have been a number of advances in data-processing tools. In

2001, we launched Scrubber, which significantly automated data processing. Briefly, Scrubber allows one to zero data before injections, crop
data, perform x-alignment, subtract reference data, and perform double
referencing. Double referencing, which we introduced in 1999, is the
process in which buffer is injected over the surfaces to determine the
systematic differences between reference and reaction surfaces (27). By
subtracting out this difference data quality can be significantly improved,
particular when responses are very low. Artifacts in data that are poorly
processed are misinterpreted too often as interesting binding events.

The next level of challenge in using biosensors is data analysis. The
two common types of analysis are equilibrium analysis, to extract affinities, and kinetic analysis to extract reaction rates. Firstly, equilibrium
analysis. The key word in equilibrium analysis is "equilibrium". When
an interaction is at equilibrium, which happens when the same number
of complexes are forming as are breaking down, the binding response
is flat. Figure 1.8a is an excellent example of an equilibrium analysis.
The responses (left panel) for every concentration reach a plateau before
the end of the injection, so each response reached equilibrium and can
be fit to a binding isotherm (right panel) to determine K_D. The biggest
problem we see in the literature regarding equilibrium analysis is that
users do not allow the interaction to come to equilibrium before taking a
measurement; a few examples are shown in Figure 1.8b. An equilibrium
analysis cannot be done unless the responses are at equilibrium. We call
this problem "end-of-injection analysis" and we see it in the literature
all the time.

Kinetic analysis is more involved than equilibrium analysis but it starts
by visualizing the data. As shown in Figure 1.9, even child psychologists
begin with images to understand, in this case, family dynamics. Interpretation of these data is a bit subjective. For example, when analyzing this
drawing of a family at play, one viewer may focus on the mother and
daughter playing catch while another sees the son appearing to throw
knives at his father. But unlike kinetic family drawings, biosensor responses are not open to interpretation. If two people analyse the same
data set, they should get the same results. But this was not always the
case because older methods of data analysis were very subjective.

In the early days of biosensor data analysis people used what is referred
to as linear analysis. Firstly, the binding response, which is normally a
curve (Figure 1.10a, left panel), would be transformed to create a plot to
which a line was then drawn (Figure 1.10a, right panel) and then these
slopes were plotted in a third plot to which another line was drawn.
From this third plot, the slope gave the on rate and the intercept gave

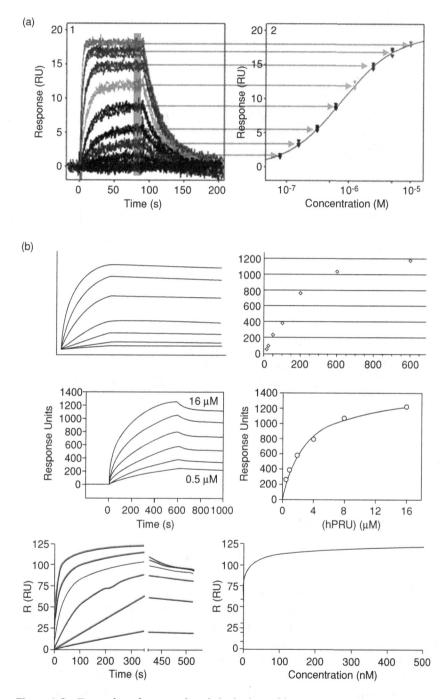

Figure 1.8 Examples of (a) good and (b) bad equilibrium analyses. (Panels in (b) reproduced from (28–30) with permission from Elsevier © 2009.)

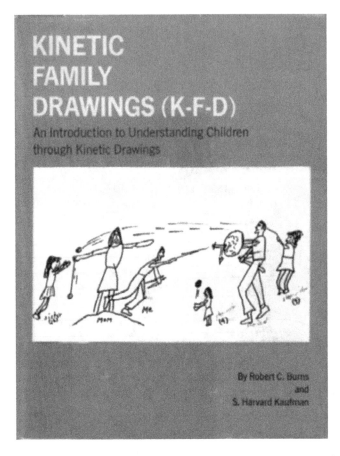

Figure 1.9 Book cover that demonstrates the variable interpretations of a kinetic drawing.

the off rate (Figure 1.10a, inset in right panel). Confusing and slow, we know.

The really big problem with linear analysis is that when binding responses are complex due to mass transport, heterogeneity or drift (Figure 1.10b, left panel), deciding which region is linear becomes subjective: one person might pick a different region to fit than someone else (the authors' selection of which region to fit is shown in Figure 1.10b, right panel). Figure 1.10c illustrates that, in many cases, linear transformation of the dissociation phase could also produce a curve instead of a straight line. Here the authors reported two dissociation rates for this complex but it could easily be argued that there was a third rate which was completely ignored. So, when users found their data could not conform to

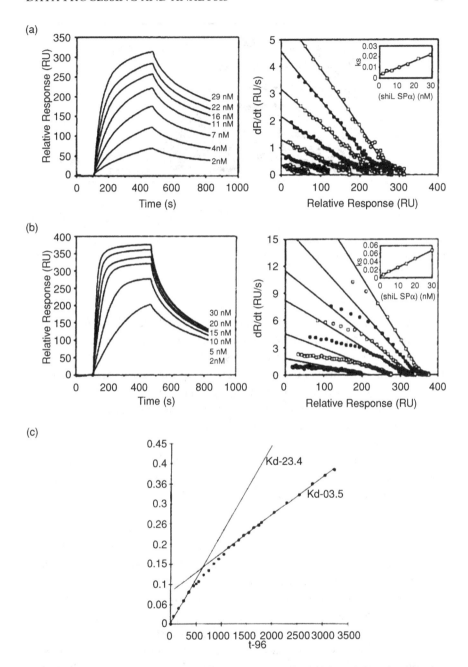

Figure 1.10 Linear analyses of biosensor data from (a) simple and (b and c) complex interactions. In (a) and (b), responses in the left panels were transformed to the linear plots in the right panels, with slope/intercept plots to determine rate constants shown in the insets. In (c), the nonlinear plot was fit to two rate constants. [(a) and (b) reprinted with permission from [31] Copyright 1994 John Wiley and Sons, Ltd and (c) reprinted from [32] with permission from Elsevier]

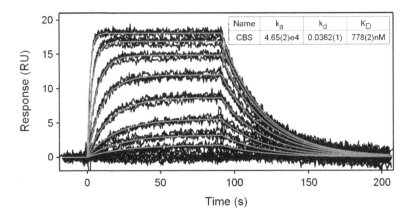

Figure 1.11 Global analysis of an interaction. The light gray lines depict the fit of the responses (black lines) to a 1:1 interaction model. Binding parameters determined from the fit are shown in the inset.

a straight line, everyone got wrapped up in developing binding scenarios that involved multiple rate constants. Unfortunately, the complexity was not due to interesting biology. Instead the experimental design was sub-optimal. That brings us back to setting up the experiment carefully.

We were always bothered by the fact that scientists were choosing which portions of their data to analyze. Some would argue to take the early phase of binding, and some the late. So in the mid 1990s we introduced the concept of globally fitting all of the data at the same time with a software program called CLAMP (33). With this approach, all the data (at each concentration and during both association and dissociation) are fit simultaneously to a single reaction model. Figure 1.11 depicts a global analysis of a small molecule binding to an immobilized target. The fit of a 1:1 interaction model (shown as the light gray lines) is overlaid on the binding responses (measured in triplicate; black lines). The overlay of the data and fit indicate this interaction is well described by the parameters listed in the inset.

One of the beauties and challenges with global analysis is that it requires very high quality data. Artifacts due to poor experimental design and processing become very apparent when you try to fit the data globally. Maybe this is why so many people do not publish their biosensor data but instead just report the rate constants they determine. Pictures really are better than words and certainly more revealing than a table of numbers. Ideally, every article describing a biosensor kinetic analysis would include at least one figure of replicate responses that span a

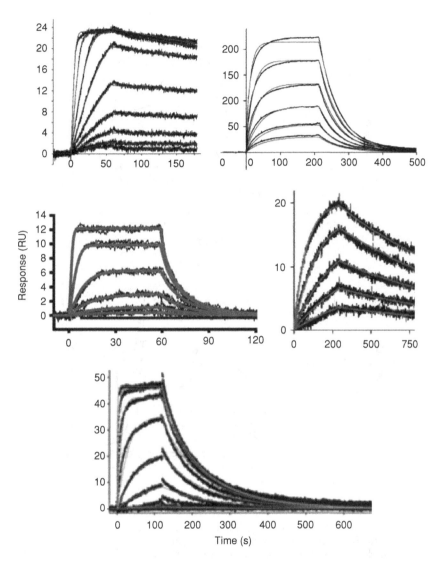

Figure 1.12 Published examples of high quality kinetic analyses. Reprinted from [Refs: 33, 34, 36 and 37] with permission from Elsevier, European Molecular Biology Organization, and National Academy of Sciences.

wide concentration range overlaid with the model fit (like those shown in Figure 1.12). But too often in the literature we see no figures of data – so we cannot trust the reported constants – or we see data that is not interpreted correctly. Figure 1.13 shows two examples from articles that included a figure of responses and reported rate constants but did not show the model fit. Since we doubted the reported rate constants really

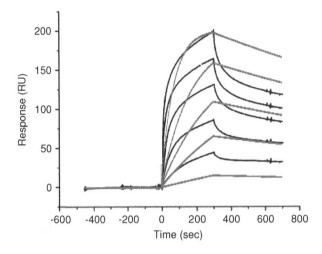

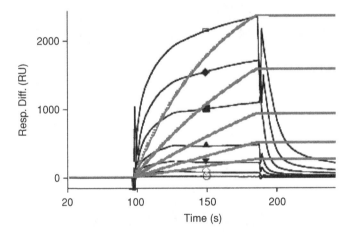

Figure 1.13 Published data sets (black lines) that do not match the accompanying reported rate constants. Fits simulated from the rate constants are shown in light gray overlaid with the responses. Reprinted with permission from [39] Copyright 2007 American Chemical Society., and Reprinted from [40] with kind permission from Springer Science + Business Media.

described these responses, we simulated data derived by the rate constants and overlaid it atop the responses. Our simulated fits (overlaid smooth lines in Figure 1.13) do not even come close to mimicking the responses, so we wonder how these data were actually analysed.

For several years now, we have been asking anyone who reports rate constants to show a data set overlaid with the model they used to fit it.

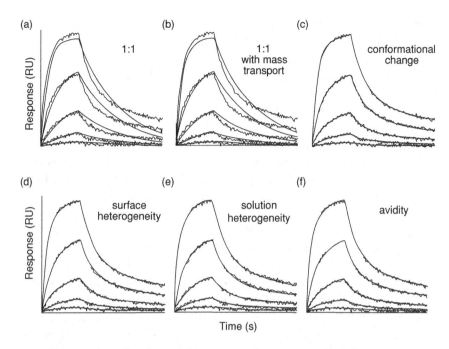

Figure 1.14 A complex data set fit to (a) simple 1:1 interaction, (b) 1:1 interaction that includes a mass transport parameter, (c) conformational change, (d) surface heterogeneity, (e) solution heterogeneity, and (f) avidity models.

But as people have begun to publish their data with model fits, we have discovered the next level of trouble: using complex reaction models. Too often users fit their data with a complex model simply because it fits the data better than a simple model does. Sometimes authors will even state this in the paper "We used this conformational change model because it fit the data." The funny thing is that you cannot prove a model is correct based on how well it fits the data. We know this sounds counterintuitive, so the data in Figure 1.14 help to illustrate the point.

We can all agree that a simple 1:1 interaction model (Figure 1.14a) and a 1:1 model that includes mass transport (Figure 1.14b) do not describe the data. Therefore, we can unequivocally state that these two models are wrong. What you often see people doing next is to apply a more complex model like a two-step conformational change model (Figure 1.14c), which appears to fit the data well. Then they run off and publish that their interaction undergoes a conformational change. A more prudent scientist would try other models as well. For example, it turns out this data set is fit equally well by a surface- and a solution-heterogeneity model (Figures 1.14d and 1.14e, respectively), as well as an avidity model (Figure 1.14f). So which model is correct? You actually cannot tell using modeling. The only way to prove a mechanism is through experimentation. And actually deconvoluting through experimentation is not easy given the fact that most users cannot set up a single sensor experiment properly. And now you are expecting them to set up multiple experiments under different conditions to help define the correct mechanism.

Even worse, the conformational change model seems to be inattentive users' favorite choice when fitting complex data. "Hey look at me, I got a conformational change." Keep in mind the biosensor measures events on the time scale of minutes. So if you apply this conformation change model and take the time to really think about the rate constants that come out of the analysis, you will find that they correspond to half-lives of minutes – sometimes up to forty minutes. It is unlikely that events on this time scale are biologically relevant. The proponents of using the conformational change model have never explained to us why an entire protein can refold on a millisecond time scale and yet their binding undergoes a conformational change with a half-life of forty minutes – seems a bit odd. Unless, of course, you consider that the complexity they see in the biosensor data is due to aggregation or nonspecific binding, which could be described by much slower events.

Finally, do not be fooled by people who use a crystal structure showing conformational change as evidence to justify fitting complex sensorgrams to a conformational change model. The crystal structure and biosensor data are completely unrelated pieces of information. Until someone shows us time resolved structural data with a conformational change that matches the slow conformational change supposedly observed in their biosensor data, we will stick to improving the quality of the biosensor experiment and remove the artifact.

1.5 THE GOOD NEWS

Now we are left to discuss the third, and our most favorite, group of scientists (Figure 1.2c), users who believe in the technology and want to use it properly to get high quality data. While their numbers may be small, fortunately this is the most rapidly growing group. The first thing we teach them at our workshops is the shape of an exponential binding response (Figure 1.15a). This "shark fin" profile is not some random shape. True binding data should conform to an exponential in

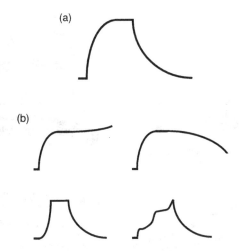

Figure 1.15 Example shapes of published responses. The shape in (A) depicts a plausible binding response, while those in (B) are due to experimental artifacts.

the association and dissociation phase. The association phase is second order, meaning it is concentration dependent. The higher the concentration of analyte, the faster the apparent binding rate. The dissociation phase is independent of concentration. No matter where you start with the response, the rate of decay should be the same. It is like radioactive decay. One ton and one gram of plutonium-238 decay at the same rate. In either case, in 88 years you still have half of a mess to clean up.

With a little practice, everyone can learn to recognize plausible binding signals (Figure 1.15a) and those responses that don't make much sense (Figure 1.15b). Unfortunately, we can find examples of all of the shapes depicted in Figure 1.15b published in the literature. Figure 1.16 shows data sets that display the signature shark fin shape (other examples are shown in Figures 1.5, 1.6, 1.11, and 1.12). Although the shark fin shape varies based on the kinetics of the interaction, by now you should be getting an idea of what a reasonable binding profile looks like. Because these are all simple exponential curves, they are well described by a 1:1 model (light gray lines in each data set).

We don't always get super data the first time we study some interaction and all users need to realize that getting good quality data is often an iterative process. Our initial studies are focused on firstly just seeing some binding between two partners. Once we can confirm that the molecules interact, then we optimize the immobilization chemistry, surface density,

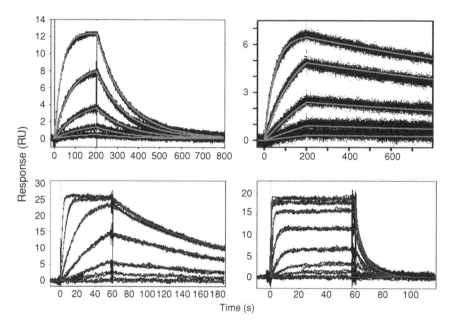

Figure 1.16 Responses of different sharkfin shapes all fit to a 1:1 interaction model. Reproduced from references 41 and 42 with permission from Elsevier © 2004 and 2006.

flow rates, regeneration conditions, and running buffer to produce better data. It is important to realize that the process of generating good data does take time and effort. In fact, a trait that defines the best biosensor users is that they recognize when data are not simple exponentials and they work hard to improve it.

The fact that biosensors are now readily available and easier to use has been one of the biggest problems with the technology as well. Users need to take a step back and really think about what they are doing. They need to be skeptical about their own data and keep an open mind about what the biosensor may be telling them. We have a saying "the biosensor doesn't lie". If you have poor quality reagents, the biosensor will show you that. If you design the experiment incorrectly, it will show you that too. The reason we need to get on top of this problem now is that the number of instruments, as well as the throughput of the technology, keeps increasing, which makes it easier to generate a lot of really poor quality data, and no one wants to see that. By alerting all users now about this problem, we are confident the technology has an exceptionally bright future.

REFERENCES

1. S. Löfås and B. Johnsson, *J. Chem. Soc. Chem. Comm.* **21**, 1526 (1990).
2. Y. S. N. Day, et al., *Protein Sci.* **11**, 1017 (2002).
3. D. G. Myszka et al., *J. Biomolec. Techniq.* **14**, 247 (2003).
4. M. J. Cannon et al., *Anal. Biochem.* **330**, 98 (2004).
5. D. G. Myszka, *Anal. Biochem.* **329**, 316 (2004).
6. T. Bravman et al., *Anal. Biochem.* **358**, 281 (2006).
7. G. A. Papalia et al., *Anal. Biochem.* **359**, 94 (2006).
8. I. Navratilova et al., *Anal. Biochem.* **364**, 67 (2007).
9. P. S. Katsamba et al., *Anal. Biochem.* **352**, 208 (2006).
10. R. L. Rich et al., *Anal. Biochem.* **386**, 194 (2009).
11. A. W. Drake, D. G. Myszka and S. L. Klakamp, *Anal. Biochem.* **328**, 35 (2004).
12. G. A. Papalia et al., *Anal. Biochem.* **383**, 255 (2008).
13. D. G. Myszka, *J. Mol. Recog.* **12**, 390 (1999).
14. R. L. Rich and D. G. Myszka, *J. Mol. Recog.* **13**, 388 (2000).
15. R. L. Rich and D. G. Myszka, *J. Mol. Recog.* **14**, 273 (2001).
16. R. L. Rich and D. G. Myszka, *J. Mol. Recog.* **15**, 352 (2002).
17. R. L. Rich and D. G. Myszka, *J. Mol. Recog.* **16**, 351 (2003).
18. R. L. Rich and D. G. Myszka, *J. Mol. Recog.* **18**, 1 (2005).
19. R. L. Rich and D. G. Myszka, *J. Mol. Recog.* **18**, 431 (2005).
20. R. L. Rich and D. G. Myszka, *J. Mol. Recog.* **19**, 478 (2006).
21. R. L. Rich and D. G. Myszka, *J. Mol. Recog.* **20**, 300 (2007).
22. R. L. Rich and D. G. Myszka, *J. Mol. Recog.* **21**, 355 (2008).
23. D. G. Myszka et al., *Prot. Sci.* **5**, 2468 (1996).
24. D. G. Myszka et al., *Biophys. Chem.* **64**, 127 (1997).
25. D. G. Myszka, *Curr. Opin. Biotechnol.* **8**, 50 (1997).
26. T. A. Morton and D. G. Myszka, *Meth. Enzymol.* **295**, 268 (1998).
27. D. G. Myszka, *J. Mol. Recog.* **12**, 279 (1999).
28. M. Thaler et al., *Clin. Chem.* **51**, 401 (2005).
29. T. Liu et al., *Bioorg. Med. Chem.* **17**, 1026 (2009).
30. D. J. Yoon et al., *J. Control. Release* **133**, 178 (2009).
31. T. A. Morton et al., *J. Mol. Recognit.* **7**, 47 (1994).
32. T. E. Ramsdale et al., *FEBS Lett.* **333**, 217 (1993).
33. D. G. Myszka and T. A. Morton, *Trends Biochem. Sci.* **23**, 149 (1998).
34. M. A. Wear and M. D. Walkinshaw, *Anal. Biochem.* **371**, 250 (2007).
35. F. Yang et al., *Biochemistry* **47**, 4237 (2008).
36. B. T. Seet et al., *EMBO Journal* **26**, 678 (2007).
37. J. S. Klein et al, *Proc. Natl Acad. Sci. USA* **106**, 7385 (2009).
38. P. J. Schmidt et al., *Cell Metab.* **7**, 205 (2008).
39. O. Srinivas et al., *Bioconjug. Chem.* **18**, 1547 (2007).
40. W-J. Jung et al., *Anal. Biochem.* **359**, 112 (2007).
41. D. Casper, M. Bukhtiyarova and E. B. Springman, *Anal. Biochem.* **325**, 126 (2004).

2

Design and Implementation of Vertically Emitting Distributed Feedback Lasers for Biological Sensing

Meng Lu[1], Steven S. Choi[1], Chun Ge[1], Clark J. Wagner[2], J. Gary Eden[2], and Brian T. Cunningham[1]
[1]*Micro and Nanotechnology Laboratory*
[2]*Laboratory for Optical Physics and Engineering Department of Electrical and Computer Engineering, University of Illinois at Urbana-Champaign, Urbana, IL, USA*

Label-Free Technologies for Drug Discovery Edited by Matthew Cooper and Lorenz M. Mayr
© 2011 John Wiley & Sons, Ltd

2.1 INTRODUCTION

Label-free optical biosensors enable the detection of small drug compounds, DNA, proteins, viral particles, bacteria, and cells through their
intrinsic dielectric permittivity. Because label-free detection methods do
not require attachment of fluorescent dye molecules or other enzyme-
based tags to the analyte being detected, it is possible to perform relatively simple detection protocols that facilitate assay development and
enhance the performance of detection procedures outside the laboratory.
Optical resonator-based, label-free biosensors have become an effective
and commercially viable means of characterizing bimolecular interactions for applications in drug discovery research, protein biomarker diagnostic testing, pharmaceutical manufacturing, and environmental monitoring (1, 2). Desirable properties for such sensors include ease of fabrication over large surface areas, robust noncontact illumination/detection
optics, the ability to perform many independent assays in parallel, and the
ability to incorporate the sensor into common biochemical assay formats,
such as microplates or microfluidic channels (3–5). Although label-free
detection methods afford detection resolutions below 1 pg/mm^2, they
have not replaced fluorescence and enzyme-based assays, which offer
higher levels of sensitivity (6). The ability to resolve exceedingly small
changes in the adsorbed mass density is particularly important for assays
requiring the detection of samples at low concentration, or the detection
of biomolecules with low molecular weight (such as drug compounds).
To address these challenges, researchers have designed label-free biosensor structures with passive optical resonators that provide Q-factors up
to 10^8 (7–11), so that smaller wavelength shifts may be resolved (12,
13). The drawbacks of extremely high Q-factor passive resonators include the requirement for precise optical alignment with the illumination
source, and retaining a sufficient dynamic range of wavelength shift to
accommodate the detection of surface functionalization layers, immo
bilized ligands and analytes (14). Recently, active optical resonators,
such as the microdisk laser (15), the photonic crystal laser (16), and the
distributed feedback (DFB) laser (17), have been integrated into label-
free biosensors. These laser-based sensors can produce their own narrow
linewidth radiation, which results in simplified coupling to the excitation
source and collection optics for detecting small changes in wavelength,
while retaining excellent sensitivity, as exhibited by the magnitude of

the wavelength shift induced by changes in surface dielectric permittivity resulting from the adsorption of biomolecules.

Semiconductor DFB lasers have been studied extensively since their first demonstration in 1971, due to interest in wavelength division multiplexing (WDM) (18) and other aspects of optical communications. Recently developed embossing and imprinting techniques have simplified grating fabrication, and have thus reduced the cost of organic DFB lasers (19–21). DFB lasers are typically designed to operate with a single narrow line width mode (22–24), making them attractive for biosensor applications. In earlier investigations, this team demonstrated a DFB laser biosensor utilizing a nano-replica molded grating with a dye-doped organic film as an optically pumped gain material. The DFB laser biosensor was successfully used to detect thin layers of deposited polymer monolayers applied to the sensor surface. In Section 2.1, the sensor structure is thoroughly analysed, thus enabling optimization of the sensitivity, and the sensitivity achieved with the modeled structure is experimentally demonstrated.

Section 2.2 describes the design criteria for the DFB laser biosensor. Section 2.3 discusses the fabrication procedure, and the experimental results concerning sensor performance for chemical and biomolecular detection are presented in Section 2.4, with conclusions summarized in Section 2.5.

2.2 DFB LASER BIOSENSOR DESIGN

Most optical resonator-based, label-free biosensors detect biomolecular adsorption on the sensor surface by monitoring changes in the resonant mode, as measured by shifts in resonant wavelength, coupling angle, or coupling efficiency. In a similar fashion, the DFB laser biosensor system reported here monitors adsorption of biomaterial through detection of shifts in the laser emission wavelength. The tracking of peak emission wavelength reveals the temporal evolution of the material mass density accumulated on the laser sensor surface. The optical cavity for the DFB laser adopted for the present experiments is a Bragg surface grating resonator in which the resonant wavelength of the cavity satisfies the Bragg condition, $\lambda = 2n_{eff} \Lambda/m$, where m is the diffraction order, Λ denotes the grating period, and n_{eff} represents the effective refractive index (RI). To facilitate the extraction of the laser radiation, the DFB laser sensor incorporates a second order Bragg grating that results in radiation output normal to the device surface by first order diffraction (25). A cross-sectional diagram (not to scale) of the DFB laser structure is shown in Figure 2.1.

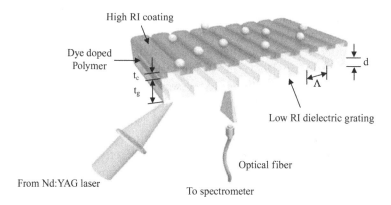

Figure 2.1 Cross-sectional diagram (not to scale) of the DFB laser-based biosensor structure and optical pumping and detection instrumental arrangement. The period and depth of the grating structure are Λ and d, respectively. The thickness of the high RI coating and gain layer are t_c and t_g, respectively.

The second order grating is formed on the surface of a dielectric substrate with an RI of n_{sub}. Upon the dielectric grating is a laser dye-doped polymer layer whose thickness and RI are t_g and n_g, respectively. This active polymer layer provides amplification, confinement, and feedback to the resonant mode. A high RI thin film is deposited on the top surface. The DFB laser sensor may be optically pumped at any incident angle, and the resulting stimulated emission is monitored by a fiber-coupled spectrometer along an axis nearly orthogonal to the surface.

The design of a sensitive DFB laser biosensor requires an understanding of the mechanisms by which the structural parameters and material properties of the device dictate its performance. The emission wavelength shift of a second order DFB laser sensor can be expressed as $\Delta\lambda = \Delta n_{eff}\Lambda$, where Δn_{eff} is caused by the interaction of detected biomaterial with the evanescent portion of the resonant mode. By manipulating the spatial distribution of the resonant mode, it is possible to improve the interaction between the biomaterials and the evanescent field, thereby enhancing the sensor sensitivity (26). The general goal is to increase the overlap between the resonance mode and the detected biomaterial (27), while maintaining a substantial part of the mode within the gain medium to facilitate lasing. Rigorous coupled wave analysis (RCWA; DiffractMOD, R-Soft) was used to numerically predict the resonant wavelength and the associated electric field distribution for different device designs. To simplify the simulation, the DFB laser sensor was modeled as a passive optical cavity.

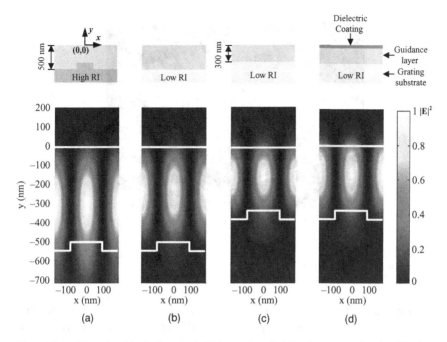

Figure 2.2 The simulated electric field intensity distributions associated with the resonant mode within a single period of the grating structure. The sensor surfaces are aligned at $y = 0$ for all of the images: (a) the substrate grating layer is formed within an epoxy material; (b) the epoxy material used in (a) is replaced with a low RI nanoporous glass material and the mode moves closer to the sensor surface; (c) t_g is reduced from 500 nm to 350 nm; (d) a HfO$_2$ film with a thickness of $t_g = 40$ nm is coated on top of the guidance layer.

Schematic diagrams and calculated electric field intensity distributions within one period of the grating are compared in Figures 2.2a–2.2d for four exemplary sensor designs. The top panel of Figure 2.2a shows a sensor design in which the grating is replica molded with an epoxy substrate of $n_{sub} = 1.45$, $\Lambda = 360$ nm and the epoxy layer has $t_g = 500$ nm and $n_g = 1.5$. The lower panel of Figure 2.2a illustrates the normalized distribution of the electric field intensity at the resonant wavelength. In all four plots, the sensor's top horizontal surface is located at $y = 0$ and is indicated by the upper horizontal white line. Using the initial sensor structure as a baseline (2a), the effect of variations in the material properties and the effect of additional deposited layers on the mode profile and sensitivity of this structure were investigated. As the first modification, the epoxy substrate is replaced by a lower RI ($n_{sub} = 1.17$) nanoporous glass substrate (Figure 2.2b). Compared to the mode profile given in

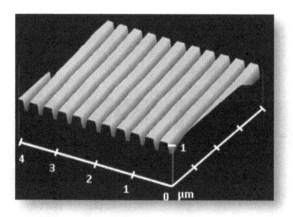

Figure 2.3 Atomic force microscope image of a replicated grating with a period of 360 nm and depth of 80 nm.

Figure 2.2a, the resonant mode shown in Figure 2.2b is closer to the sensor surface. As discussed elsewhere (28), using a low RI substrate can increase the sensor sensitivity by a factor of two. The second improvement involves reduction of the polymer layer thickness from $t_g = 500$ nm to $t_g = 350$ nm. Figure 2.2c shows the extension of the resonant mode above the sensor surface when this modification to the cavity is implemented. An additional optimization is achieved by adding a high RI thin film coating, such as hafnium dioxide (HfO_2; $n_c \sim 2.0$ at $\lambda = 500$ nm). Coating the sensor surface with a 40 nm thick hafnium dioxide film draws the mode closer to the sensor surface and improves the mode's spatial overlap with the biomolecule adsorption region.

To verify the modal analysis, the resonant wavelength shift induced by small changes in the RI of the bulk medium in contact with the sensor surface was studied for this device with different thicknesses of the polymer layer and the hafnium dioxide coating. RCWA simulations and experimental measurements are compared in Section 2.4.2.

2.3 FABRICATION AND INSTRUMENTATION

Nanoreplica molding was used to pattern the sol-gel, low RI porous silica into a one dimensional grating on a glass substrate (18, 28). The process begins with production of an eight-inch diameter silicon "master" wafer that contains a positive surface profile of the final device. The silicon wafer was patterned with a linear grating ($\Lambda = 360$ nm, 50% duty cycle, and 80 nm depth) by deep-UV photolithography and reactive ion etching. The silicon "master" grating structure can be used to produce multiple "daughter" grating replicas from polydimethylsiloxane (PDMS; Sylgard 184, Dow), which forms a negative surface image of the master. To fabricate the daughter mold, PDMS was poured into a rectangular metal frame placed on top of the master wafer. The PDMS mold was thermally cured (90 °C, 4 h) and then peeled from the silicon master. To facilitate release of the cured PDMS mold from the silicon wafer, the wafer surface was treated with a release layer of dimethyldichlorosilane (Repel Silane, Amersham Biosciences). Replica molding of the sol-gel silica film on a rigid glass substrate is performed with the daughter PDMS grating serving as a molding tool. After spin casting a 1 µm thick film of sol-gel silica (Nanoglass, Honeywell Electronic Materials) onto a glass substrate with a surface area of 10.8×7.2 cm^2, the PDMS mold was gradually applied from one end of the substrate to the other. With the PDMS stamp in contact with the sol-gel layer, the porous dielectric was cured on a hotplate at 110 °C for two minutes. Once the sol-gel porous dielectric becomes rigid, the flexible PDMS and the dielectric replica of the grating were separated by peeling the PDMS mold away from the device, and the sol-gel porous dielectric was fully cured by further baking. As verified by atomic force microscopy (Figure 2.3), the replicated porous dielectric gratings have a 360 nm period and an imprint depth of 80 nm.

The gain medium comprises a thin film of a laser dye/polymer mixture on the surface of the grating. For a 360 nm period DFB cavity, the calculated resonance wavelength will occur within a wavelength range of 480–520 nm, depending on the choice of the substrate RI. In this work, Coumarin 503 dye (Exciton) with a maximum fluorescence emission wavelength at 503 nm, was used. Coumarin 503 powder was first dissolved in methylchloride to a concentration of 10 mg/ml. The solution was mixed with poly(methyl methacrylate) (PMMA) solution (4% PMMA solid dissolved in chlorobenzene) to a volume percentage of 10%. The mixture was sonicated for improved homogenization and subsequently spin coated onto the dielectric grating/substrate assembly at 4000 rpm for 30 seconds. The device was baked on a 110 °C hotplate for 1.5 minutes to vaporize the solvent and to densify the film. The spun-on polymer thickness and RI were verified by ellipsometry (VASE, J.A. Woollam). The sensor was finally coated with a hafnium dioxide film using an electron beam evaporator (Denton Vacuum). The fabricated sensor was attached to a standard format, bottomless 96-well microplate with double-sided adhesive, so that the DFB laser biosensor surface formed the bottom surface of each well within the microplate.

The laser sensor was excited by ∼8 ns pulses from a frequency-tripled, Q-switched Nd:YAG (neodymium:yttrium aluminum garnet; Continuum) laser ($\lambda = 355$ nm) in the single pulse mode. The pump light was focused to illuminate a ∼2 mm diameter spot on the sensor surface. The output signal from the DFB laser was coupled through an optical fiber to a spectrometer (HR 4000, Ocean Optics) having a resolution (in first order) of 0.05 nm full width at half maximum (FWHM). An optical fiber oriented perpendicular to the sensor surface, and coupled to the spectrometer, captures detected emission from the DFB laser. The trigger of the Nd:YAG pump laser was synchronized to the spectrometer by a PC controller. To achieve wavelength accuracy better than the spectrometer resolution, the recorded laser spectrum was fitted to a Lorentzian profile, and the peak laser emission wavelength was determined mathematically. The peak laser emission wavelengths were recorded and plotted as a function of time to dynamically quantify biomolecule adsorption on the sensor surface.

2.4 EXPERIMENTAL RESULTS

2.4.1 Vertically Emitting DFB Laser

The tested device incorporates a nanoporous SiO_2 grating, Coumarin 503 doped PMMA ($t_g = 350$ nm, $n_g = 1.5$), and a hafnium dioxide coating ($t_c = 45$ nm). Figure 2.4a shows the laser emission spectrum recorded when the sensor surface is exposed to air and the pump fluence was maintained at 7.5 mJ-cm^{-2}. From the best fit of the Lorentzian (shown in gray in Figure 2.4a) to the spectrum, the laser emission wavelength was determined to be 497.52 nm, with a line width of 0.07 nm. Figure 2.4b shows the dependence of the DFB laser pulse energy on the pump fluence. A linear least-squares fit to the data yields a threshold pump fluence of 2.0 mJ-cm^{-2} for lasing in air, while a threshold of 2.5 mJ-cm^{-2} was measured when the sensor surface was covered with deionized water.

2.4.2 Bulk Material Sensing

Initially the dependence of the laser emission wavelength on changes in the RI of the media exposed to the sensor surface was studied by observing the wavelength shift induced by changing the material on the sensor

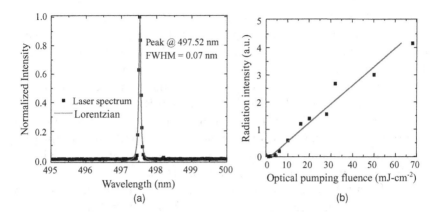

Figure 2.4 (a) Laser spectrum for pump energies above threshold for a device operated with water in contact with the sensor surface; the best fit of a Lorentzian to the data is also presented. (b) The dependence of the relative laser output power on the pump fluence. From these data, the threshold pump fluence is calculated to be $2.0\,\mathrm{mJ\text{-}cm^{-2}}$.

surface from air (RI $= 1.0$) to water (RI ~ 1.33). All of the tested devices were fabricated upon nanoporous glass gratings ($n_{sub} = 1.17$) with Coumarin 503 doped PMMA and a hafnium dioxide coating ranging between zero and 60 nm in thickness. Devices with polymer thicknesses of $t_g = 345\,\mathrm{nm}$, 385 nm, 460 nm, and 502 nm were evaluated by measuring the water-induced shift of the peak lasing wavelength at five locations on each device. The measured results are compared with the values predicted by RCWA simulations in Figure 2.5a. By reducing t_g from 500 nm to 345 nm, the wavelength shift for an air–water superstrate transition

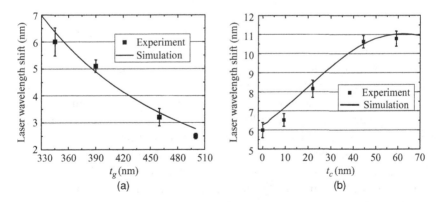

Figure 2.5 (a) Data acquired for the shift in the peak laser wavelength when the sensor surface was exposed to air and subsequently to deionized water. For these measurements, t_g was varied from 340 nm to 500 nm. (b) The same laser wavelength shifts were investigated for t_c between 0 and 70 nm.

is increased from ~ 2.5 nm to ~ 6 nm. To explore the impact of hafnium dioxide film thickness on sensor performance, devices having a 345 nm thick polymer layer and a hafnium dioxide film thickness of $t_g = 0$ nm, 10 nm, 22 nm, 45 nm, or 60 nm were fabricated. As before, five spots on each sensor were tested and results are shown and compared with numerical predictions (Figure 2.5b). Adding the high RI dielectric film results in the laser wavelength shift for the transition from air to water increasing from 6 to 11 nm. On the other hand, excessive reduction of the gain layer thickness or a thick hafnium dioxide coating results in a high lasing threshold and multiple mode emission. By reducing t_g from 502 nm to 345 nm for a 60 nm thick hafnium dioxide film, the DFB laser sensor's sensitivity was enhanced by a factor of 4.2. The bulk RI sensitivity is calculated to be $S_b = \Delta PWV/\Delta n = 33.4$ nm/RIU (refractive index unit).

2.4.3 Sensitivity Resolution

The other criterion by which sensor performance is evaluated is the sensitivity of wavelength emission to surface adsorbed mass density. In bulk material sensing, the analyte is a homogeneous solution and any species on or above the sensor surface contributes to the laser emission wavelength shift. For surface adsorbed mass detection, only surface-bound material contributes to the final laser emission wavelength shift, while nonbound material is removed from the sensor by a washing procedure. Surface sensitivity is the most important criterion for the detection of protein–protein or protein–small molecule binding interactions.

Sensitivity to surface mass adsorption was characterized by introducing a solution of the protein polymer poly(Lys, Phe) (PPL) to the laser surface. PPL (Sigma-Aldrich) was dissolved in phosphate-buffered saline (PBS) at a concentration of 0.5 mg/ml, which has been shown to deposit a self-limiting monolayer with a mass density of 2.5 ng/mm^2 (29). Figure 2.6 shows the dynamic detection of a PPL layer on the sensor surface. Initially, a baseline value for the laser wavelength was established with the sensor surface soaked in a PBS solution. After four minutes, the PBS solution was replaced with a PPL solution and stabilized for 10 minutes. Next, the sensor surface was rinsed with PBS solution to remove any PPL that was not firmly attached to the sensor. The sensor produced a wavelength shift of 0.64 nm for PPL monolayer adsorption, and exhibited no detectable drift over periods of up to one hour.

To determine the sensor detection limit, the minimum detectable laser wavelength shift was first ascertained by exposing the sensor to deionized

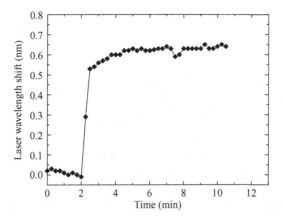

Figure 2.6 Kinetic plot of lasing wavelength shift for a PPL monolayer deposited onto the DFB laser sensor surface. The pump fluence was kept constant at 12.5 mJ-cm^{-2}. The stabilized surface shift for the DFB laser based biosensor under these conditions is 0.64 nm.

water and measuring the wavelength every second for a total period of one minute. As shown in Figure 2.7, the wavelength shift ranges between +1 and −4 pm, with a standard deviation (σ) of 1.05 pm. Thus, the system resolution was found to be $\delta\lambda = 3\sigma = 3.15$ pm. The bulk RI and surface mass resolutions were calculated to be $\delta\lambda/S_b = 9.4 \times 10^{-5}$ RIU and 12.3 pg/mm^2, respectively.

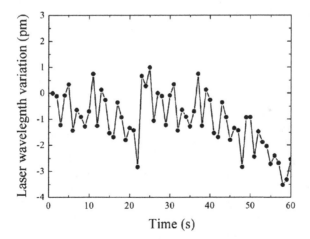

Figure 2.7 The time dependent laser wavelength variation when the sensor was immersed in deionized water and pumped at 10.2 mJ-cm^{-2}.

2.4.4 Small Molecule Binding Detection

A common test for characterizing biosensor performance is to immobilize a large molecule that subsequently captures selectively a much smaller molecule with a 1:1 binding ratio. In these experiments, the avidin–biotin system was used owing to its high affinity constant (10^{15} M^{-1}). To immobilize strepavidin (SA, MW = 60 kDa, Sigma-Aldrich), the HfO_2-coated sensor was first immersed in a proprietary amine polymer solution for 24 hours, followed by deionized water washing. Next, the amine polymer surface was exposed to glutaraldehyde (GA; $C_5H_8O_2$; 25% in deionized water) for 3.5 hours. The GA is a bifunctional linker that functionalizes the amine groups in the amine polymer film and enables the subsequent attachment of SA. SA (0.5 mg/ml in deionized water) was added to the sensor surface as a precursor to the detection of biotin (MW = 244 Da; Sigma-Aldrich) and allowed to incubate for 30 hours at 4 °C.

The DFB laser wavelength was monitored during the first 16 minutes of the SA immobilization process; the results are shown in Figure 2.8a. By making several measurements of the sensor as a function of time, the kinetic characteristics of mass adsorption can be determined (Figure 2.8a). After 30 hours of SA incubation, the sensor was rinsed with deionized water. While immersed in 100 μl of deionized water, the sensor was stabilized for five minutes. Upon adding 5 μl biotin solution (0.25 mg/ml; in deionized water), the kinetic binding process shown in Figure 2.8b was observed. The binding of biotin to SA produced a laser wavelength shift of ~54 pm. In a reference well where the sensor surface is not immobilized with SA, nonspecific binding of biotin at the

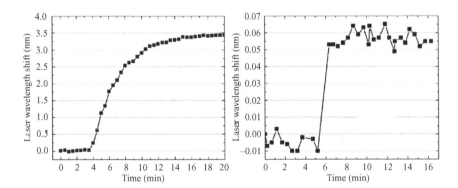

Figure 2.8 Detection of biotin–avidin binding. (a) Kinetic peak laser wavelength plot of the streptavidin immobilization process onto the sensor surface that was pretreated with a specific surface chemistry protocol. (b) Detection of biotin binding with immobilized SA; the stabilized shift of the peak laser wavelength is 55 pm.

same concentration was monitored. The subsequent wavelength shift is smaller than the wavelength resolution of the sensor.

The expected laser wavelength shift caused by biotin binding can be estimated as follows. Since every SA molecule can capture up to four biotin molecules, biotin binding can result in a laser wavelength shift of $\Delta\lambda_{biotin} = 4 \times MW_{biotin}/MW_{SA} \times \Delta\lambda_{SA}$, where MW represents molecular weight. According to the kinetic measurement of SA immobilization, the laser emission wavelength shift of SA absorption is $\sim$3.5 nm. From the above equation, the calculated biotin shift is $\sim$57 pm, which agrees well with experiment.

2.5 CONCLUSIONS

In summary, this chapter describes the use of a DFB laser for label-free optical bioassay detection. The DFB laser reported here exhibits single mode operation and a spectral line width of 0.07 nm. The DFB laser sensor demonstrates a surface adsorbed mass detection limit of 28 pg/mm^2. As a result of biotin binding on a SA immobilized sensor surface, the DFB laser sensor kinetically detects a shift of $\sim$54 pm. The major limitation on resolution results from the minimum detectable laser wavelength shift. Since the narrow laser emission spectrum is detected by 4–5 pixels on the spectrometer, the calculated laser emission wavelength has a significant uncertainty. Bypassing this limitation by using alternate wavelength measurement methods, such as a higher resolution spectrometer or a recently developed graded wavelength filter detector, is under investigation. Because the replica molding process is inexpensive and scalable to large areas, and the DFB grating structure is amenable to simple yet robust excitation and output detection methods, this type of sensor is expected to become practical for applications demanding high sensitivity in life science research, diagnostic testing, and environmental detection.

ACKNOWLEDGEMENTS

This work was supported by SRU Biosystems and the US Air Force Office of Scientific Research. The authors gratefully acknowledge Honeywell Electronic Materials for providing Nanoglass low-k dielectric material. The authors also wish to thank the staff of the Micro and Nanotechnology Laboratory at the University of Illinois at Urbana-Champaign.

REFERENCES

1. B. Cunningham, B. Lin, C. Baird, *et al.*, *Sensors and Actuators B-Chemical* **85**, 219 (2002).
2. U. Jonsson, L. Fägerstam, B. Ivarsson, *et al.*, *Biotechniques* **11** (5), 620 (1991).
3. C. J. Choi and B. T. Cunningham, *Lab on a Chip* **7**, 550 (2007).
4. B. T. Cunningham, P. Li, S. Schulz, *et al.*, *Journal of Biomolecular Screening* **9**, 481 (2004).
5. S. Mandal and D. Erickson, *Optics Express* **16**, 1623 (2008).
6. W. E. Moerner, *Proceedings of the National Academy of Sciences of the United States of America* **104**, 15584 (2007).
7. A. M. Armani and K. J. Vahala, *Optics Letters* **31**, 1896 (2006).
8. L. Rindorf and O. Bang, *Optics Letters* **33**, 563 (2008).
9. I. M. White, H. Oveys and X. D. Fan, *Optics Letters* **31**, 1319 (2006).
10. A. Yalcin, K.C. Popat, J.C. Aldridge, *et al.*, *Ieee Journal of Selected Topics in Quantum Electronics* **12**, 148 (2006).
11. N. M. Hanumegowda, C. J. Stica, B. C. Patel *et al. Applied Physics Letters* **87**, (2005).
12. W. C. Karl and H. H. Pien, *IEEE Transactions on Signal Processing* **53**, 4631 2005).
13. I. M. White and X. D. Fan, *Optics Express* **16**, 1020 (2008).
14. C. Y. Chao, W. Fung, and L. J. Guo, *Ieee Journal of Selected Topics in Quantum Electronics* **12**, 134 (2006).
15. W. Fang, D.B. Buchholz, R.C. Bailey, *et al.*, *Applied Physics Letters* **85**, 3666 (2004).
16. M. Loncar, A. Scherer, and Y. M. Qiu, *Applied Physics Letters* **82**, 4648 (2003).
17. M. Lu, S. Choi, C. J. Wagner *et al. Applied Physics Letters* **92**, (2008).
18. J. A. Rogers, M. Meier, A. Dodabalapur *et al. Applied Physics Letters* **74**, 3257 (1999).
19. Y. Chen, Z. Li, Z. Zhang, D. Psaltis, and A. Scherer, *Applied Physics Letters* **91**, (2007).
20. L. J. Guo, *Journal of Physics D – Applied Physics* **37**, R123 (2004).
21. M. Gaal, C. Gadermaier, H. Plank, *et al. Advanced Materials* **15**, 1165 (2003).
22. N. Naki, M. Fukuda, and K. Mito, *Japaneses Journal of Applied Physics* **45**, 998 (2006).
23. S. Balslev, T. Rasmussen, P. Shi, and A. Kristensen *Journal of Micromechanics and Microengineering* **15**, 2456 (2005).
24. M. Berggren, A. Dodabalapur, R. E. Slusher *et al. Applied Physics Letters* **72**, 410 (1998).
25. R. F. Kazarinov and C. H. Henry, *Ieee Journal of Quantum Electronics* **21**, 144 (1985).
26. I. D. Block, N. Ganesh, M. Lu, and B. T. Cunningham, *Ieee Sensors Journal* **8**, 274 (2008).
27. L. Rindorf and O. Bang, *Journal of the Optical Society of America B-Optical Physics* **25**, 310 (2008).
28. I. D. Block, L. L. Chan, and B. T. Cunningham, *Sensors and Actuators B-Chemical* **120**, 187 (2006).
29. J. Voros, *Biophysical Journal* **87**, 553 (2004).

3

SPR Screening of Chemical Microarrays for Fragment-Based Discovery

Thomas Neumann and Renate Sekul
Graffinity Pharmaceuticals GmbH, Heidelberg, Germany

Label-Free Technologies for Drug Discovery   Edited by Matthew Cooper and Lorenz M. Màyr
© 2011 John Wiley & Sons, Ltd

3.1 INTRODUCTION

Surface plasmon resonance (SPR) is known to be a versatile tool for the study of biomolecular interactions that can generate affinity data in a highly sensitive and label-free detection format. This chapter focuses on the application of SPR imaging technology to the high throughput screening (HTS) of immobilized small molecule libraries for fragment-based discovery.

3.2 KEY FEATURES OF FRAGMENT SCREENING

Fragments are considered as substructures of drug-like substances that interact with individual protein epitopes or subsites. In contrast to typical HTS screening compounds, fragments are smaller (MW >300 Da) and chemically less complex, therefore more likely to match a given binding site (1). Despite weaker protein–ligand interactions (in the high micromolar to millimolar range), fragments bind with higher ligand efficiencies (binding energy per number of heavy atoms) (2). These properties increase the chance of discovering new chemotypes which may be missed with conventional technologies. Furthermore, small and simple molecules open up more opportunities for further optimization (Figure 3.1).

3.3 SPR FRAGMENT SCREENING

A prerequisite for successful fragment-based screening is the availability of highly sensitive screening technologies for the detection of initially weak protein fragment interactions. In addition to approaches such as X-ray, NMR or MS, a promising solution is to immobilize fragments

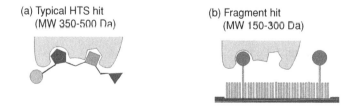

Figure 3.1   The essence of fragment-based screening.

on sensor surfaces and monitor the interaction with soluble protein by surface plasmon resonance (SPR) (Figure 3.1b). In particular, SPR imaging of chemical microarrays can simultaneously generate affinity data for up to 9216 immobilized fragments per array and allows screening of protein targets against compound libraries of 110 000 small molecules in a high throughput fashion (3–6).

For the construction of arrayed fragment libraries, small organic molecules are covalently immobilized on a chemically modified chip surface. Soluble protein is then allowed to interact with the ligands constituting the chemical microarrays. Protein binding events can be monitored by means of Plasmon Imager® instrumentation. Immobilizing the ligands instead of the target protein itself has the advantage of minimizing the risk of denaturing the protein. Also, the immobilized compounds to be screened do not need to be extremely soluble at high concentrations, as in reverse approaches where the screening compound is floated over the chip surface. Furthermore, proteins typically cause larger local changes in refractive index when bound to the chip surface. Hence, the sensitivity and detection limit of the SPR imaging readout allows even small protein targets to be conveniently screened with a good signal to noise ratio.

SPR technology has the capability to detect protein/ligand affinities up to the μM to mM range. Being primarily independent of further reporter assays, the approach can also be applied to the identification of novel binding sites for difficult targets, such as protein–protein interaction targets, which are often not easily addressed with conventional types of assays.

3.4 SYNTHESIS OF LIBRARY COMPOUNDS

Library compounds are synthesized using parallel high throughput chemistry approaches (7). A linker molecule, the so-called ChemTag®, is coupled to a solid phase synthesis (SPS) support in a batch process (Figure 3.2a). In the case of the directly immobilized fragment array compounds, individual fragments are attached to the ChemTag® linker. For binary libraries, the building blocks are organized such that each row and column share one specific motif. This allows the coordinated parallel synthesis of up to 9216 array compounds per batch (Figure 3.2b).

After synthesis, ChemTag®-compound conjugates (Figure 3.7a) are cleaved from the synthesis resin and stored in 384-well microtiterplates for quality control, storage and array production (Figure 3.2c). These

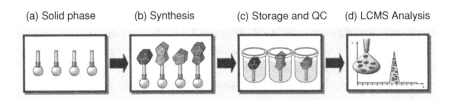

Figure 3.2   Parallel synthesis of library compounds.

tagged structures, referred to as array compounds, are then rigorously quality controlled by parallel quantitative LC/MS for their yield and purity (Figure 3.2d). Purity acceptance levels are >75% for lead-like compounds and >90% for fragments. Compounds failing the quality control criteria are flagged and not considered during data analysis.

The ChemTag® (Figure 3.7) is a long, flexible and hydrophilic linker, designed to be resistant to unspecific protein binding and to allow penetration into even deep protein binding pockets. Different types of spacer molecules contain diverse sets of terminal functionalities (e.g. amino group in Figure 3.7), which enable a large range of chemistries for fragment attachment and library synthesis. The common element of all linkers is a thiol group located at the opposite terminus; this is needed for the immobilization of the construct on the functionalized sensor surface.

As the synthesis of array compounds is conducted on a miniaturized scale (50 nmol/compound), the consumption of educts is reduced to a minimum and, hence, allows rare building blocks to also be included into the library.

3.5 LIBRARY DESIGN AND ARRAY CONTENT

Graffinity's compound collection comprises a total of ~110 000 fragment and lead-like compounds available for screening as indicated in Figure 3.3. Besides using common medicinal chemistry and biophysical property design rules, filters were also applied to exclude undesired toxic or reactive functional groups (8). To increase the probability of hit identification, diversity selection criteria and available biological information influenced the library design. Additionally, the design was aimed at an enrichment of privileged motifs and pharmacophores. By using in-house combinatorial chemistry approaches, unique one- and two-dimensional

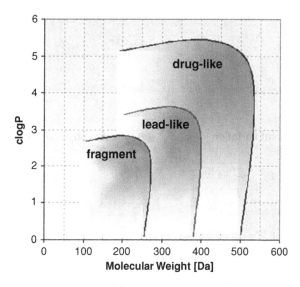

Figure 3.3 Classification of Graffinity's fragment and lead-like collection according molecular weight and clogP.

libraries with an average molecular weight of ~320 Da were developed, which can be subdivided into the following groups:

(1) *Lead-like libraries*: This library contains 87 000 compounds, which mostly consist of combinations of two building blocks displayed on various small scaffolds and molecular weight >300 Da. Such arrays are also referred to as binary or two-dimensional arrays.

(2) *Fragment libraries*: Fragment libraries consist of 23 000 small molecule compounds largely complying with the 'rule of three' (9), which defines the molecular properties of fragments such as molecular weights of <300 Da or cLogP of ≤3 and so on. They contain directly immobilized synthesized fragments and modified building blocks, as well as displayed fragments on privileged scaffolds. A large fraction of these structures are unique, *de novo* synthesized fragments.

Typical fragment design and immoblilization strategies are summarized in Figure 3.4. In addition to directly immobilized fragments and building blocks (Figure 3.4a), a substitution pattern variation was applied for each compound to obtain decorated fragments. This facilitates

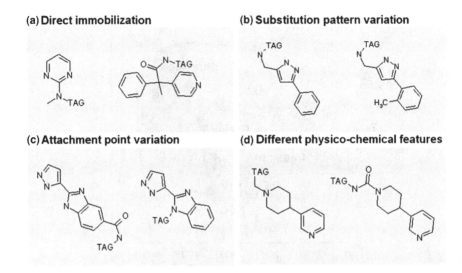

Figure 3.4 Fragment library design.

the generation of structure affinity relationships from identified binder series (Figure 3.4b).

To account for orientational constraints introduced by the attachment of the small molecules to the sensor surface, the position of the linker attachment point was varied for part of the fragment space if chemically possible (Figure 3.4c). This variation can help to estimate the orientation of the fragment in the protein binding pocket. The attachment point can be seen as a chemical handle for the further optimization of identified fragments. Also, by applying a variety of available surface chemistries, fragment linkers with different physico-chemical features can be generated (Figure 3.4d).

3.6 CHEMICAL MICROARRAY PRODUCTION

Graffinity has developed high density chemical microarrays consisting of small molecules immobilized onto gold chips. The chips are based on maleimide-thiol coupling chemistry in combination with high density pin-tool spotting, as summarized in Figure 3.5.

Glass plates are microstructured by photolithographical methods in order to define up to 9216 sensor fields per array (Figure 3.5a). A gold coating applied subsequently provides the basis for the SPR effect and enables the formation of a binary, mixed self-assembled monolayer (SAM)

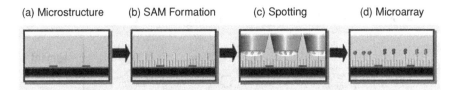

(a) Microstructure   (b) SAM Formation   (c) Spotting   (d) Microarray

Figure 3.5   Microarray production.

of two different thiols (Figure 3.5b). One thiol, the diluent molecule, does not contain any further functionality. The other thiol exhibits a reactive maleimide moiety to which the tagged array compounds (Figure 3.7) can couple to during spotting. By varying the ratio of both thiols the number of binding sites per sensor field can be precisely adjusted. To reduce background generation in the SPR experiment, the SAM surface was designed to minimize unspecific protein binding to the chip surface.

Chemical microarrays (Figure 3.5d) are produced by using proprietary pin-tool spotting technology (Figure 3.5c). The custom-built pin-tool spotter (Figure 3.6) is capable of producing 100 arrays per day. During spotting, a camera controlled spotting head, containing 384 steel needles (Figure 3.6a), transfers nanolitre droplets of compound solution from the microwell plates onto individually addressable sensor fields. After thiol-tagged array compounds are allowed to covalently react, potentially unreacted maleinimide groups are capped and the saturation of the sensor fields is tested by internal quality control measurements. The resulting microarrays (Figure 3.5d and Figure 3.6b) comprise 9216 sensor fields, each containing multiple copies of a defined and quality

(a) Pin Tool   (b) Microarray

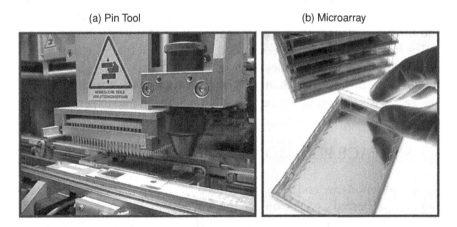

Figure 3.6   Spotting technology.

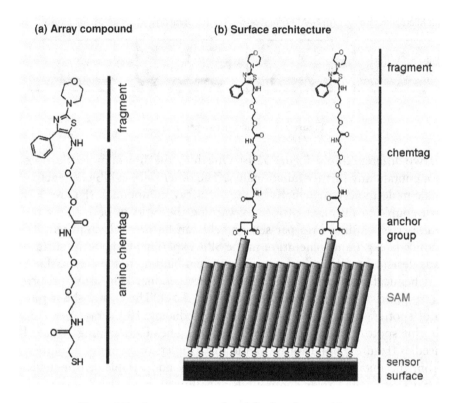

Figure 3.7 Array compound and final surface architecture.

controlled array compound. The final surface architecture is shown in Figure 3.7. The resulting highly defined surface architecture consists of the gold layer, the binary SAM monolayer, including the anchor thiol, and the fragments covalently attached to the SAM via the ChemTag®.

The ligand density can be controlled precisely and is adjusted depending on the protein's properties, such as its molecular weight. Long-term studies have proved that chemical microarrays can be stored for up to one year without loss of data quality in the SPR binding experiments.

3.7 SURFACE PLASMON RESONANCE

Surface plasmons are collective oscillations of electrons at a metal surface and can be viewed as electromagnetic waves confined to the interfacial plane between a metal (e.g. gold) and a dielectric. They can be resonantly excited by coupling polarized light to the surface modes of the metal surface in a variety of optical setups. In the most commonly applied prism coupling, incident light is reflected at the base plate of a prism, which is in optical contact with a thin metal layer. At incidence angles larger than the critical angle (total reflection conditions), incoming light waves and surface bound plasmon waves can be tuned to resonate by varying the light wavelength at constant incidence angle (or vice versa). At surface plasmon resonance conditions, energy from incident light is transferred to the surface plasmon mode and the reflected light intensity exhibits a sharp attenuation (SPR minimum). The angle and wavelength position of this reflectance minimum are, among other parameters, strongly dependent on the refractive index of the medium adjacent to the metal surface. The latter is sensed by the surface plasmon field exponentially decaying into the dielectric medium. Processes which alter the local refractive index in close proximity to the metal surface can, therefore, be monitored by recording the shift of the resonance minimum.

3.8 SPR IMAGING

Chemical microarrays are read using Graffinity's proprietary Plasmon Imager® for label-free imaging in a highly parallel, wavelength dependent measuring mode. In contrast to channel-based systems, the SPR imaging approach uses an expanded beam of parallel light to illuminate the entire microarray sensor area at a fixed angle. The reflected light is then captured by means of a charged coupled device camera. While scanning over a range of wavelengths covering the SPR resonance conditions, reflection images are recorded step-by-step. A close-up of a greyscale picture is given in Figure 3.8a for a specific wavelength. Automated spot finding routines and subsequent greyscale analysis of the obtained pictures lead to SPR resonance curves for all 9216 individual sensor fields in parallel (Figure 3.8b).

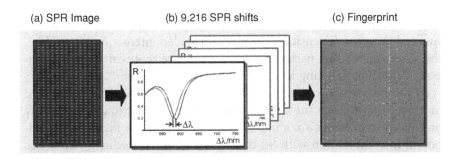

Figure 3.8 Analysis of SPR images.

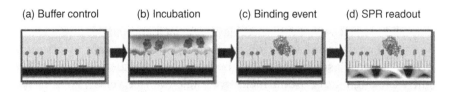

Figure 3.9   SPR measurement protocol.

Measurement data can be visualized as two dimensional colour-coded fingerprints containing all recorded SPR shifts (Figure 3.8c). In total, up to four microarrays can be mounted onto a set of prism blocks simultaneously. This gives the capability of measuring almost 37 000 interactions per day per reader, and thus facilitates a high throughput SPR read out of the chemical microarrays.

Figure 3.9 schematically describes the workflow for a routine SPR equilibrium measurement. Before monitoring protein binding to the array, a reference scan is performed with a screening buffer (Figure 3.9a). Thereafter, the array is incubated with the target protein under optimized screening conditions (Figure 3.9b). As the targets binds to the immobilized fragments, a change in the local refractive index alters the resonance conditions for the respective sensor field (Figure 3.9c). A shift in the wavelength dependent SPR minimum (referred to as the SPR shift) occurs with respect to the buffer control (see also Figure 3.8b) and thus indicates protein–ligand interaction (Figure 3.9d). The SPR wavelength shift (recorded in nanometres) increases with the change in refractive index at the sensor surface and correlates to surface coverage and amount of protein bound to the sensor fields.

3.9 ARRAY VISUALIZATION AND ANALYSIS

SPR measurement data of the affinity fingerprint experiments can be visualized in a two dimensional false colour-coded interaction map. Here, the wavelength shifts within a certain range are represented by a 'rainbow' colouring denoting low to high SPR shifts (Figure 3.10).

In the binary array design, microarray plate views can be arranged in a way that reflects the combinatorial synthesis approach. Each row or column represents a common fragment within the final array compound in combination with 96 other diversities. Accordingly, hit series for binary libraries appear as coloured lines in the fingerprints. The

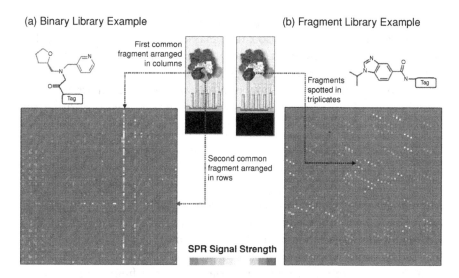

Figure 3.10 Visualization of fingerprint data.

fragment arrays, however, consist of individually selected and synthesized compounds and, thus, are not organized in rows and columns. Due to spotting of fragments in multiplicates, hits clearly show up as triplicate patterns. All arrays contain a limited number of specific control ligands used for internal quality control, distributed across the physical array layout. These ligands are displayed either as grey fields or are blanked out in the screen shots of each array.

For manual analysis, evaluation software is used to provide access to the experimental data (SPR shifts) linked to structural information on the array compounds and quality control data generated during array compound synthesis (e.g. molecular weight, purity, yield), array production quality control (e.g spotting batches, saturation of ligands) and protein target quality control (molecular weight, purity, concentration). The manual array-by-array analysis provides a first overview of the affinity fingerprints, reveals initial SAR trends, and is used for selection of preliminary hits series.

After completion of the screening campaign, all data are collected and analysed using a program package based on Spotfire™, Oracle™, Isis™ and scripts developed in-house. A range of compound properties and descriptors are pre-computed for all library compounds by in-house data mining routines and fed into an Oracle project database. After SPR data processing, actual screening SPR data, as well as structural data and quality control parameters, are included. The chemical interpretation of the microarray affinity fingerprints is based on dividing the entire data set into chemical families – also called classes or subsets. Following the mapping of the background-corrected experimental SPR data onto the subsets, they can be annotated using statistical properties such as number of compounds, ratio of hits and non-hits or mean signal strength. A combination of such properties is used to rank the classes in order to focus further analysis on chemically related array hit series.

3.10 FOLLOW-UP

After fingerprinting and hit identification, soluble hit compounds are resynthesized without the linker used for the immobilization on the chip. Such compounds can then be used in biochemical assays, if available, or for studies using biophysical methods, such as NMR, X-ray crystallography or calorimetry. In addition, from the initial fingerprinting SAR pattern, new structure series and focused libraries can be designed and explored along more traditional medicinal chemistry routes.

3.11 APPLICATIONS: MMP CASE STUDY

The matrixmetalloprotease (MMP) study is a representative example of successful SPR screening and demonstrates the kind of information that can be gained by SPR imaging. The MMP protein family consists of zinc dependent endopeptidases that degrade extracellular matrix proteins. MMPs are thought to play an important role in cell proliferation, migration and are considered as drug targets in oncology and immunology. Small molecule inhibitors generally contain chelating groups, such as carboxylates or hydroxamates, which bind the catalytic zinc atom at the active site. However, these polar inhibitors have shown unfavourable pharmacological properties and low selectivities (10, 11). Therefore, within the scope of this case study, it was investigated whether alternative site binders for MMPs could be identified by SPR screening and whether early selectivity information could be generated by screening a number of enzymes from the same target class.

3.11.1 Search for New Binding Modes

The SPR screening of MMP X against the chemical microarrays revealed a couple of diverse hit series. One fingerprint is shown in Figure 3.11a, where the spots represent individual sensor fields to which protein

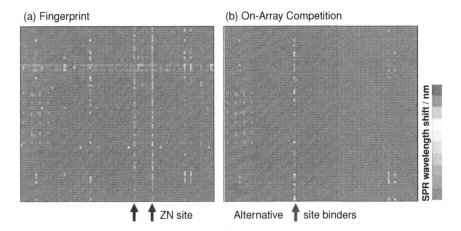

(a) Fingerprint   (b) On-Array Competition

↑ ↑ ZN site   Alternative ↑ site binders

Figure 3.11 Fingerprinting affinity map of matrixmetalloprotease X screened against a library of small molecules. (a) Interaction map of unblocked protein. (b) Competition experiment using known zinc site binder.

binding occurred. Structurally related hit series are arranged in rows and columns. In a second experiment the actual binding site mapping was subsequently performed by on-array competition studies. For this purpose, MMP X was preincubated with acetohydroxamate (a known zinc site ligand for MMPs) before the target inhibitor mixture was applied to the microarray. Blocking the enzyme's zinc site prevented binding to several initially identified hit series. The remaining signals were interpreted to represent alternative site binders (Figure 3.11b).

Members of this hit series were synthesized and tested for inhibition in a MMP activity assay. Here, the best lead-like compound (molecular weight 420 Da) showed an IC_{50} of 1 μM, which dropped to 3 nM when determined in the presence of acetohydroxamate. The most active fragment (molecular weight 250 Da) had an IC_{50} of 10 μM, which decreased to 400 nM in the presence of acetohydroxamate. In summary, these results confirm the zinc independent binding mode of the identified structures.

3.11.2 Selectivity Studies

Selectivity studies were performed with two members of the MMP family (here, MMP Y and MMP Z), which were screened against the same library. As shown in Figure 3.12, clear differences in the binding pattern were observed for both proteins. For hit confirmation, identified hits were

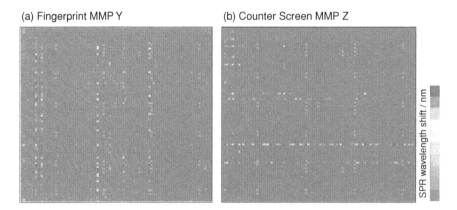

Figure 3.12 Selectivity studies for MMPs. Two members of the MMP family were screened against the same library, which revealed clear differences in the obtained binding patterns.

tested in a solution-based enzymatic assay. While MMP Y specific motifs inhibited MMP Y at micromolar concentrations ($IC_{50} = 5 - 40\,\mu M$), they were less active or inactive against MMP Z ($IC_{50} \gg 100\,\mu M$). These data clearly show the feasibility of generating early selectivity information by SPR imaging.

3.12 OTHER TARGET CLASSES

Graffinity's SPR screening technology is compatible with all types of soluble proteins. As of today, the fragment-based discovery platform has been successfully applied to more than 90 drug targets from various protein classes, such as proteases, kinases, phosphodiesterases, metabolic enzymes, RNA polymerases and protein–protein interaction domains. Further case studies have been published elsewhere, describing the discovery of chemotypes with novel binding modes for thrombin (5) and array informed fragment to lead optimization for PDE5 (6).

3.13 CONCLUSION

SPR imaging of chemical microarrays represents a promising tool for fragment-based discovery. The technology is based on a unique combination of an appropriate sensor surface chemistry, a suitable compound library and a sensitive SPR imaging device capable of simultaneously screening thousands of fragment–protein interactions. In addition to identifying novel fragment motifs, the approach can deliver selectivity data and binding site information by on-array competition studies.

REFERENCES

1. D. C. Rees, M. Congreve, C. W. Murray, and R. Carr, *Nature Reviews Drug Discovery* **3**, 660 (2004).
2. A. L. Hopkins, C. R. Groom, and A. Alex, *Drug Discovery Today* **9**, 430 (2004).
3. D. Vetter, *Journal of Cellular Biochemistry*, 79 (2002).
4. S. Dickopf, M. Frank, H.D. Junker *et al.*, *Analytical Biochemistry* **335**, 50 (2004).
5. T. Neumann, H.D. Junker, O. Keil *et al.*, *Letters in Drug Design & Discovery* **2**, 590 (Dec, 2005).
6. T. Neumann, H. D. Junker, K. Schmidt, and R. Sekul, *Current Topics in Medicinal Chemistry* **7**, 1630 (2007).
7. S. Maier, M. Frank, H. Rau *et al.*, *Qsar & Combinatorial Science* **25**, 1047 (2006).
8. T. Mitchell, and G. A. Showell, *Curr Opin Drug Discov Devel* **4**, 314 (2001).
9. M. Congreve, R. Carr, C. Murray, and H. Jhoti, *Drug Discovery Today* **8**, 876 (2003).
10. H. Matter, and M. Schudok, *Current Opinion in Drug Discovery & Development* **7**, 513 (2004).
11. Q.-X. A. Sang, Y. Jin, R.G. Newcomer *et al.*, *Current Topics in Medicinal Chemistry* **6**, 289 (2006).

4

The CellKey® System: A Label-Free Cell-Based Assay Platform for Early Drug Discovery Applications

Ryan P. McGuinness, Debra L. Gallant, Yen-Wen Chen, Trisha A. Tutana, Donna L. Wilson, John M. Proctor, and H. Roger Tang
Molecular Devices Inc., Sunnyvale, CA, USA

4.1 INTRODUCTION

More than two decades of investment in high throughput screening and infrastructure has produced an underwhelming number of new,

Label-Free Technologies for Drug Discovery   Edited by Matthew Cooper and Lorenz M. Mayr
© 2011 John Wiley & Sons, Ltd

clinically successful compounds (1–3). Novel technologies and greater biological understanding are required to break through the recent barriers to the development of innovative therapies. Label-free cell-based assays are now widely considered to be among the most promising technologies for ushering in a new generation of drug discovery successes (4). With the positive attributes of tissue-based assays in high density formats, these technologies represent a unique balance of biological relevance and industrial throughput. Their application to drug discovery will likely enhance the understanding of complex biology whilst also meeting requirements for high throughput campaigns.

As described throughout this book and elsewhere, there has been intense interest in, and development of, label-free approaches for both biochemical and live-cell investigation (4). Label-free technologies, such as the impedance-based CellKey® System, are free from the liabilities associated with the use of radioactive or fluorescent labels and are exquisitely sensitive to cellular changes induced by receptor mediated signal transduction. Unlike most other cell-based assay technologies, this high sensitivity permits independence from tagged or chimeric reporter proteins, or other engineered mediators which enhance receptor activity for the sake of detection. Impedance assays are universal, making forced coupling unnecessary to monitor diverse families of receptors. Finally, impedance assays enable the use of an expanded repertoire of cell lines beyond the immortalized workhorses such as CHO and HEK293, thus providing access to more biorelevant cellular models for screening.

A few specific examples of the benefits impedance assays have brought to drug discovery relate to the investigation of adenylate cyclase (AC)-dependent G-protein coupled receptors (GPCRs), especially those coupled to Gαi, expanded access to assay suspension cells and the ability to monitor complex states of receptor biology.

Impedance technology has overcome traditional challenges in the measurement of Gαi receptors by enabling a simple, direct and functional live-cell assay less than 15 minutes in duration (5, 6). In most other cAMP assays involving Gαi-coupled receptors, there is a functional requirement for external upregulation of AC by indirect means (such as the biochemical modulator, forskolin) in order to be measurably suppressed by activation of Gαi-coupled GPCRs. These assays present researchers with many practical problems, such as stimulation windows too narrow to reliably screen for antagonists, undesired artifacts of indirect measurement and a total dependence on overexpressed heterologous systems (7–9).

Suspension (nonadherent) cells are highly amenable to analysis on the system (6). This capability permits the use of a wide range of important cell lines and primary cells from the lymphoid, myeloid and erythroid cell lineages. These cell types are highly relevant models for a number of disease states involving inflammation, autoimmunity and malignancy (10). An important aspect of CellKey assays for nonadherent cells is the ability to interrogate these cell types without attachment factors coated over the assay plates. Attaching nonadherent cells to a cell culture substrate via cell adhesion molecules does have impact on the biology of signaling pathways (11–13). By not requiring this methodology, it can be argued that impedance assays maintain a more natural state of cell biology when compared to protocols requiring manipulated adhesion.

As the complexity of GPCR behavior is better understood and the need for probing multiple outputs becomes standard, universal assays like those performed with the CellKey system become beneficial (14, 15). Full evaluation for certain receptor families could involve as many as three distinct assay platforms in order to measure only the most proximal events of activation (16). For example, members of the Edg family of GPCRs and the related orphan GPCRs GPR3, 6 and 12 are understood to functionally couple to up to three different G-protein pathways dependent on cell type and activating ligand (17–19). Impedance-based assays very conveniently capture the downstream effects of receptor activation for these target families and even report on the complex interplay in temporal and dose dependent ways.

This chapter contains a detailed description of this label-free impedance-based assay platform. The underlying technology, its ability to monitor native states of receptor mediated signal transduction, its application to a wide range of drug discovery experimentation and the benefits the technology brings to drug discovery research are discussed.

4.2 CELLULAR IMPEDANCE TECHNOLOGY

The principals underlying the CellKey system have been described previously (20, 21) and are outlined in Figure 4.1. Briefly, an alternating voltage of a set frequency is applied to a cell monolayer via planar electrodes patterned at the base of culture wells, and the resultant electrical current is measured. This is repeated for a series of 24 frequencies from 1 kHz to 110 MHz. The total time to scan all wells for all frequencies is two seconds for the 96-well CellKey system and four seconds for the CellKey®384 System. The cell monolayer, by its presence in the electric field, resists (impedes) the flow of current. This interaction can be described in a basic sense by Ohm's Law, where impedance (Z) is the ratio

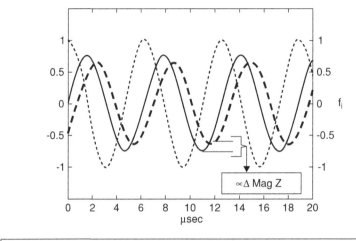

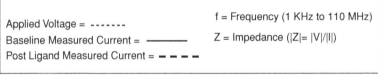

Figure 4.1 Bioimpedance measurements with the CellKey system. Alternating voltage (V) (dotted line) at set frequencies (f_i) is applied in a circuit that includes a monolayer of cells. The resultant electrical current (I) is measured for a short period to generate a baseline (solid line). This is repeated for a series of 24 frequencies from 1 kHz to 110 MHz. At the end of the baseline period, ligand is added to the cells and the change in the amplitude of the measured current (dashed line) is recorded. This change is proportional to the change in the magnitude of the impedance, which is then calculated and displayed. This process is repeated over time to generate kinetic information about cellular changes resulting from receptor activation.

of applied voltage to measured current (Z = V/I) (22, 23). At low frequencies, the applied voltages induce extracellular currents (iec) that pass around individual cells in the monolayer. At high frequencies, the voltages induce transcellular currents (itc) that penetrate the cellular membranes (21). Changes in impedance due to extracellular currents (dZiec) and to transcellular currents (dZitc) are reported for each well. When cells are exposed to a stimulus, such as a receptor ligand, signal transduction events occur that lead to cellular changes. These cellular changes individually or collectively affect the flow of iec and itc, and, therefore, affect the magnitude and characteristics of the measured impedance.

A set of example data is provided in Figure 4.2. Displayed are CellKey response profiles generated by activating CHOm$_1$ cells (Chinese hamster ovary cells stably transfected with the m$_1$ muscarinic AchR) with ligands

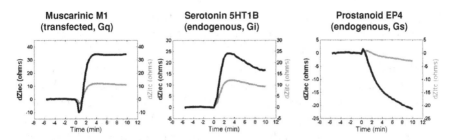

Figure 4.2 Sample CellKey response profiles. Algorithms within the CellKey Software interpret the raw impedance data to generate kinetic response profiles. Displayed here are typical profiles for three different families of GPCRs expressed in CHOm₁ cells. Left: transfected Gαq-coupled muscarininc m₁ receptor. Middle: endogenous Gαi-coupled 5HT1B receptor. Right: endogenous Gαs-coupled prostanoid EP4 receptor.

for one transfected and two endogenous GPCRs. Kinetic response profiles allow quantitative measurement of receptor activation, as well as an indication of the response pathways activated. The left-hand panel of Figure 4.2 displays the response of CHOm₁ cells to administration of the m₁ muscarinic AchR agonist, carbachol. The feature set that resulted can be considered a typical Gαq-coupled response profile, with an early dip in impedance followed by a sustained rise. Typical Gαi and Gαs-coupled response profiles are displayed in the center and right of Figure 4.2, respectively. The endogenous serotonin 5HT1B receptor was activated with the agonist serotonin to generate the Gαi-coupled response profile of an immediate and sustained rise in impedance. The endogenous prostanoid EP4 receptor was activated with the agonist PGE₂ to generate the Gαs response profile of an immediate and sustained decrease in impedance. While kinetic data generated across individual GPCRs and cell types cannot be mapped directly over one another, the features of the response profiles do hold largely true. Many of the key pathway mediators related to the features in the kinetic response profiles have been investigated previously, and include well known second messenger molecules such as Ca^{2+} and cAMP (6, 24).

From a cellular perspective, the impedance readout is dependent on downstream events in receptor signaling pathways, particularly changes in the cytoskeleton (25). Entire classes of cellular receptors are known to modulate the cytoskeleton as a downstream event in signal transduction (26–28). GPCR families and their proximal second messengers have linkage to cytoskeletal reorganization through many pathways, most often converging on the Rho or MAP kinase cascades (29). These include the

$G\alpha_{12/13}$-coupled receptors that signal directly through Rho kinases (30, 31), $G\alpha q$ that connects with Ca^{2+} dependant PKC activity (32) and the adenynlate cyclase-coupled GPCRs, $G\alpha i$ and $G\alpha s$, that signal via PKA to MAP kinase (33–35). G-protein dependent and independent β-Arrestin signaling is also linked to cytoskeletal modulation via RhoA/ROCK and ERK mediators, respectively (36, 37). Finally, some ion channels have been demonstrated to link their signal directly to the cytoskeleton and/or via cross-talk and access to the pathways mentioned above (38–40). Accordingly, to date, essentially all receptors families that are known to signal through these well characterized pathways have been successfully measured on impedance systems. The CellKey system therefore represents a highly sensitive and flexible assay platform that is capable of contributing to a wide range of experimentation in the drug discovery workflow.

4.3 TARGET IDENTIFICATION AND VALIDATION

Due to its sensitivity to endogenous levels of cellular receptors and its cell-type independence, the CellKey system is well suited for target identification and validation. Included in this process is a technique known as receptor panning. As described previously (6, 25, 41), receptor panning is a rapid approach for cataloging active endogenous receptors in living cells. It involves testing a panel of activating ligands and pathway modulators on any cell type of interest (whether adherent or suspension, primary or immortalized) and monitoring impedance changes that result. The kinetic data gathered not only indicate the presence of an active target, but also give some indication of the response pathway accessed (Figure 4.2). In this way, endogenous receptor targets and pathways can be discovered quickly and in a highly relevant state.

Once an endogenous target is found to be active it can be validated pharmacologically with reference agonists and antagonists when they exist (25). In cases where no antagonist tool compounds are available, impedance assays can be paired with small inhibitory RNA (siRNA) technology to knock down expression of the receptor target and demonstrate receptor specificity. RNA interference (RNAi) has been widely adopted as a drug discovery tool in the areas of target identification and validation, assay validation, compound selectivity and mechanism of action studies (42–44). To provide an example of matching impedance assays with RNAi for analysis of endogenous receptor specificity, the histamine H1 receptor (H1) expressed in HeLa cells was evaluated. H1 was previously determined to be active in HeLa cells via receptor panning (25). In the studies described here, cells were transfected with pools of siRNA through a convenient and efficient "reverse transfection" method optimized by Ambion Inc. (Austin, TX). Using this protocol cells were transfected at the same time they were plated onto the CellKey Standard 96W microplates. As siRNA expression increased over time post-transfection, the gene silencing effect also increased. When working with RNAi, determining the time at which maximal knock down occurs is important, and is typically done through a laborious process of cell lysis, nucleic acid isolation, purification and reverse transcription polymerase chain reaction (RT PCR) or Western blotting. This process was greatly simplified with the CellKey system. Using the noninvasive impedance measurement, the same cells were tested repeatedly at sequential time points to collect functional responses. In practice, at various time points culture media was replaced with assay buffer and cellular responses to activating ligand were monitored. Once each measurement was completed, cells were washed back into culture media and returned to the incubator until the next time point.

By applying three different pools of siRNA to HeLa cells it was possible to identify a single pool that effectively and specifically knocked down expression of H1. Figure 4.3 shows the resulting data. HeLa cell H1 receptor responses to the native agonist, histamine (at EC_{80} concentration), were repeatedly recorded on the same cells at different points in time post-transfection (24, 48 and 72 hours). The magnitudes of responses were quantified and displayed in the bar graph at the top of Figure 4.3 (data were n = 4 and error bars represent ±SD). From this data, it was determined that siRNA pool 2 was the most effective of the three pools tested, and that maximal knock down was reached at about 48 hours. It was also observed that gene expression and receptor function were on the increase by 72 hours. The bottom of Figure 4.3 shows the kinetic response profiles from which the bar graphs were derived. Each panel represents four individual wells from a single plate overlaid with error bars representing ±SD. As can be seen, the kinetic responses were very reproducible over time and across wells. The data demonstrated the degree to which each pool inhibited functional expression of H1 and the specificity of the experiment. A pool of random/nonspecific siRNA had no impact on the function of the receptor (E). Pool 2 demonstrated a maximal effect (B). Pools 1 and 3 (A and C) knocked down functional expression significantly, but not entirely. These data provide a good example of utilizing a label-free impedance assay for the RNAi mediated interrogation of cellular processes like receptor signal

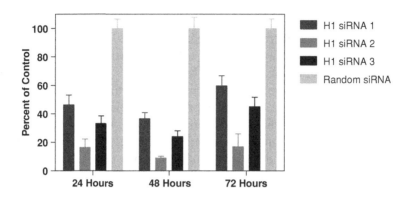

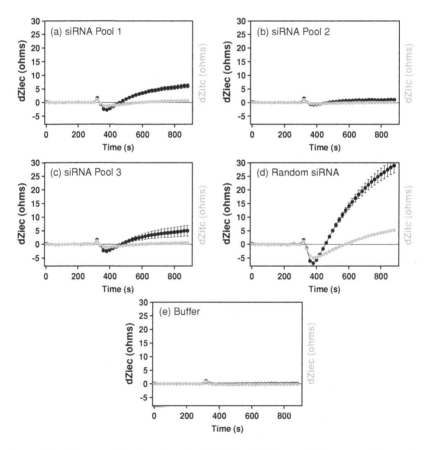

Figure 4.3 Target validation through siRNA knockdown – Endogenous Histamine H1 receptor in HeLa cells. Top: time course of siRNA dependent gene silencing in HeLa cells over three days for three different pools of siRNA and a random siRNA control. Bottom: kinetic response profiles at Day 2 post-transfection. All data are $n = 4 \pm SD$.

transduction. These data also provide proof of concept for expanded work with RNAi, which could include the knock down of key intracellular kinases involved in many response pathways to aid drug discovery for these important targets.

4.4 SCREENING AND LEAD OPTIMIZATION

Having identified active H1 on HeLa cells by receptor panning and validating the target through RNA interference, a pilot screen of the library of pharmacologically active compounds (LOPAC1280 from Sigma, St Louis, MO) was performed using the CellKey384 system. The CellKey384 system is an assay platform capable of monitoring real-time impedance changes in 384-well format. The instrument has the same features of the 96-well system, with the inclusion of 384-well pipettor and an onboard tip washing unit for increased unattended throughput in screening mode.

Important benefits of screening in the endogenous setting include access to natural expression levels of receptor targets attached to their native response pathways in relevant cell types to the disease under study. This is in contrast to typical highly engineered cell/receptor systems in which heterologous receptor genes are overexpressed in cell types chosen for their convenience as screening tools (3).

In these studies, HeLa cells were plated onto CellKey Standard 384W microplates at a density of 9000 cells per well. Cell plates were incubated overnight in a 37 °C incubator with 5% carbon dioxide atmosphere. Immediately prior to experimentation, cell plates were washed three times with assay buffer, HBSS supplemented with 20 mM HEPES and 0.1% BSA (referred to hereafter as HH) using onboard fluidics. Twenty μl of HH were left in the wells after the final exchange. Baseline measurements were then gathered for a period of 90 seconds. Using onboard fluidics, ligands at 3X concentration were added to all 384 wells simultaneously while the instrument actively measured the impedance in each well. Measurement continued for 10 minutes after ligand addition to monitor cellular responses. All experiments were performed at 32 °C.

Figure 4.4 displays a dot plot of HeLa responses after administration of the LOPAC1280 compounds. Data analysis was performed by directing the CellKey384 Software to export the maximum minus minimum value for each well. All responses were then normalized to the average 1 μM histamine response (positive control) and multiplied by 100. Data were graphed in Prism 5.0 (GraphPad, San Diego, CA). By setting a threshold

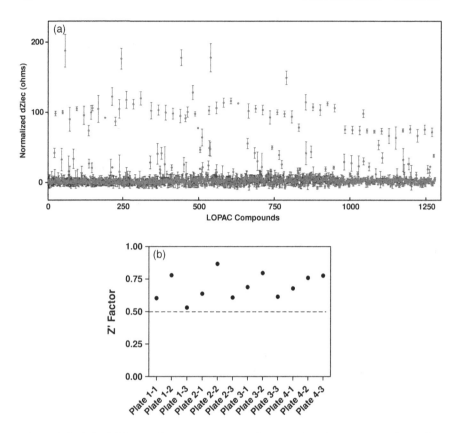

Figure 4.4 LOPAC1280 pilot screen: HeLa cells. Top: Agonist screen results in dot plot format. 1280 compounds were assayed for activity on endogenous receptors expressed on HeLa cells. Data were normalized using the average response to 10 μM histamine as a positive control. Each value on the plot is n = 3 ±SD, compiled from single data points on each of three replicate plates. Bottom: Z' Factors for each of 12 individual agonist screening plates. Values of 0.50 and greater are indicative of a highly robust assay.

at 50% of positive control, 67 activating hits were identified in the initial screen. Hits were generated by ligands known to activate a variety of endogenous receptors on HeLa cells, including H1, dopaminergic and adrenergic receptors. As well, a number of biochemical modulators present in the LOPAC1280 library were active in a nonreceptor mediated fashion. Each value on the plot represents n = 3 ±SD, compiled from single data points on each of three replicate plates. In this pilot screen the average signal to background across all plates was 12.9 and the Z' factor was 0.7 (45).

The LOPAC1280 was also screened in antagonist mode on HeLa cells (data not shown) by using the onboard fluidics to apply 1X compounds (at 10 μM) to all wells after the final HH wash step. Ligands were allowed to bind for a period of 30 minutes. Similar to the agonist screen described above, a 90-second baseline was measured, after which an EC_{80} concentration (430 nM) of histamine was added (experiment temperature was 32 °C). Ten minutes of post-addition data were collected. Data was again analysed in Prism, and by setting a threshold of 50% inhibition, 77 hits were identified. Average signal to background at EC_{80} across all plates was 6.5 and the Z' factor was 0.56. Further study is required to validate all of the antagonist hits from this initial screen; however, several LOPAC1280 compounds known to block histaminergic receptors (H1 and other subtypes) were identified, as well as compounds known to disrupt cytoskeletal dynamics, or inhibit key intracellular kinases involved in the H1 pathway.

Screening endogenously provides shortcuts that could prove to be quite significant in certain situations. In a typical cell-based assay scenario, a recombinant cDNA version of a receptor target must first be available through ownership or license. Labeled cell-based assays then require that the target be transfected into a cell line known to efficiently incorporate heterologous DNA and express it at high levels (such as CHO or HEK293 cells). This part of the process is very laborious, and can require many months to a year to complete (46). At this point a screenable assay can be developed. If the screening campaign requires a cross-species evaluation of leads prior to *in vivo* experimentation, the cell line development must begin again in the proper species' background. When working with impedance technology, endogenous targets are routinely detectable, thus eliminating the requirement for proprietary cDNA constructs. Also, as shown here, natural levels of receptor expression are sufficient for detection. There is no need to sub-clone or overexpress targets, eliminating lengthy and laborious cell line development. Because label-free assays are cell line independent, the list of potential cell lines and primary cell types is very large and includes many different species.

After screening, the earliest steps in lead optimization include deriving the potencies of the identified hits. In this example of the H1 receptor screen in HeLa cells, a small panel of antagonist hits was followed up by performing concentration response curves (Figure 4.5). The data demonstrate potency ranking of the compounds chosen and could serve as the basis for further lead optimization and structure–activity relationship (SAR). SAR is commonly focused on increasing the potency and efficacy

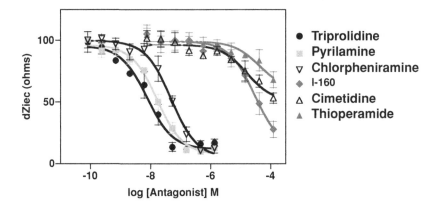

Figure 4.5 Concentration response curves for selected antagonist hits. Potency was derived for six antagonist compounds chosen from a screen against the endogenous H1 receptor expressed in HeLa cells. Cells were pre-incubated with $10\,\mu M$ compounds and challenged with an EC_{80} dose of histamine (480 nM). Data are n = 4 $\pm SD$. I-160: 3-(1H-Imidazol-4-yl)propyl di(p-fluorophenyl)methyl ether.

of lead candidates from the perspective of a bioassay dependent on a single point in complex signaling pathways, like cAMP, or even through radioligand binding assays. The CellKey system enables enhanced selectivity screening and an expanded view of bioassay SAR because of its ability to detect integrated cellular responses (24, 47). In fully developed impedance assays response profiles are highly reproducible, enabling a more comprehensive view of the ligand-directed signaling induced by variations on lead chemistries. Indeed, impedance assays can resolve the nuanced signaling of pathway biased ligands which would otherwise be missed in single-point assays. Label-free cell-based assays and their integrated cellular responses are sensitive to greater biological texture and should allow an expanded and more informative approach to SAR.

4.5 CONCLUSION

Here, the benefits of applying label-free impedance assays to the early drug discovery process, including experimentation in target identification and validation, compound screening and lead optimization, have been discussed. Label-free assays carry drug discovery an important step closer towards reintroducing biology to the early stages of the process by allowing identification of key screening targets expressed at natural endogenous levels in highly relevant cell types (10). The CellKey system, with its noninvasive detection method can be flexibly paired with other powerful techniques, such as RNAi-mediated gene silencing, to validate targets in a functional and relevant fashion. The CellKey384 system is the first impedance-based assay technology to reach 384-well density for automated screening. This high throughput instrument enables simultaneous access to quantitative measures of receptor activation and highly informative kinetic data about the signaling pathways involved. Screening follow-up and lead optimization is possible with impedance systems and benefits from the integrated cellular responses generated (48). Ultimately, technologies such as the CellKey system will support an expanded view of biological SAR, capturing not only increases in potency and efficacy, but also the subtleties in receptor signaling and pathway diversity. Growing knowledge and appreciation of complex receptor target states will be complemented by the information derived from label-free cell-based assays. Importantly, unlike times past, this rich cellular assay information is now available in assay formats and protocols that conform to high throughput infrastructure.

REFERENCES

1. M. Williams, *Curr Opin Pharmacol* **3**, 571 (2003).
2. L. E. Sundstrom, *EMBO Rep* **8**, S40 (2007).
3. M. A. Walker, T. B. Barrett and L. J. Guppy, *Drug Discovery Today: Targets* **3**, 208 (2004).
4. L. K. Minor, *Comb Chem High Throughput Screen* **11**, 573 (2008).
5. M. F. Peters, K. S. Knappenberger, D. Wilkins, *et al.*, *J Biomol Screen* **12**, 312 (2007).
6. G. Leung, H. R. Tang, M. Ryan, *et al.*, *Journal of the Association for Laboratory Automation* **10**, 258 (2005).
7. P. J. Greasley and F. J. Jansen, *Drug Discovery Today: Technologies* **2**, 163 (2005).
8. S. W. Robinson and M. G. Caron, *Mol Pharmacol* **52**, 508 (Sep, 1997).
9. S. Titus, S. Neumann, W. Zheng, *et al.*, *J Biomol Screen* **13**, 120 (Feb, 2008).
10. R. M. Eglen, A. Gilchrist and T. Reisine, *Comb Chem High Throughput Screen* **11**, 566 (2008).
11. A. Guilherme, K. Torres and M. P. Czech, *J Biol Chem* **273**, 22899 (1998).
12. Y. Li, N. Clough, X. Sun, *et al.*, *J Cell Sci* **120**, 1436 (2007).
13. X. Huang, W. Dai and Z. Darzynkiewicz, *Cell Cycle* **4**, 801 (2005).
14. A. Christopoulos and T. Kenakin, *Pharmacol Rev* **54**, 323 (2002).
15. W. Tan, D. Martin and J. S. Gutkind, *J Biol Chem* **281**, 39542 (2006).
16. W. C. Horne, J. F. Shyu, M. Chakraborty and R. Baron, *Trends Endocrinol Metab* **5**, 395 (1994).
17. A. Ignatov, J. Lintzel, I. Hermans-Borgmeyer, *et al.*, *J Neurosci* **23**, 907 (2003).
18. K. Uhlenbrock, H. Gassenhuber and E. Kostenis, *Cell Signal* **14**, 941 (2002).
19. M. H. Graler, R. Grosse, A. Kusch, *et al.*, *J Cell Biochem* **89**, 507 (2003).

20. G. J. Ciambrone, V. F. Liu, D. C. Lin, *et al.*, *J Biomol Screen* **9**, 467 (2004).
21. R. McGuinness and E. Verdonk, in *Label-Free Biosensors: Techniques and Applications* (ed. M. A. Cooper,) Cambridge University Press, Cambridge, UK (2009), pp. 251–278.
22. E. Gheorghiu, *Bioelectromagnetics* **17**, 475 (1996).
23. S. Grimnes and O. Martinsen, *Bioimpedance and Bioelectricity Basics*, Academic Press, (2000), pp. 51–83.
24. M. F. Peters and C. W. Scott, *J Biomol Screen* **14**, 246 (2009).
25. E. Verdonk, K. Johnson, R. McGuinness, *et al.*, *Assay Drug Dev Technol* **4**, 609 (2006).
26. R. Maddala, V. N. Reddy, D. L. Epstein and V. Rao, *Mol Vis* **9**, 329 (2003).
27. E. A. Papakonstanti, E. A. Vardaki and C. Stournaras, *Cell Physiol Biochem* **10**, 257 (2000).
28. C. J. Caunt, A. R. Finch, K. R. Sedgley and C. A. McArdle, *Trends Endocrinol Metab* **17**, 276 (2006).
29. S. Vogt, R. Grosse, G. Schultz and S. Offermanns, *J Biol Chem* **278**, 28743 (2003).
30. J. E. Lauckner, J. B. Jensen, H. Y. Chen, *et al.*, *Proc. Natl Acad. Sci. USA* **105**, 2699 (2008).
31. B. H. Meyer, F. Freuler, D. Guerini and S. Siehler, *J Cell Biochem* **104**, 1660 (2008).
32. M. Street, S. J. Marsh, P. R. Stabach, *et al.*, *J Cell Sci* **119**, 1528 (2006).
33. N. J. Lamb, A. Fernandez, M. A. Conti, *et al.*, *J Cell Biol* **106**, 1955 (1988).
34. N. Gerits, T. Mikalsen, S. Kostenko, *et al.*, *J Biol Chem* **282**, 37232 (2007).
35. M. Bouaboula, L. Bianchini, F. R. McKenzie *et al.* *FEBS Lett* **449**, 61 (1999).
36. S. M. DeWire, S. Ahn, R. J. Lefkowitz and S. K. Shenoy, *Annu Rev Physiol* **69**, 483 (2007).
37. W. G. Barnes, E. Reiter, J. D. Violin, *et al.*, *J Biol Chem* **280**, 8041 (2005).
38. S. Loebrich, R. Bahring, T. Katsuno, *et al.* *Embo J* **25**, 987 (2006).
39. M. Kneussel, S. Haverkamp, J. C. Fuhrmann, *et al.*, *Proc. Natl Acad. Sci. USA* **97**, 8594 (2000).
40. C. Goswami, M. Dreger, R. Jahnel, *et al.*, *J Neurochem* **91**, 1092 (2004).
41. R. McGuinness, *Curr Opin Pharmacol* **7**, 535 (2007).
42. C. Sachse, E. Krausz, A. Kronke, *et al.*, *Methods Enzymol* **392**, 242 (2005).
43. D. Vanhecke and M. Janitz, *Drug Discov Today* **10**, 205 (2005).
44. N. M. Wolters and J. P. MacKeigan, *Cell Death Differ* **15**, 809 (2008).
45. J. H. Zhang, T. D. Chung and K. R. Oldenburg, *J Biomol Screen* **4**, 67 (1999).
46. L. K. Minor, *Handbook of Assay Development in Drug Discovery*, Drug Discovery Series (ed. A. Carmen) (2006), pp. 488.
47. R. P. McGuinness, J. M. Proctor, D. L. Gallant, *et al.*, *Comb Chem High Throughput Screen* (2009).
48. E. N. Johnson, *American Drug Discovery* **3**, 12 (2008).

5

Dynamic and Label-Free Cell-Based Assays Using the xCELLigence System

Yama A. Abassi[1], Alexander Sieler[2], Manfred Watzele[2], Xiaobo Wang[1], and Xiao Xu[1]

[1]*ACEA Biosciences Inc., San Diego, CA, USA*
[2]*Roche Diagnostics GmbH, Penzberg, Germany*

Label-Free Technologies for Drug Discovery   Edited by Matthew Cooper and Lorenz M. Mayr
© 2011 John Wiley & Sons, Ltd

5.1 INTRODUCTION

Cell-based assays have become an increasingly important part of the preclinical drug discovery process (1, 2) – allowing for insight into the efficacy, specificity, permeability, solubility, stability, toxicity and mechanism of drug interaction with target cells. The data collected from cell-based assays are pertinent for go/no go decisions and can help guide and determine lead candidate progression to subsequent phases in the preclinical pipeline of drug development processes, such as animal studies and ADME analysis (1, 2). It is, therefore, of utmost importance that the appropriate cell-based assay technology platforms are implemented in order to fully and thoroughly exploit the potentials of drug libraries and reduce the attrition rate of candidates during preclinical animal studies and early stage clinical trials.

Label-free cell-based technologies have recently received considerable attention for implementation in the preclinical drug discovery setting (3–8). As the name implies, the preclusion of label allows for assessment of cells in their native and physiologically relevant environment, circumventing the potential negative impact of label on cellular processes. The inclusion of certain labels and reporters, particularly labels for live cells, has been shown to impact various aspects of cellular behavior. For example, it has been shown that the live cell fluorescent dye 2',7'-bis-(2-carboxyethyl)-5-(and 6)-carboxyfluorescein (BCECF-AM) and rhodamine 6G (R6G) can dose dependently block the migration of macrophage and mononuclear cells, respectively, urging caution when utilizing these dyes for cell-based assays (9, 10). Label-free technologies have the added advantage of being noninvasive and, therefore, live cells present in tissue culture wells can be continuously interrogated. This feature directly leads to one of the main advantages of label-free technologies, which is real-time kinetic measurement (3, 5, 6, 11, 12). Real-time monitoring of cellular processes offers distinct and important advantages over traditional end-point assays. Firstly, comprehensive representation of the entire length of the assay is possible, allowing the user to make informed decisions regarding timing of manipulations or treatments. Secondly, the actual kinetic response of cells provides important information regarding the biological status of the cells, such as growth, arrest and morphological changes. In this chapter, the xCELLigence System, co-developed by Roche Applied Science and ACEA Biosciences, is introduced and the principles of the technology and its applications for cell-based assays are discussed. A number of applications, including cell proliferation and cytotoxicity, cell adhesion, barrier function, and functional monitoring of membrane receptors, has been developed on the system (a comprehensive review is given elsewhere [8]). The discussion focuses primarily on cell proliferation and cytotoxicity assays as well as functional monitoring of G-protein coupled receptor (GPCR) responses.

5.2 THE XCELLIGENCE SYSTEM

The xCELLigence Real-Time Cell Analysis (RT-CA) system is a series of three instruments that differ primarily in throughput capacity (Figure 5.1). The RT-CA SP system is composed of four main components: the electronic microtiter plates (E-Plate^{TM}); the RT-CA SP station, which

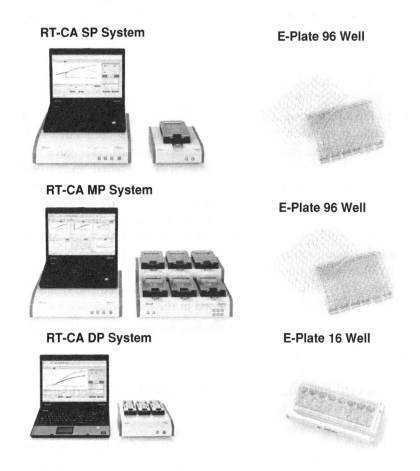

RT-CA SP System

E-Plate 96 Well

RT-CA MP System

E-Plate 96 Well

RT-CA DP System

E-Plate 16 Well

Figure 5.1 The xCELLigence System includes the RT-CA SP system, the RT-CA MP system and the RT-CA DP system. The SP and MP systems utilize 96 well E-Plates while the DP system utilizes 16 well E-Plates.

accommodates one E-Plate and is placed inside a tissue culture incubator; the RT-CA Analyzer for sending and receiving the electronic signals; and the RT-CA Control Unit, which operates the software and continuously acquires and displays the data. The RT-CA MP system is a higher throughput version, where the MP station can accommodate up to six E-Plates at the same time or alternate times by up to six different users. Each of the six modules of the RT-CA MP system can be independently operated. The RT-CA DP system is a lower throughput version which accommodates up to three 16 well E-Plates at the same time or different time. Importantly, aside from throughput capacity, one of the other key features of the RT-CA DP system is that it is able to operate the 16 well Cell Invasion and Migration (CIM) device, which is a modified Boyden chamber and can monitor cell migration and invasion in real time and in an automatic fashion.

5.3 PRINCIPLE OF DETECTION

The xCELLigence system utilizes impedance readout to noninvasively quantify cellular status in real time (12–14). The cells are seeded in E-Plates^{TM} that are integrated with gold microelectrode arrays (Figure 5.2). Application of a low voltage (less than 20 mV) AC signal leads to the generation of an electric field between the electrodes; this interacts with the ionic environment inside the wells of the E-Plates and is differentially modulated by the number of cells in the well, the morphology of the cells and the strength of cell attachment (12, 13). The impedance readout harnesses and quantifies these unique changes in cell morphology and adhesion, allowing for an unbiased detection of specific cellular processes in real time. The specific cell-based applications developed and validated on the xCELLigence system are discussed in the following.

5.4 APPLICATIONS

5.4.1 Cell Proliferation, Cytotoxicity and Time Dependent Cellular Response Profiling

One of the fundamental characteristics for cancer cells is their ability to grow and proliferate unconstrained from the regulatory mechanisms that are in place inside the cell (15). The xCELLigence system can be used to quantitatively and dynamically monitor cell proliferation (14, 16). As opposed to single point assays, there are several

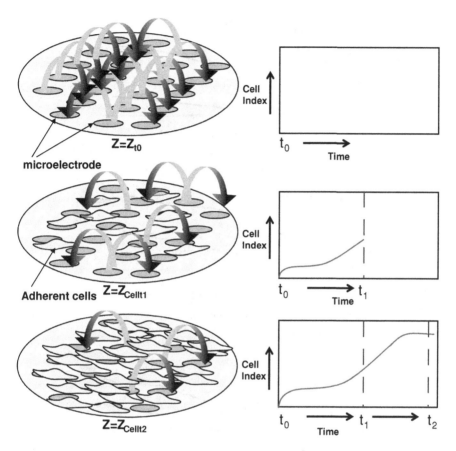

Figure 5.2 Schematic drawing of the interdigitated gold microelectrodes fabricated on the bottom of each well of the E-Plates. Application of low voltage AC signal leads to the generation of currents, which can be impeded by the presence of cells, between the electrodes. The interaction of adherent mammalian cells with the microelectrodes leads to the generation of cell substrate impedance response that is proportional to the number of cells seeded in the wells, the morphology of the cells and the quality of cell attachment. The signal generated is displayed by the arbitrary unit of cell index (CI). Adapted with permission from Elsevier. Copyright 2009.

fundamental advantages that are offered by dynamically monitoring cells in real time.

Primarily, in addition to cell number, the impedance readout used by the xCELLigence system is also affected by cell size and morphology as well as by adhesion characteristics of each cell line or cell type. Therefore, each cell displays a very unique proliferation pattern based on the cell density seeded. Figure 5.3 shows the unique growth profile of four cancer cell lines. These profiles can be very reproducible and predictive, depending on the passage number of the cells. This characteristic growth

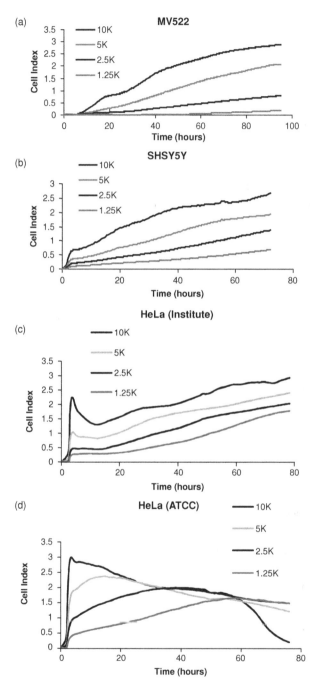

Figure 5.3 Dynamic monitoring of cell proliferation in real time using the xCEL-Ligence system. (a) MV 522, (b) SHSY5Y and (c) (d) HeLa cells obtained from two different sources were seeded in E-Plates and continuously monitored on the RT-CA SP system. Each cell type displays a unique time dependent proliferation pattern.

signature pattern can be used as a measure of quality control for the cell line of interest, to ensure consistency in the same experiment and between different experiments (17). Interestingly, cell type (c) and (d) are both HeLa cells. Cell type (c) was obtained from a research institute and cell type (d) was obtained directly from American Type Culture Collection (ATCC). The data clearly show that the growth characteristics of the cell line obtained from the research institute have significantly deviated from that supplied by ATCC. Therefore, it is imperative to be aware of such variations and have a quality control procedure in place to detect these differences. Secondly, impedance monitoring of cell proliferation can also be used to define and observe very distinct biological or cellular stages throughout the assay, such as cell attachment and spreading (a characteristic lag phase unique to each cell type), exponential growth phase and, finally, confluence. All the kinetic data provided by the xCEL-Ligence system are crucial for cell-based assay development by helping to optimize different assay parameters, such as seeding density and time of treatment.

As mentioned previously, the impedance readout utilized by the xCEL-Ligence system is affected by multiple parameters, including cell number, adhesion and morphology. Each of these features is uniquely affected by cytotoxic compounds depending on the mechanism of action of the compounds (14, 16). Compound treatment in combination with real-time monitoring on the xCELLigence system results in unique Time Dependent Cellular Response Profiles (TCRPs) that can be used in a predictive manner for elucidating mechanism of compound action. As an example, Figure 5.4a shows the TCRP for MDA-MB-231 cells treated with compounds having different mechanisms of action. Each compound displays unique time dependent profiles that are dependent on mechanism of action of the compound. Compounds with similar mechanisms result in similar TCRPs, as shown for two DNA damaging agents, etoposide and cytosine-arabinofuranoside (Figures 4b and 4c). These distinctive TCRPs can be used as a screening tool to identify compounds with unknown function (18). Due to the kinetic nature of the profiling approach both short term and long term compound activities can be measured, allowing for detection of temporally isolated but distinct activities of small molecules and potentially off-target effects. These findings indicate that using impedance-based monitoring and profiling of cellular response upon exposure to biologically active compounds can provide incisive and quantitative information and novel mechanisms for existing drugs as well as experimental biological compounds; it can also be used to complement other profiling approaches using the time resolution in

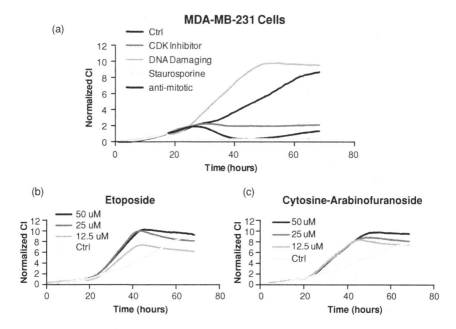

Figure 5.4 Dynamic monitoring of biologically active compounds using the xCEL-Ligence system. (a) MDA-MB-231 cells were seeded in E-Plates and, at the indicated time, treated with compounds with different mechanisms. Each compound results in unique time dependent cellular response profiles (TCRP). (b) (c) MDA-MB-231cells were treated with either etoposide (topoisomerase inhibitor) and cytosine-arabinofuranoside (anti-metabolite), both of which lead to DNA damage leading to similar TCRPs.

the assay. In addition to compound mediated cytotoxicity, impedance readout can also be utilized to monitor cytotoxicity induced by other nonchemical agents, such as immune cells and viruses (19, 20).

5.5 FUNCTIONAL ASSAYS FOR G-PROTEIN COUPLED RECEPTORS

Approximately, 50% of the current drugs on the market are targeted against G-protein coupled receptors (GPCRs) (21, 22), making them an important target for pharmaceutical drug development. The vast majority of GPCRs couple to and activate heterotrimeric G-proteins and subsequently stimulate second messenger systems (22). The heterotrimeric G-protein consists of a $G\alpha$ subunit and $G\beta/\gamma$ complex, both of which can activate downstream effectors depending on the receptors being activated (22). More recently, it has become apparent that GPCR signaling either through or in addition to heterotrimeric G-proteins also activates Rho family of small GTPases (23, 24). Rho family GTPases participate in a number of cellular processes, the main one being regulation and maintenance of specific structures within the actin cytoskeleton framework (25). GPCRs have been shown to modulate the actin cytoskeleton, and hence cell morphology, in a very specific manner depending on the Rho family GTPase being activated (25). Since GPCRs couple to the actin cytoskeletal network and induce very defined morphological changes, it is possible to harness this information as a functional and biologically relevant readout for GPCRs using the xCELLigence system (26).

As shown in Figure 5.5, Chinese Hamster Ovary (CHO) cell and HeLa cervical carcinoma cells were seeded in E-Plates and at the indicated time stimulated with increasing concentrations of ATP and histamine,

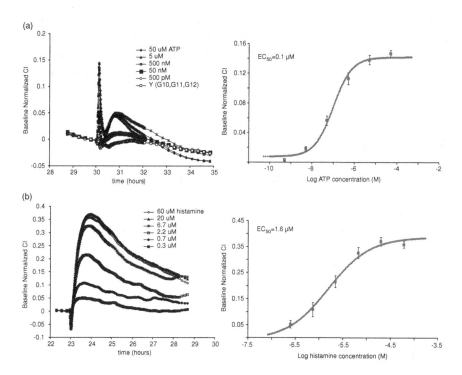

Figure 5.5 Functional monitoring of Gq coupled GPCR activation. (a) Serum starved CHO-K1 cells (3 h in 0.5% FCS) were treated with ATP (500 pM – 50 μM) and the cellular response was detected by impedance measurement on an xCELLigence cell analyser (left panel). The respective $EC_{50} = 0.1$ μM was determined by a sigmoidal dose response curve (right panel). (b) Analysis of GPCR stimulation by histamine (60 μM – 250 nM) in HeLa cells reveals an $EC_{50} = 1.6$ μM.

respectively. The receptors for ATP and histamine are expressed endogenously in these cell types and are coupled to the Gq pathway. Plotting the log of the agonist concentration versus the maximal cellular response allows for the generation of a dose–response curve with an EC_{50} value that is comparable to standard assays. In addition to the Gq pathway, it has been demonstrated that the xCELLigence system can detect functional responses of receptors coupled to the Gi and Gs pathways (26). The important contribution of the xCELLigence system for GPCR cell-based assays is several fold. Firstly, since the readout is noninvasive, the cells can be stimulated multiple times in order to assess desensitization or cross-talk with other receptor types (26). Secondly, the xCELLigence system can be used to functionally monitor GPCRs coupled to different signaling pathways, including Gq, Gs, Gi and $G\alpha12/13$ (26). Traditionally, several different technologies would be required to carry out assays for GPCRs depending on the signaling pathways (21). Thirdly, and most importantly, cells expressing endogenous GPCRs, including primary cells, can also be used with the xCELLigence system, precluding the need for overexpression of exogenous GPCRs or engineering the cells to express promiscuous G-proteins (26). This allows the evaluation of the receptors in physiologically appropriate cell types.

5.6 CONCLUSION

In summary, the xCELLigence system offers an innovative solution to a number of limitations with current cell-based assay systems. The convergence of label-free technology coupled with a noninvasive readout and kinetic data culminates in obtaining information rich and high content data. Real-time cell electronic sensing applications cover a large span of cell-based assays, including proliferation, cytotoxicity, receptor–ligand interactions, cell adhesion, endothelial barrier function, CTL and NK assays, and cell migration and invasion.

REFERENCES

1. K. Moore and S. Rees, *J Biomol Screen* **6**, 69 (2001).
2. R. S. Hauptschein, B. K. Eustace and D. G. Jay, *Exp Hematol* **30**, 381 (2002).
3. J. M. Atienza *et al.*, *Assay Drug Dev Technol* **4**, 597 (2006).
4. G. J. Ciambrone *et al.*, *J Biomol Screen* **9**, 467 (2004).
5. Y. Fang, *Assay Drug Dev Technol* **4**, 583 (2006).

6. R. McGuinness, *Curr Opin Pharmacol* **7**, 535 (2007).
7. E. Verdonk *et al.*, *Assay Drug Dev Technol* **4**, 609 (2006).
8. B. Xi *et al.*, *Biotechnol J* **3**, 484 (2008).
9. E. M. Denholm and G. P. Stankus, *Cytometry* **19**, 366 (1995).
10. K. B. Abbitt, G. E. Rainger and G. B. Nash, *J Immunol Methods* **239**, 109 (2000).
11. M. A. Cooper, *Drug Discov Today* **11**, 1068 (2006).
12. I. Giaever and C. R. Keese, *Nature* **366**, 591 (1993).
13. I. Giaever and C. R. Keese, *IEEE Trans Biomed Eng* **33**, 242 (1986).
14. K. Solly *et al.*, *Assay Drug Dev Technol* **2**, 363 (2004).
15. D. Hanahan and R. A. Weinberg, *Cell* **100**, 57 (2000).
16. J. Z. Xing *et al.*, *Chem Res Toxicol* **18**, 154 (2005).
17. S. L. Kirstein *et al.*, *Assay Drug Dev Technol* **4**, 545 (2006).
18. Y.A. Abassi, *et al. Chem Biol* **16**, 712 (2009).
19. J. Glamann and A. J. Hansen, *Assay Drug Dev Technol* **4**, 555 (2006).
20. Y. A. Abassi *et al.*, *J Immunol Methods* **292**, 195 (2004).
21. P. Nambi and N. Aiyar, *Assay Drug Dev Technol* **1**, 305 (2003).
22. S. Siehler, *Biotechnol J* **3**, 471 (2008).
23. R. A. Hall, R. T. Premont and R. J. Lefkowitz, *J Cell Biol* **145**, 927 (1999).
24. M. Bhattacharya, A. V. Babwah and S. S. Ferguson, *Biochem Soc Trans* **32**, 1040 (2004).
25. S. Etienne-Manneville and A. Hall, *Nature* **420**, 629 (2002).
26. N. Yu *et al.*, *Anal Chem* **78**, 35 (2006).

.

6

Selecting the Best HTS Hits to Move Forward: ITC Ligand Binding Characterization Provides Guidance

Ronan O'Brien and Richard Brown

GE Healthcare, MicroCal Products Group, Northampton, MA, USA

Label-Free Technologies for Drug Discovery   Edited by Matthew Cooper and Lorenz M. Mayr
© 2011 John Wiley & Sons, Ltd

6.1 INTRODUCTION

Isothermal titration calorimetry (ITC) has become the "gold standard" for the accurate determination of the affinity of biomolecular interactions. It uses the heat that is either generated or absorbed upon binding as a probe to determine the dissociation constant, K_D, of an interaction (1). The change in temperature that occurs when molecules associate is, for all practical purposes, a universal phenomenon and is one of the cornerstones of classical thermodynamics. The magnitude of this event is related to the enthalpy which, with the K_D, can be used to calculate the entropy of the process (1). This thermodynamic datum gives insight into the noncovalent forces responsible for the binding. It can be used to direct structure–activity relationship (SAR) programs and help reveal the energetic "hot spots" that are key for molecular recognition and which need to be retained throughout lead optimization (2, 3).

The universal nature of this thermal response means that ITC has been used to study a wide variety of biomolecular interactions. These include, but are not limited to, protein–small molecule, protein–protein, protein–nucleic acid, protein–metal ion, protein–carbohydrate, nucleic acid–nucleic acid and ion–ion interactions.

The latest developments in ITC, namely the iTC$_{200}$ and the AutoiTC$_{200}$, have made huge advances in the speed of measurement, throughput and protein consumption (4, 5). In addition to the improvements in hardware, there have been significant methodological developments in recent years which have resulted in:

- an increase in the range of affinities that can be determined from 10^3–10^9 to 10^2–10^{12} M (6–9);
- an approximately threefold increase in the speed of the measurement (4);
- measurement of enzymatic activity (with only picograms of material) (10, 11).

The combination of all these factors has meant that ITC can be used further downstream, at key points of decision making, in the drug discovery process.

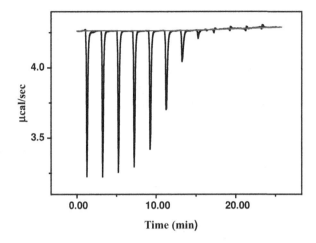

Figure 6.1 Typical raw data output for an ITC titration. A series of injections of a ligand are injected into a binding partner, typically a protein. The light gray line is a computer generated baseline which is used for peak integration.

6.2 PRINCIPLES OF ISOTHERMAL TITRATION CALORIMETRY (ITC)

Isothermal titration calorimeters measure the temperature changes that occur when two molecules interact. The heat arises from the redistribution of the noncovalent bonds when the interacting molecules go from the free to the bound state. The resultant 10^{-9} °C changes are monitored using a differential system that monitors changes in temperature between a reference cell and a reaction cell. This difference is then compensated for, so as to bring the two cells back to thermal parity. It is the power needed to maintain this parity that generates the output signal for ITC (Figure 6.1).

The reference cell will usually contain water, whilst the sample cell will have one of the binding partners (often a protein) and a stirring syringe which holds the ligand. The ligand is injected into the sample cell, typically in 0.5–2 µl aliquots until the ligand concentration in the cell is two to threefold greater than the protein. Each injection of ligand results in a heat pulse, which is then integrated with respect to time to generate a binding isotherm from which the affinity (K_D), enthalpy (ΔH) and stoichiometry (N) can be determined (Figure 6.2).

6.3 APPLICATIONS OF ITC IN HIT VALIDATION

Typically, the iTC_{200} can be used to generate a binding isotherm in approximately 20 minutes. This single experiment can be used to confirm

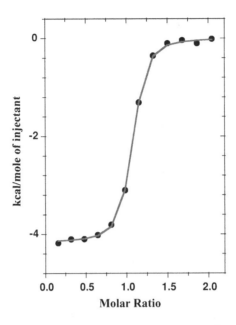

Figure 6.2 The integrated heat change per injection from the raw ITC data. The light gray line is the best fit curve to a binding algorithm from which the affinity, enthalpy and stoichiometry of the reaction are derived.

binding, measure the affinity and determine the specificity of an interaction, and all with minimal assay design. The universal nature of the probe means that ITC is applicable to a wide variety of pharmaceutically relevant targets. The automated version of this product, the AutoiTC$_{200}$, allows for about 35 measurements per day in a traditional, multiple injection mode and close to 75 measurements per day in the high speed, single injection mode.

Protein requirements have been considerably reduced with the latest technology developments, and, for high throughput screening (HTS) hits, that typically have affinities no weaker than 10 μM, 50 μg of material per validated K_D should be sufficient for a 20 kD protein. For many projects, many hundreds of hits could be tested in this way in a matter of days.

6.3.1 Assay Design for Hit Confirmation and Affinity Determination

Figure 6.3 shows the binding isotherms for binding of AMBSA and ACZA to bovine carbonic anhydrase. Both experiments were performed

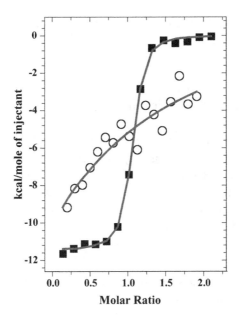

Figure 6.3 The ITC binding isotherms for the interaction of Bovine Anhydrase (~10 μM) with AMBSA and ACZA (~100 μM). Both experiments were performed in 5% DMSO. The affinities were 10 μM and 35 nM for the AMBSA (open circles) and ACZA (black squares), respectively.

with approximately 10 μM of protein and 100 μM of the ligand in 5% DMSO. The K_Ds for these two interactions were 10 μM and 35 nm for the AMBSA and ACZA, respectively.

These clearly demonstrate that a single concentration regime can be used in the ITC experiment to validate hits with affinities typically identified in a HTS assay. ITC can be used to determine affinities between 10^{-2} and 10^{-12} M. However, any given single experiment has an affinity determination "window" of about three orders of magnitude (1, 12). The weakest affinity that can be measured is equal to the concentration of material used, that is, if the calorimetric cell contains 10 μM protein then the weakest K_D that can be determined is 10 μM. At the other extreme, the highest affinity that can be measured is about 1000 times lower than the concentration, 10^{-6} M/1000 = 10 nM (12) in this example. It follows that an ITC hit validation assay should be set up with the [target] at the "cut off" K_D, above which is considered too weak to be interesting for further characterization or lead optimization. The ligand concentration normally used is 10–20 times higher than the [target].

A typical experiment for hit validation would, therefore, have starting concentrations of ~10 μM protein and ~150 μM ligand.

6.3.2 Identification of Nonspecific Binders, Unstable Protein Targets and Multiple Binding Sites

The isotherm for the interaction of BCAII to ACZA (Figure 6.3) has an inflection at a molar ratio of [ligand]/[target] close to one, clearly demonstrating the specific, stoichiometric binding of the ligand to the target. Because ITC titrations are typically performed at target concentrations above the K_D they yield very accurate stoichiometric data, allowing for the rapid and facile identification of:

- nonspecific binders
- targets with multiple binding sites
- unstable protein targets.

These elements need to be identified if false positives are to be eliminated and SAR data are to be interpreted unambiguously. Stoichiometries of two or more reveal the presence of multiple binding sites. Stoichiometries of less than one indicate that a portion of the protein is inactive and is, therefore, unstable under the condition used. Nonspecific binders clearly reveal themselves to be "super stoichiometric" in "reverse" ITC experiments where the protein is injected into the ligand.

6.3.3 High Speed ITC Hit Characterization Assays

In 2004, Markova and Hallen (13) described what they termed as "continuous ITC", which involved a slow, single injection of ligand. They demonstrated that this method was quicker and could deliver quantitatively similar results to those obtained through the traditional, multiple injection approach.

The motivation behind most ITC experiments has been to obtain high quality affinity data with little or no emphasis on the speed of the experiments. Time was not the issue and, as such, there has been little uptake of the method in the literature. However, the reduction in protein consumption and the development of robust automation has meant that the emphasis is changing somewhat. Now, using the iTC$_{200}$ with automation

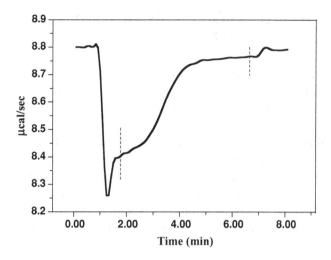

Figure 6.4 Typical Single Injection Method (SIM) ITC data. The data either side of the dashed lines are truncated before fitting to the binding algorithm.

and the high speed ITC methodology, 200 K_Ds can be determined in 2–3 days with 13 mg of a 20 kD protein – a vast improvement over previous models and a very attractive prospect, especially when one considers that the method is label-free, requires no immobilization and has minimal assay design.

Figure 6.4 shows the raw data output for the "high speed" single injection mode (SIM), and Table 6.1 shows a comparison of the K_Ds for the binding of a series of ligands to bovine carbonic anhyrase II determined in the standard, multi-injection mode and using SIM. The agreement is excellent, demonstrating the utility of this approach when increased throughput is desirable.

Table 6.1 Comparison of the affinities determined for the binding of bovine carbonic anhydrase to a series of ligands using the single and multi-injection (classical) methods.

	Single injection (High Speed Mode) K_D (nM)	Multi-injection (Standard Mode) K_D (nM)
AMBSA	4700	5500
BSA	760	650
2H	72	64
3H	60	27
ACZA	29	40

6.4 APPLICATIONS OF ITC IN FRAGMENT-BASED DRUG DISCOVERY

The "fragment-based" strategy for ligand design is now well established in the pharmaceutical industry, in particular in situations where high throughput screening campaigns have failed to identify a suitable lead compound.

The challenge has been to measure weak affinities with good accuracy, not a trivial exercise especially considering that the community has focused efforts over the last 10 to 15 years on optimizing methods for the determination of very tight interactions, nanomolar and lower. It has led to a complete switch in the way biochemists have approached affinity assays, and the same is true of thought leaders in ITC method development.

6.4.1 Measuring Weak Affinities by ITC

"Classical" ITC measurements of 50 μM and weaker interactions require too high a protein consumption to be a practicable solution if many systems are to be studied. However, straightforward new ITC strategies for reducing protein consumption have been developed and used in successful fragment-based drug discovery programs. These include competition experiments and a direct binding assay, known as the "low c" method.

6.4.1.1 "Low c" ITC

The relationship between the K_D and the protein concentration requirement for ITC has been formalized and described in terms of a unit-less parameter known as the "c" value (1):

$$c = [Protein]/K_D \times N$$

where c should be 1–1000 for a valid "classical" ITC experiment. The requirement to have the protein concentration equal to or higher than the K_D (c > 1) can be relaxed if the value for the stoichiometry can be assumed and, therefore, fixed in the fitting procedure. Fixing the stoichiometry to one (or any other value) allows c values of 0.01 to be used, reducing the protein requirements by two to three orders of magnitude for weak binding measurements (6).

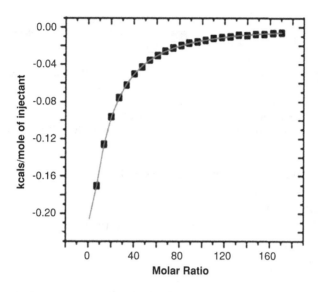

Figure 6.5 A "low c" titration for the binding of a GalBOMe to CTB. The affinity was 15 mM.

Figure 6.5 shows the "low c" titration for the binding of the monosaccharide to the B subunit of the cholera toxin (CTB) (3). The affinity of 15 mM was determined with 145 μM protein ($c = 0.03$) and 100 mM ligand ($\sim 7 \times K_D$). It is clear, from the figure, that these low c isotherms are hyperbolic and, as such, there is no inflection (as in classical ITC) from which to independently determine the stoichiometry. An interaction of 1 mM could be determined with a protein concentration of 10 μM ($c = 0.01$, ~ 60 μg of a 20 kD protein) and a ligand concentration of 5 mM.

6.4.1.2 Competition Experiments

The second approach for reducing protein consumption in the determination of weak binding is known as either the displacement or competition method. This method involves pre-incubating a protein with a weak binding ligand and then displacing it with one of higher affinity that binds to the same site (Figure 6.6).

The titration of the higher affinity ligand should be "well behaved", that is, the experiment should be able to be performed at usual "c" values, so as to obtain a sigmoidal binding isotherm. The presence of

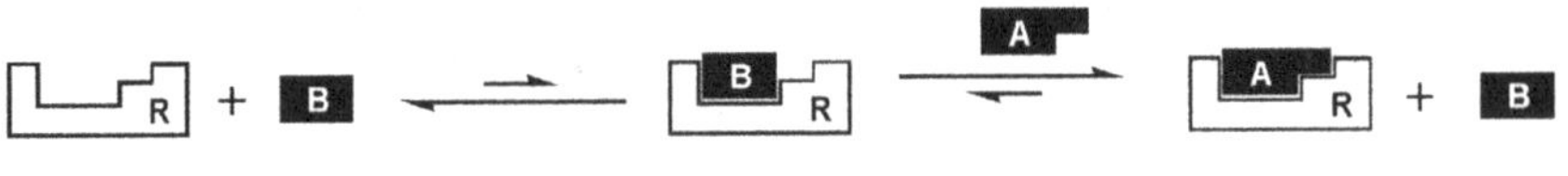

1. Premix low affinity ligand B with receptor R   **2.** Titrate in high affinity ligand A to displace ligand B

Figure 6.6   Representation of an ITC competition experiment. A receptor molecule (R) is pre-incubated with a weak ligand (B). A higher affinity ligand (A) is then titrated into the mixture to displace the weaker one. Figure courtesy of W. B. Turnbull.

the weak, competitive inhibitor in a second experiment will perturb the resultant isotherm by an extent that can be used to determine the affinity of the weak ligand (Figure 6.7).

The extent of the perturbation is related to the relative affinities of the two ligands and their concentrations. The simplest way to describe this relationship is: (9)

$$K_{app} = K_S/1 + K_W[W] \qquad (6.1)(9)$$

where K_{app} is the apparent affinity, K_s and K_w are the association constants for the high and low affinity ligands, respectively, and [W] is the concentration of the weak ligand pre-incubated with the protein. It is clear, from this expression, that using a concentration of the weaker ligand equal to the K_D will reduce the apparent affinity by half. Therefore, when screening for, or validating fragment hits, the concentration that should be premixed with the protein should be set at the K_D "cut off", above which the affinities are considered too weak to act as starting points for hit growth and optimization. This method would be the

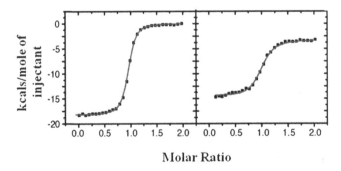

Figure 6.7   The left hand panel is the ITC binding curve for the interaction of CTB with the GM1 pentasaccharide. The right hand panel is the ITC data for the same interaction performed in the presence of a weaker binding ligand. The weaker affinity can be determined by the extent of perturbation. Figure courtesy of W. B. Turnbull.

preferred choice if targeting a particular site on the protein and/or ligand solubility is limiting.

It should be noted that the relationship described in Equation 6.1 is a very useful tool for experimental design. However, it does not hold true over all concentrations and affinity regimes and, as such, the more rigourous and complex description of the relationship described by Sigurskjold (7) is used in the MicroCal curve fitting package provided with the instrument.

6.5 APPLICATIONS OF ITC IN MECHANISM OF ACTION STUDIES

The simplest mechanism by which a drug molecule can modulate the activity of a protein is by competing directly with the natural ligand for the same site. However, targets can rarely be considered solely in these terms. Many targets have active sites that are influenced by external factors, such as allosteric effects, change in oligomerization state and complexation with proteins downstream in the pathway. These external influences can change the properties of the active site, meaning that it can no longer be considered a single target for molecular intervention. This, in turn, opens up the possibility of modulating protein function using different mechanistic approaches. This has not only opened up novel biochemical approaches to drug discovery programs, but has given pharmaceutical companies the opportunity to widen intellectual property space and to compete for "best in class" status in crowded markets.

Kinases are a perfect example of a therapeutically important class of enzymes that offer multiple opportunities for intervention. During a catalytic cycle any given kinase will bind, at least, a substrate, ATP and product (14). Each one of these enzyme forms may exist in a different conformation. Hits identified by enzyme based or other biochemical assays will reflect this diversity of targets. This has both problems and opportunities associated with it. Misleading SAR and conflicting IC_{50} will result when, unknowingly, comparing hits with different mechanisms of action but once they are identified then a number of different active pharmocophores become accessible for optimizing safety and efficacy This is where ITC can have a big impact in a drug discovery program.

Unlike enzyme assays, ITC experiments can be set up where only a single population of the enzyme form is populated. The simplest case is to perform titrations with the free enzyme but is also possible to investigate binding to the enzyme–substrate, enzyme–ATP, enzyme–ADP, enzyme–product complexes, allowing for detailed analysis of each population. The Lead Generation Group of Astra Zeneca, at Alderley Park, UK, did just that on a therapeutically important kinase. It used ITC to identify three ligands with different mechanisms of action:

- noncompetitive binding with respect to ATP;
- uncompetitive binding with respect to ATP;
- binding to a kinase:substrate complex.

Figure 6.8 (top panel) shows the titration of a ligand with the kinase in the presence and absence of ATP. The K_D was shown to be identical in both cases, demonstrating the noncompetitive nature of the interaction with respect to ATP. Interestingly, the heat of the interactions differed, indicating that the structure of the binding site had been altered without changing the affinity. This has implications for SAR and acts as a warning for using structural information in the absence of supporting thermodynamic data. Figure 6.8 (lower panel) shows the binding isotherm for a similar test that showed uncompetitive inhibition. In this case, the ligand did not bind unless there was ATP present. The third experiment in this series was to measure the affinity of a ligand to the isolated kinase and to the kinase:kinase substrate complex. The ITC data clearly show that the ligand preferentially binds the complex.

6.6 APPLICATIONS OF ITC IN LEAD OPTIMIZATION

ITC can facilitate the decision making of medicinal chemists for improving the affinity of a lead while ensuring "rule of five" compliance (15, 16). This is a direct consequence of the ability of the technique to determine thermodynamic quantities, namely the Gibb's free energy (ΔG), the enthalpy (ΔH) and the entropy (ΔS), all of which can be determined in a single experiment.

How the K_d, the enthalpy and the stoichiometry are determined from an ITC binding isotherm was described earlier in this chapter. The other thermodynamic parameters are calculated using the expressions:

$$\Delta G = RT \ln K_D \qquad (6.2)$$

and

$$\Delta G = \Delta H - T\Delta S \qquad (6.3)$$

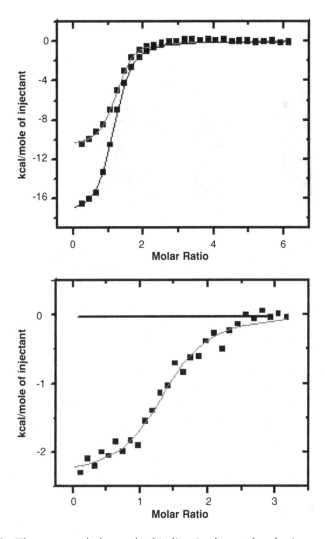

Figure 6.8 The top panel shows the binding isotherms for the interaction of a ligand to a kinase in the presence and absence of ATP. The affinities were the same, indicating that the ligand was noncompetitive with respect to ATP. The lower panel shows an example of uncompetitive inhibition. The ligand did bind the kinase in the presence of ATP (black squares) but not in the absence (black line). Figure courtesy of G. Holdgate.

where R is the gas constant and T is the absolute temperature in Kelvin (K). It is clear from these expressions that the affinity is made up of an enthalpic and an entropic component that can either drive or oppose the interaction. The more negative the ΔG the tighter the interaction. The relevance to the drug designer being that the way the affinity is parsed between these two is central to understanding the mechanism of binding

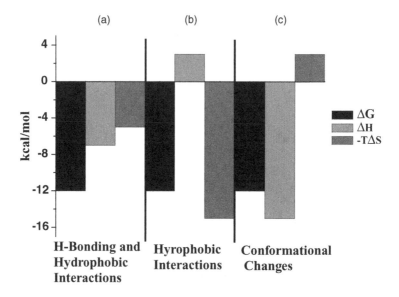

Figure 6.9   The thermodynamic signatures for three different interactions. All three have the same affinity but different thermodynamic profiles, indicating that each relies on different noncovalent bonds for binding.

and for revealing strategies for improving the affinity and "drug-like" properties of a lead (15–18).

ITC data are often shown in the form of a bar chart, graphically depicting the "thermodynamic signature" of an interaction. Three such representations are shown in Figure 6.9. Each has the same affinity, that is, the ΔG (left hand bar) is the same in all cases. However, each has vastly differing contributions from the enthalpic and entropic components. Represented in Figure 6.9a is an interaction that is both enthalpically and entropically favorable and this signifies that binding is driven by a mixture of polar and nonpolar interactions. Represented in Figure 6.9b is an interaction that relies on an entropic force and, most likely, is driven by the release of water from hydrophobic surfaces. Figure 6.9c is the thermodynamic signature of an interaction that makes excellent polar contacts (large negative enthalpy) but which is entropically opposed due to binding induced conformational changes.

These simple rules can be used to assess the success of a given optimization iteration, not only in terms of the affinity but also the mechanism by which it was achieved. In parallel to this, Lipinski's "rule of five" (19) dictates that a drug should not be too hydrophobic or hydrophilic. Using thermodynamic signatures, ITC is uniquely positioned to be able to help guide the medicinal chemist to a new chemical entity with a high affinity while maintaining a good balance between these forces, such as that shown in Figure 6.9c. Compounds that do not rely heavily on either hydrophobic or polar interaction are more likely to obey Lipinski's rules. If they do not, then ITC driven SAR can be used to identify those moieties that have the least impact on the affinity and are can be readily sacrificed.

The strategy proposed by the Freire laboratory at Johns Hopkins University, based on their work on anti HIV 1, statins and antimalarial inhibitors (18, 20, 21), is that a compound with a large negative enthalpy should be used as the scaffold for a lead optimization program regardless of the affinity. The hydrogen bonding network that this represents is the most difficult to engineer and should be retained. Strategically positioned hydrophobic groups can then be added with a good chance of increasing the affinity. The net result is a high affinity compound with few nonproductive moieties and with good drug properties (16).

6.7 ITC AS AN ENZYME ACTIVITY MONITOR

ITC can also be used as a universal monitor of enzyme reactions (10, 11, 22). There is no need for any specific assay development or for coupling of reactions. The ubiquitous nature of heat as a probe means that ITC can be used to monitor virtually all enzyme reactions (10). It can be used quantitatively to measure K_M, V_{max}, and K_i of an inhibitor, semi-quantitatively to determine IC_{50} or qualitatively to measure whether an enzyme is active or not in the presence or absence of an inhibitor.

The quantitative measurements typically take about 20 minutes (10, 22). The semi-quantitative and qualitative measurements can often be performed faster (Figure 6.10) and will be less dependent on the kinetic parameters with most measurements requiring only picograms of protein.

The applications most suited to these approaches fall into three major categories:

- As a replacement to slow, complex and expensive assays where high throughput is not a requirement.
- As an assay method for enzymes where no assay has been developed.
- As an orthogonal enzyme assay for hit confirmation/validation and SAR.

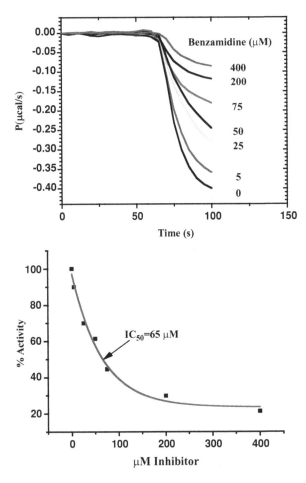

Figure 6.10   The upper panel shows the ITC outputs generated for the catalysis of BAEE by trypsin in the presence of varying concentrations of benzamidine. The lower panel represents the IC_{50} data generated from these data.

6.8 CONCLUSION

ITC can generate high quality, label-free, affinity data that require minimal assay development and sample preparation. It can be used to validate hits, generate high quality SAR data and help decision making in the advancement of hits and leads. The latest developments, resulting in reduced protein consumption and higher throughput, mean that ITC can be now be used to accelerate the drug discovery time-lines for a wide range of targets.

REFERENCES

1. T. Wiseman, S. Williston, J. F. Brandts, and L. N. Lin, *Anal. Biochem.* **179**, 131 (1989).
2. A. Ciulli, G. Williams, A. G. Smith, *et al. J. Med. Chem*, **49**, 4992 (2006).
3. W. B. Turnbull, B.L. Precious, and S.W. Homans, *J. Am. Chem. Soc.* **126**, 1047 (2004).
4. R. Brown, J. M. Brandts, R. O'Brien, and W.B. Peters, in *Label-Free Biosensors: Techniques and Applications* (Ed. M. Cooper), Cambridge University Press (2009).
5. E. Freire, *E. Pharm. Rev.*, **5**, 73 (2007).
6. W. B. Turnbull and A.H. Daranas, *J. Am. Chem. Soc.* **125**, 14859 (2003).
7. B. W. Sigurskjold, *Anal. Biochem.* **277**, 260 (2000).
8. Y. L. Zhang and Z. Y. Zhang, Anal. Biochem. **261**, 139 (1998).
9. A. Velazquez-Campoy, Y. Kiso, and E. Freire, *Arch. Biochem. Biophys.* **390**, 169 (2001).
10. M. J. Todd and J. Gomez, *Anal. Biochem.* **296**, 179 (2001).
11. T. Lonhienne, E. Baise, G. Feller, *et al. Biochim. et Biophys. Acta* **1545**, 349 (2000).
12. J. Tellinghuisen, *J. Phys. Chem. B.* **109**, 20027 (2005).
13. N. Markova and D. Hallen, *Anal. Biochem.* **331**, 77 (2004).
14. G. Holdgate, MicroCal Application Note (2007).
15. A. J. Ruben and Y. Kiso, *Chem. Biol. Drug Des.* **67**, 2 (2006).
16. E. Freire, *Drug Discov. Today*, **13** (19–20), 869 (2008).
17. R. W. Sarver, J. Peevers, W.L. Cody, *et al.*, *Anal. Biochem.* **360**, 30 (2007).
18. V. Lafont, A. A. Armstrong, H. Ohtaka, *et al. Chem Biol Drug Des* **69**, 413 (2007).
19. C.A. Lipinski, F. Lombardo, B.W Dominy, and P.J. Feeney, *Adv. Drug Deliv.*, **46**, 3 (2001).
20. T. Carbonell and E. Friere, *Biochemistry*, **44**, 11741 (2005).
21. U. Bacha, J. Barrila, A. Velazquez-Campoy *et al. Biochemistry* **43**, 4906 (2004).
22. M. L. Bianconi, *Biophys. Chem.* **126** (1-3), 59 (2007).

7

Incorporating Transmitted Light Modalities into High-Content Analysis Assays

Robert Graves
GE Healthcare Life Sciences, Piscataway, NJ, USA

7.1 INTRODUCTION

The increased use of high content cell-based assays in research and pharmaceutical drug discovery, has been enabled by developments in automated fluorescent microscope hardware (rapid auto-focusing and stage movement), and dedicated analysis software capable of batch processing large numbers of images [1, 2]. The assays run on these instruments are

Label-Free Technologies for Drug Discovery   Edited by Matthew Cooper and Lorenz M. Mayr
© 2011 John Wiley & Sons, Ltd

typically performed in 96- or 384-well microplates and use combinations of fluorescent probes, such as cell permeable stains, labeled antibodies for fixed cell assays, or they use cells expressing fluorescent proteins such as GFP [3].

High content image analysis software generates data for each cell analyzed, including various measurements related to object intensity and numerous morphology descriptors. As a consequence of this rich data output at the single cell level, high content analysis is particularly suited to the study of heterogeneous cellular responses. This heterogeneity of response can simply be a consequence of an inherent variation in gene expression, can be related to the cell cycle status of each cell, or can be experimentally introduced in transient expression assays or those with mixed cell populations.

The most commonly used image analysis strategy for the identification of individual cells is to use an image of nuclei fluorescently stained with dyes such as Hoechst or DAPI. In the analysis of multicolor assays, once the nuclear location has been assigned in the image, it is then used as the seed for the image analysis processing to identify associated features, such as adjacent cytoplasm, and subcellular structures, such as organelles. Fluorescently labeled nuclei typically present the easiest targets for the analysis "de-clumping" of closely spaced cells, especially under conditions of cell confluency. However, fluorescent DNA stains have associated long term exposure toxicity, limiting their use to fixed end-point assays or to short duration live cell assays, and they are therefore not suitable for monitoring live cells over a period of several days [4]. Cell compartments such as nuclei can be fluorescently tagged with suitable reporters in transient or stable expression systems, but there is considerable assay development and validation required, and such methods are often not suitable for primary cell cultures.

An alternative approach is to incorporate transmitted light imaging into high content analysis. The IN Cell Analyzer 1000 automated microscope from GE Healthcare provides full fluorescent imaging capability coupled with the transmitted light imaging modalities of bright field, phase contrast and differential interference contrast [5]. The supplied image analysis software (IN Cell Investigator) can be used to achieve comparable cell detection efficiency from phase contrast images compared to fluorescent images. This chapter reviews the use of transmitted light modalities alone (label-free mode), or in conjunction with fluorescent microscopy, for high content analysis applications including cell counting and the determination of cell viability.

7.2 TRANSMITTED LIGHT (BRIGHT FIELD) IMAGING

An example $10\times$ IN Cell Analyzer 1000 image of fluorescent nuclei labeled with Hoechst dye, and of the same cells imaged in bright field or phase contrast mode, is shown in Figure 7.1. The phase contrast image is generated from the image pre-processing of three bright field images, one in-focus, one over-focus and one under-focus, using software developed by Iatia Imaging Pty Ltd (Victoria, Australia). This application, which is an integral component of the IN Cell Analyzer image acquisition software, uses a proprietary algorithm to generate phase maps showing how much light was delayed at each point in the sample. When combined with intensity (amplitude) data, the phase maps enable reconstruction of the exit wave information. Nomarski Differential Interference Contrast (DIC) images are also obtained using the in-focus (amplitude) image and the phase map.

Some challenges associated with the analysis of bright field and phase contrast images compared to images of fluorescent nuclei are highlighted in Figures 7.2a–7.2c. MCID image analysis software (InterFocus Imaging Ltd, Cambridge, UK) was used to generate pixel value profile plots across the images in Figure 7.1. The fluorescent nuclei show as distinct peaks above the image background, the height and slope of the peaks in part defining the contrast and sharpness of the objects in the image (Figure 7.2a). Bright field images show a much less distinct pattern of peaks associated with the cell locations (Figure 7.2b) and phase contrast images typically show more background variation and an inverted pixel value profile pattern when compared with the profile from an equivalent fluorescent image (Figure 7.2c). Image analysis algorithms are typically optimized to work with the pixel value distributions seen in images of fluorescently stained objects, as represented by Figure 7.2a.

7.3 IMAGE ANALYSIS OF PHASE CONTRAST IMAGES

The IN Cell Investigator analysis software available with the IN Cell Analyzer 1000 includes the Developer toolbox, which allows the end-user to create custom analysis routines. These user-defined protocols can incorporate advanced image pre-processing to enhance the identification (segmentation) of the features of interest in the images. This strategy is used to identify the cell locations in phase contrast images (Figure 7.3c)

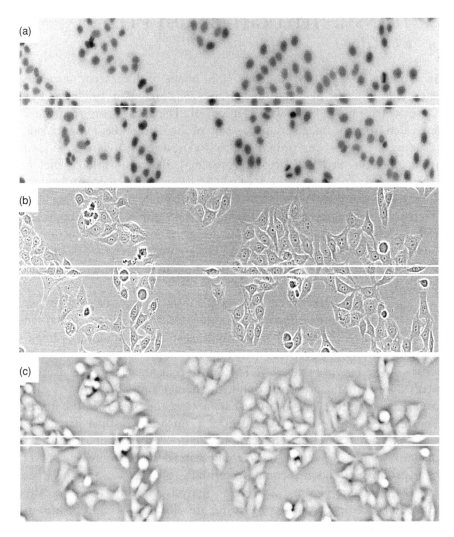

Figure 7.1 Example 10× images from the IN Cell Analyzer 1000 showing partial field of view of nuclei fluorescently stained with Hoechst dye (a), the same cells imaged in bright field mode (b) and the same cells imaged in phase contrast mode (c). The acquisition times were 500 ms for image (a) and 10 ms for image (b). The phase contrast image (c) is obtained by the acquisition and image pre-processing of three bright field images. The horizontal transect lines were used to define sampling areas for pixel intensity profiles across the image (Figure 7.2).

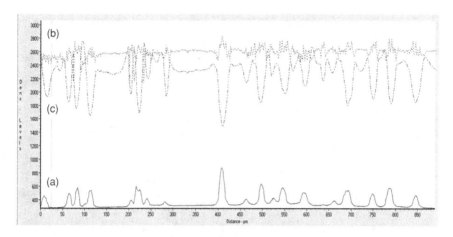

Figure 7.2 Mean pixel intensity profiles along the area defined by the horizontal transect lines in Figure 7.1 for the image of nuclei fluorescently stained with Hoechst dye (a), the same cells imaged in bright field mode (b) and the same cells imaged in phase contrast mode (c). For each set of data the X axis displays the distance across the transect line and the Y axis displays the mean pixel values at each location.

by incorporating a contrast enhancement step (Figure 7.3d) followed by image inversion (Figure 7.3e).

Figures 7.4a–7.4d shows the use of the Developer pre-processed phase contrast image in an application for cell counting. Depending on the data required by the investigator, analysis of the phase contrast image generates an object segmentation bitmap, which can report basic measurements such as the proportion of an image field occupied by cells (Figure 7.4b) or, following additional post-processing and object de-clumping, the resulting bitmap can be used to report the location and morphology of individual cells (Figure 7.4c). The segmentation bitmaps are also used to define the sampling regions for pixel intensity values from the original images. Example results of cell count per image field from a variety of image fields spread across several wells of an assay plate are shown in Figure 7.4d. The cell counts derived from analysis of the phase contrast images compare favorably with the corresponding counts of fluorescently stained nuclei from the same cells.

High content analysis is being increasingly used to study cell health and the mechanisms associated with chemically induced cell toxicity, an area of particular importance for drug discovery. Figures 7.5a–7.5d show example images of control HeLa cells (Figures 7.5a and 7.5b) or cells showing signs of chemically induced toxicity after treatment with 200 nM nocodazole for 48 hours (Figures 7.5c and 7.5d). The cells

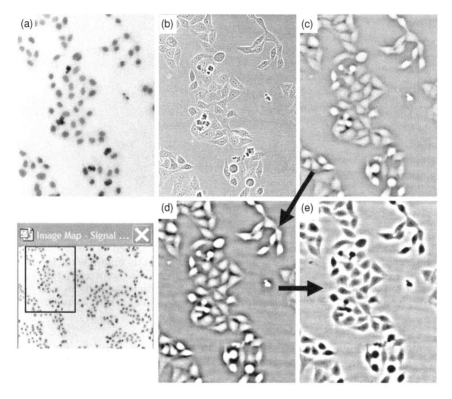

Figure 7.3 10× images from IN Cell Analyzer 1000 showing partial field of view of nuclei fluorescently stained with Hoechst dye (a), the same cells imaged in bright field mode (c) and the same cells imaged in phase contrast mode (c). The Developer analysis protocol used to identify the cell location in image (c) incorporates a pre-processing step to contrast enhance the phase contrast image (d) followed by image inversion (e).

were stained with MitoTracker Red (Life Technologies Corporation, CA, USA), a cell permeable fluorescent dye used to monitor mitochondrial status (Figures 7.5a and 7.5c), and the same cells were also imaged using phase contrast (Figures 7.5b and 7.5d). It is evident from the images that the treated cells are fewer in number, and there is a significant increase in the number of treated cells showing rounded morphology and an increase in the MitoTracker Red fluorescent signal. The cell loss and change in brightness and morphology are also apparent when looking at the phase contrast images.

Figures 7.6a and 7.6b show dose response results for HeLa cells exhibiting nocodazole induced toxicity. After treatment, the cell nuclei were stained with Hoechst, the mitochondria with MitoTracker Red,

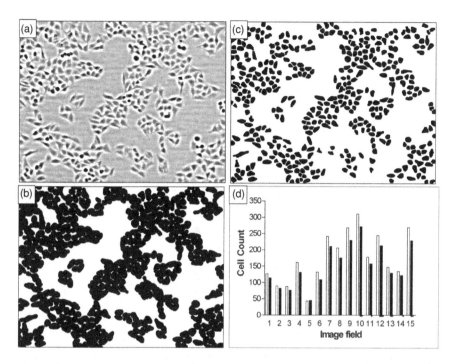

Figure 7.4 10× images from IN Cell Analyzer 1000 showing full field of view of cells imaged in phase contrast mode, after image pre-processing by Developer software (a). (b) and (c) are binary images derived from the Developer analysis of the cells in image (a) to determine the total area of the image occupied by cells (b) or to identify the location and morphology of individual cells (c). In (d) the count of cells per field from a variety of image fields is compared after Developer image analysis of nuclei fluorescently stained with Hoechst dye (□), or for the same cells imaged using phase contrast (■).

and images were taken of these fluorescent stains plus phase contrast images. Figure 7.6a shows comparable results are obtained from image analysis of the fluorescent images or phase contrast images for both cell count and total area of cells per image field. The size, intensity and number of stained mitochondria detected in the images of MitoTracker Red fluorescence are some of the measurements used with this dye to track changes in cell health in response to toxic insult. Figure 7.6b shows comparable results for the MitoTracker Red signal when the cells are located with an image analysis protocol utilizing either the image of the Hoechst-stained nuclei to determine cell location, or using the phase contrast images. In both cases the cell location derived from analysis of these images is used as the image analysis seed to determine MitoTracker Red fluorescence in the adjacent cytoplasm.

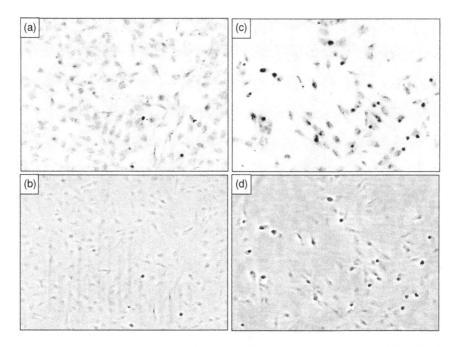

Figure 7.5 Example 10× images from IN Cell Analyzer 1000 showing full field of view of control HeLa cells fluorescently stained with MitoTracker Red (a), or from cells similarly stained and treated with 200 nM nocodazole for 48 hours (c). In the same experiment phase contrast images were also acquired of the control cells (b) and of the treated cells (d). Images were also acquired of the nuclei fluorescently stained with Hoechst dye (not shown).

7.4 CONCLUSION

High content analysis is the application of high throughput automated microscopy in concert with automated multiparameter image analysis, and is a powerful and rapidly advancing approach to the study of cellular processes. The combination of data from fluorescent probes coupled with detailed morphological analysis provides researchers with in-depth insight for study of the effects of drugs, siRNA and other perturbations on cellular functions. The use of transmitted light modalities offers additional analysis capability because it allows the investigator to avoid the use of potentially harmful fluorescent stains, such as the DNA intercalating dyes Hoechst and DAPI, commonly used to mark cell location. This is especially important for any live-cell assays requiring the same cells to be monitored over a period of several days.

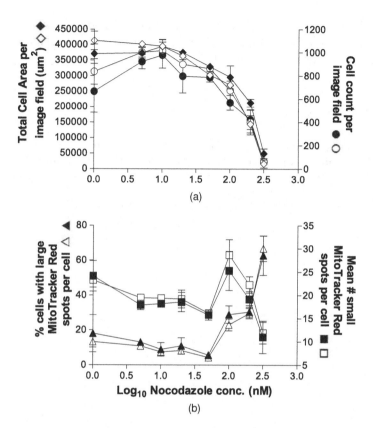

Figure 7.6 Dose response experiment for HeLa cells treated with nocodazole for 48 hours. (a) reports the image analysis results for cell count per image field (O) or total cell area per image field (◇) using images of nuclei fluorescently stained with Hoechst dye, or the cell count (●) and cell area per image field (♦) of the same cells imaged using phase contrast. (b) shows results from the same experiment in which the fluorescent MitoTtracker Red signal was analyzed for small spots per cell in the cells identified using the fluorescent nuclear marker (□) or using the phase contrast image of the whole cell (■). The fluorescent MitoTtracker Red signal was also analyzed for large spots per cell in the cells identified with the fluorescent nuclear marker (△) or using the phase contrast image of the whole cell (▲). The data represent the mean of three wells per treatment (+/–SD) with three image fields acquired per well.

The results discussed in this chapter indicate that the IN Cell Analyzer 1000 has the potential to perform entirely label-free assays using image analysis of phase contrast images to monitor cell numbers. It is also demonstrated that phase contrast imaging and analysis can be used to determine gross morphological changes such as cell rounding. However, one potential limitation of this approach is a lack of mechanistic information as to the cause of cell rounding, such as differentiating between mitotic and apoptotic cells. For enhanced analysis specificity it is likely that most studies would use a combination of well-tolerated fluorescent markers in concert with bright field and phase contrast imaging.

REFERENCES

1. O. Rausch, *Current Opinion in Chem. Biol.* **10**, 316–329 (2006).
2. A.F Hoffman and R.J. Garippa, *Methods Mol. Biol.* **356**, 19–31 (2006).
3. N. Thomas and I.D. Goodyer, *Targets*, **2**, 26–33 (2003).
4. A.Y. Chen, C. Yu and A. Bodley, *Cancer Res*; **53**, 1332–1337 (1993).
5. P. Ramm, Y. Alexandrov, A. Cholewinski *et al. J. Biomolecular Screening*, **8**, 7–18 (2003).

8

Nonradioactive Rubidium Efflux Assay Technology for Screening of Ion Channels

Georg C. Terstappen

Faculty of Pharmacy, University of Siena, Siena, Italy

8.1 INTRODUCTION

Ion channels are pore-forming integral membrane proteins which enable the fast passage of ions across cell membranes. Their ion conductivity is typically highly specific and has been used for general classification

---

Label-Free Technologies for Drug Discovery   Edited by Matthew Cooper and Lorenz M. Mayr

Na⁺ channels

K⁺ channels

Ca²⁺ channels

Cl⁻ channels

Nonselective cation channels

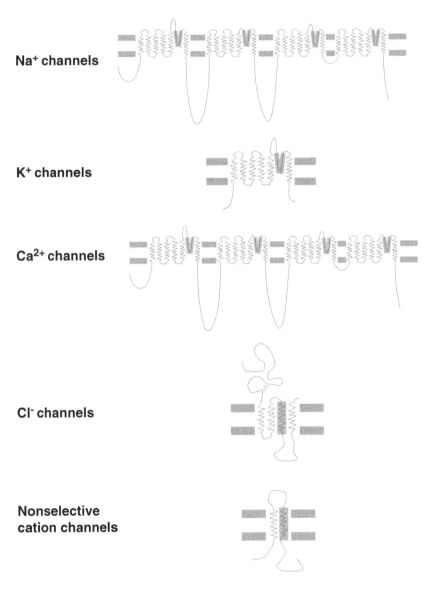

Figure 8.1 Schematic representation of different ion channel classes and their membrane topology. Adapted with permission from Elsevier. Copyright 2005.

into sodium (Na^+), potassium (K^+), calcium (Ca^{2+}), chloride (Cl^-) and nonselective cation channels (Figure 8.1). As opposed to active transport by membrane pumps such as the Na^+/K^+ ATPase, ion channel proteins allow only passive transport of ions along a concentration gradient. The opening and closing ("gating") of ion channels is regulated by a number of different stimuli, such as transmembrane voltage, ligand binding, mechanical stress and temperature. As the first two stimuli are the most common, these membrane proteins are broadly grouped into voltage-gated and ligand-gated ion channels. Ion channels are involved in many biological and disease processes and are particularly important for the regulation of electrical properties of excitable cells such as neurons and myocytes. In many other cell types they contribute to important physiological processes, such as hormonal secretion and blood pressure regulation, to name only two. Although ion channels represent a complex gene class, they are all characterized by a pore-forming region that determines ion selectivity and mediates ion flux across cell membranes.

The sequencing of the human genome has identified about 400 pore-forming ion channel genes, which corresponds to about 1.3% of the human genome (1). The pore-forming ion channel subunits comprise a minimum of two transmembrane domains (e.g., the inward rectifying K^+ channel Kir) and up to 24 transmembrane domains (e.g., the voltage-gated Na^+ and Ca^{2+} channels). Some of the K^+ channels even comprise two pore-forming regions in tandem. Functional ion channels often are homo- or heteromeric protein complexes that can co-assemble with accessory subunits, thus generating a vast number of physiological ion channel complexes with different functions and pharmacology.

8.2 ION CHANNELS AS DRUG TARGETS

Although a large number of disease relevant ion channels have been identified, drugs targeting ion channels constitute only approximately 7% of drugs currently on the market. The majority of these drugs block Ca^{2+} channels and have been registered for treatment of hypertension, angina pectoris and arrhythmia as main disease indications. Blockers of Na^+ channels are mainly prescribed for treatment of epilepsy, arrhythmia and depression. Activators of K^+ channels have major disease indications for cardiac failure and hypertension, and Cl^- channel activators for treatment of cystic fibrosis. Blockers of the nonselective cation channel 5-HT3 are mainly in use for the treatment of emesis and nausea, and K^+ channel blockers are prescribed for indications such as arrhythmia and noninsulin dependent diabetes. In 2000, ion channel drugs generated over $18 billion of world-wide revenues and constituted 10% of all prescription drug sales. Today, around 15% of the top 100 best selling drugs target ion channels. Examples are the Ca^{2+} channel blockers Norvasc and Cardizem, the 5-HT3 blocker Zofran and the Na^+ channel blocker Lamotrigene. Since only a fraction of the ion channels have been explored as drug targets, there is great potential for novel ion channel therapeutics. In conjunction with novel assay technologies and structural and mechanistic insights into channel function, the development of selective and state dependent drugs is on the horizon.

8.3   ION CHANNEL ASSAYS AND SCREENING

With the rational design of ion channel modulators still in its infancy, the emphasis for ion channel drug discovery programs remains random or focused screening (2, 3). Whereas high throughput screening (HTS) assays are well established for target classes such as G-protein coupled receptors (GPCRs) and enzymes, ion channel drug discovery is less developed due to the technical difficulties in developing such assays. The "gold standard" for functional analysis of ion channels, patch clamp electrophysiology (4), traditionally required hand-drawn glass capillary electrodes and highly skilled micromanipulation, allowing acquisition of only tens of data points per day. Recent advances in the development of functional ion channel assays, however, are currently enabling a more systematic exploitation of this important target class. Since activation of ion channels leads to a movement (flux) of charged molecular species across the cell membrane, a concomitant transient change in membrane potential is evoked (Figure 8.2). Both of these consequences of ion channel activation are being employed for the development of functional ion channel screening assays (a review has been given elsewhere, 5).

8.4   NONRADIOACTIVE RUBIDIUM EFFLUX ASSAY BASED ON ATOMIC ABSORPTION SPECTROMETRY

To avoid problems caused by the short half-life (18.65 days) and high energy emission of radioactive ^{86}Rb (β_{max} 1.77 MeV; γ_{max} 1.08 MeV) and, in consequence, safety and environmental hazards (6), the author developed a nonradioactive Rb$^+$ efflux assay for the functional analysis of native and recombinant ion channels in the early 1990s when working at the Pharma Research Center of Bayer AG, Wuppertal, Germany (7). Rubidium is an alkali metal with atomic number 37 and an ionic radius of 1.61 Å which is not present in eukaryotic cells and tissues. Its close similarity to K$^+$ results in a high permeability in K$^+$ channels and

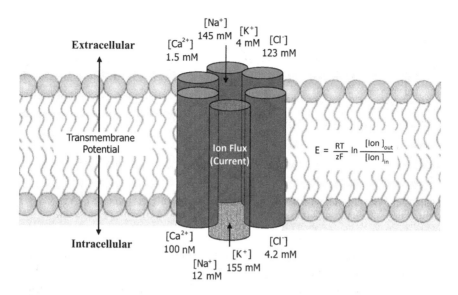

Figure 8.2 Schematic representation of an ion channel embedded in the cell membrane. Activation of the ion channels leads to flux of ions along their concentration gradients and concomitant changes in membrane potential, which can be quantified by the Nernst equation. Both of these aspects can be exploited for development of functional ion channel assays. Adapted with permission from Elsevier. Copyright 2005.

also nonselective cation channels (8). Importantly, it can easily be detected by using atomic absorption spectroscopy ("flame photometry") with a sensitivity (so-called "characteristic concentration") of 0.11 mg/l by measuring its light absorption at 780 nm. Interestingly, its name derives from the Latin word *rubidus*, which means deep red. This is the color its' salts impart to flames and which actually has led to its discovery in 1860/1861 by the German scientists Robert Bunsen and Gustav Kirchhoff.

Atomic absorption spectroscopy (AAS) is a well established technology traditionally employed for detection of trace elements in environmental, biological and medical samples. It uses thermal energy to generate free ground state atoms in a vapor phase that absorb light of a specific wavelength, which is 780 nm in the case of rubidium. In practice, atomization is usually achieved by spraying a sample into the flame of an atomic absorption spectrometer and measuring absorption of light – typically emitted by a hollow cathode lamp – with a photomultiplier (Figure 8.3). Thus, an atomic absorption spectrometer can also be imagined as a photometer where the *cuvette* is replaced by a burner generating the flame, hence the name "flame photometry". Although the law of

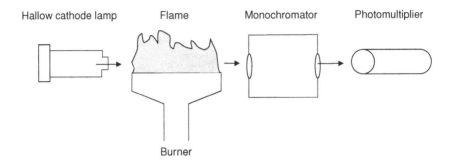

Hallow cathode lamp   Flame   Monochromator   Photomultiplier

Burner

Figure 8.3 Schematic diagram of an atomic absorption spectrometer (AAS). Copyright Wiley-VCH Verlag GmbH & Co. KGaA. Reproduced with permission.

Lambert–Beer–Bouger applies and can be employed to determine the concentration of an element by measuring its absorption, in practice this is typically accomplished by comparing the light absorption of the sample with a standard curve obtained under identical experimental conditions.

The experimental protocol for a nonradioactive Rb^+ efflux assay comprises two parts, the first concerning cell culture and manipulation and the second concerning determination of the tracer rubidium by AAS (Figure 8.4). Thus, cells expressing the ion channel under investigation, either natively or recombinantly, are cultured in cell compatible microplates and loaded with the tracer rubidium by simply exchanging potassium in a cell compatible buffer solution with the same concentration

Rb-loading of cells
- physiological buffer containing 5.4 mM RbCl; 3-4h, 37 C (e.g. 96-well microplates)

- 2-3 wash steps with physiological buffer containing 5.4 mM KCl to remove extracellular Rb

Rb determination by atomic absorption spectroscopy
- removal of supernatant and lysis of cells with 1% Triton-X 100

- Rb determination in both samples

Activation of channels
- addition of appropriate 'activator' and incubation for 10 min

Calculation of relative Rb-efflux
- $Rb_{supernatant}/ Rb_{supernatant + lysate}$

- direct measure of channel activity

Figure 8.4 Schematic representation of the experimental workflow for the nonradioactive rubidium efflux assay.

of rubidium. This loading phase, which typically takes 2–4 hours, can be blocked by cardiac glycosides like oubain, as cellular Na^+/K^+-ATPases are mainly responsible for transporting Rb^+ into the cells. Prior to starting efflux experiments, excessive RbCl needs to be removed by a series of quick wash steps with isotonic buffer The frequency and buffer volumes necessary for these wash steps mainly depend on the cell type, cell density, microplate formats and washing devices used. They need to be optimized on a case-by-case basis, which is very important, as appropriate removal of excessive Rb^+ is essential for obtaining good signal-to-background ratios, and thus the specific signal window. Activation of the ion channel under investigation leads to Rb^+ efflux into the cell supernatant as a consequence of the established concentration gradient over the cell membrane for this tracer ion (Figure 8.2). Voltage-gated potassium channels can be activated by addition of a depolarizing concentration of KCl (typically $\geq 50\,mM$) to the cells, whereas ligand-gated channels (e.g., nicotinic acetylcholine receptors) are activated by addition of an appropriate concentration of the respective activating ligand (e.g., acetylcholine). Although it is highly recommendable to optimize the incubation time empirically on a case-by-case basis in order to achieve optimal efflux results, in most cases a period of 5–10 minutes was found to be sufficient. Compounds to be screened for channel blocking effects should be added prior to channel activation for at least 10 minutes because of kinetic considerations, but also this parameter should be optimized for the very channel under investigation. Cell supernatants which contain the "effluxed" Rb^+ are removed and collected and the remaining cells are lysed and collected as well. Both of these Rb^+ containing matrices can either be used directly for AAS analysis or stored at room temperature prior to rubidium determination, which is not disturbed by cell debris.

Although, in principle, rubidium determinations can be carried out with any high quality flame atomic absorption spectrometer, the development of innovative AAS instrumentation specifically for ion channel analysis (the Ion Channel Reader, ICR, series of instruments, Aurora Biomed Inc., Vancouver, Canada; http://www.aurorabiomed.com) has largely facilitated application of this assay technology over the last few years; this is also demonstrated by many published examples (Table 8.1) after the first description of this technology was published 10 years ago (7). In fact, this assay technology has been made compatible with the throughput requirements of HTS in drug discovery with the development of the ICR 12 000, which features a sophisticated microsampling process utilizing 96- or 384-well microplates and simultaneous

Table 8.1   Published examples of ion channels that were analysed employing nonradioactive Rb^+ efflux assay technology.

Voltage-gated K^+ channels	Ca^{2+}-activated K^+ channels	Ligand-gated nonselective cation channels
Kv1.1 (7)	SK (7)	nAChR (7)
Kv1.3 (9)	BK (7, 10, 11)	P2X (79)
Kv1.4 (7)		
Kv1.5 (12)		
KCNQ1/KCNE1 (mink) (13)		
Kv7.2 (KCNQ2) (14)		
Kv7.2/3 (KCNQ 2/3) (15)		
Kv11 (hERG) (16, 17)		
Kir2.1 (18)		
Kir6.2/SUR2A (19)		

measurements of 12 samples at a time (Figure 8.5). It is claimed that this system allows measurements of up to 60 000 samples per day (http://www.aurorabiomed.com).

To determine the Rb^+ efflux, the relative amount of rubidium in the supernatant is calculated as a fraction of the total rubidium [Rb in

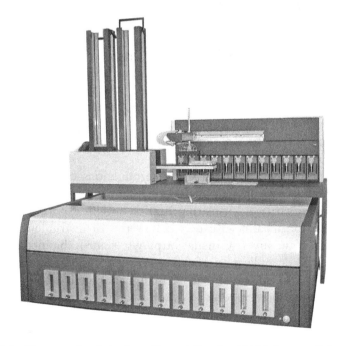

Figure 8.5   Photograph of the Ion Channel Reader 12000 for parallel rubidium efflux AAS measurements of ion channels.

supernatant / Rb in supernatant + Rb in cell lysate]. In this way, potential well-to-well differences in cell densities, cell loss during assay
process and Rb^+ loading can be eliminated. This relative rubidium efflux is a robust and direct measure of ion channel activity, both of
which are important features. In particular, the latter differentiates this
assay technology from several other fluorescence-based HTS methods
for ion channel drug discovery that measure indirect consequences of
channel modulation based on membrane potential changes (5) and are
thus much more prone to disturbances, resulting in a comparatively high
"false–positive" rate. Typically, a more than twofold increase of Rb^+
efflux upon channel activation over basal efflux levels is sufficient for the
development of good quality HTS assays (20), as standard deviations for
rubidium measurements by AAS are low (7). If sample throughput needs
to be further increased, under highly standardized experimental conditions it might be possible to measure rubidium in the supernatant only.
However, since this might compromise the quality of the screening assay
it is very important to test the reliability under these conditions very
carefully on a case-by-case basis for the ion channel under investigation.

8.5 A TYPICAL ASSAY PROTOCOL

The following assay protocol for the analysis of calcium-activated SK
channels was successfully used for screening of modulators of SK channels and can be employed using either recombinant HEK-293 cells stably
expressing SK channels or PC-12 cells, which natively express three different SK channel members (SK1, SK2 and SK3). This protocol can also
serve as a basis for the development of such efflux assays for other potassium and nonselective cation channels.

Cells are grown at $37\,^\circ$C in cell culture-compatible microplates for 48
hours to a final cell density of about 1×10^4 cells per well of a 96-well
plate for recombinant HEK-293 cells or 2×10^5 cells per well for PC-12
cells in a 24-well plate in standard cell culture medium. After aspirating
the medium, 0.2 ml (or 0.5 ml for 24-well plates) cell buffer containing
RbCl is added (5.4 mM RbCl, 150 mM NaCl, 2 mM $CaCl_2$, 0.8 mM
NaH_2PO_4, 1 mM $MgCl_2$, 5 mM glucose, 25 mM HEPES, pH 7.4) and
cells are incubated for four hours at $37\,^\circ$C. Cells are then quickly washed
three times with buffer (the same as above, but containing 5.4 mM KCl
instead of RbCl) to remove extracellular Rb^+. Subsequently, 0.2 ml
buffer containing a saturating concentration of 10 μM thapsigargin
(Figure 8.6) is added to the recombinant HEK-293 cells in order to

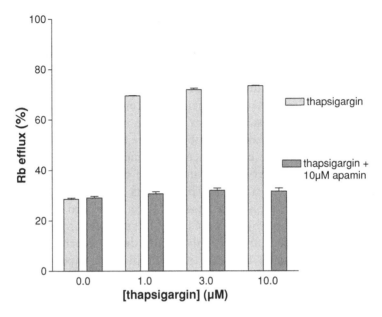

Figure 8.6   Activation of SK channels stably expressed in recombinant HEK293 cells using thapsigargin and its inhibition by the specific SK channel blocker apamin. (For details refer to the text.) Copyright Wiley-VCH Verlag GmbH & Co. KGaA. Reproduced with permission.

activate SK3 channels through release of intracellular Ca^{2+}, whereas 0.5 ml buffer containing 50 mM KCl is added to activate natively expressed SK channels in PC-12 cells (since SK channels also express voltage-sensitive L-type calcium channels, depolarization with KCl leads to calcium influx through these channels which in turn activates SK channels) (Figure 8.7). After incubation for 10 minutes the supernatant is carefully removed and collected for rubidium measurements. Cells are lysed by the addition of 0.2 ml (in the case of HEK-293 cells) or 0.5 ml (for PC-12 cells) 1% Triton X-100 and cell lysates are also collected for rubidium determinations. AAS measurements are carried out with a flame atomic absorption spectrometer. The stimulated relative Rb^+ efflux [Rb in supernatant / Rb in supernatant + Rb in cell lysate] with recombinant HEK-293 cells amounts to about 75% (Figure 8.6), while about 65% was obtained in the case of PC-12 cells (Figure 8.7). The specificity of the induced Rb^+ efflux is further demonstrated by the use of the specific SK channel blocking peptide apamin isolated from bee venom toxin (Figures 8.6 and 8.7) which blocks the channels in a concentration dependent manner with an IC_{50} of 10 nM (Figure 8.8).

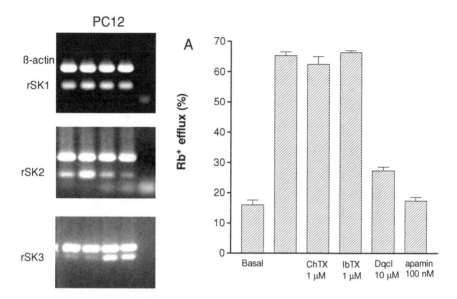

Figure 8.7 Activation of SK channels endogenously expressed in PC-12 cells. In the left-hand panel, RT-PCR with subtype-selective primers demonstrates presence of all three different SK channel members (SK1–3). In the right-hand panel, 50 mM KCl was used to activate SK channels in the presence of various blockers. Whereas the SK-specific blocker apamin completely abolishes channel activity, the BK blockers charybdotoxin (ChTX) and iberiotoxin (IbTX) have no effect. Dequalinium chloride (Dqcl), a nonspecific blocker of potassium channels, has only a weak effect. Adapted with permission from Elsevier. Copyright 1999.

If this protocol is used for the analysis of other potassium or nonselective cation channels, channel activation and specificity analysis have to be adapted on a case-by-case basis and the very ion channel under investigation.

8.6 CONCLUSIONS

After the original publication of the nonradioactive rubidium efflux assay in 1999, many pharmaceutical companies have implemented and used this assay technology in their screening cascades for ion channel drug discovery and/or general preclinical safety pharmacology tests, which include the hERG potassium channel (21). Published examples in the literature of such applications of the nonradioactive rubidium efflux assay technology comprise many different potassium and nonselective cation channels (Table 8.1). Moreover, this assay technology has also inspired others to investigate the Na^+/K^+-ATPase using rubidium and its uptake

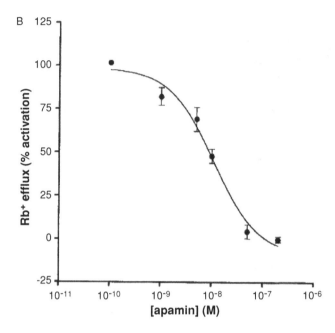

Figure 8.8   Application of the bee venom toxin peptide apamin leads to a concentration dependent block of SK channels endogenously expressed in PC-12 cells ($IC_{50} = 10\,nM$). Adapted with permission from Elsevier. Copyright 1999.

measured by AAS (22), chloride channels using silver and the formation of an AgCl complex measured by AAS (23), and sodium channels using lithium and its influx measured by AAS (24). Since functional ion flux assays with AAS as "readout" represent a direct measure of channel activity, they are robust and insensitive to disturbances. Compared to electrophysiological methods, which can be considered the "gold standard" for functional analysis of ion channels, their temporal resolution is limited to the seconds/minutes range and the membrane potential cannot be controlled precisely. Thus, these assays cannot be employed for screening of bona fide state dependent ion channel modulators. Nevertheless, owing to its ease, throughput and robustness the nonradioactive rubidium efflux assay technology has established itself as part of the standard repertoire of contemporary ion channel drug discovery.

REFERENCES

1. Venter, J.C., Adams, M.D., Myers, E.W., *et al.*, The sequence of the human genome, *Science* **291**, 1304–1351 (2001).

2. Valler, M. and Green, D., Diversity screening versus focussed screening in drug discovery, *Drug Discovery Today* 5, 286–293 (2000).

3. Terstappen, G. C. and Reggiani, In *silico* research in drug discovery, *Trends Pharmacol. Sci.* 22, 23–26 (2001).

4. Hamill, O. P., Marty, A., Neher, E., *et al.* Improved patch-clamp techniques for high-resolution current recording from cells and cell-free membrane patches. *Pflug. Arch. Eur. J. Physiol.* 391, 85–100 (1981).

5. Terstappen, G. C., Ion channel screening technologies today, *Drug Discovery Today: Technologies* 2, 133–140 (2005).

6. Weir, S. W. and Weston, A. H., The effects of BRL 34915 and nicorandil on electrical and mechanical activity and on ^{86}Rb efflux in rat blood vessels, *Brit. J. Pharmacol.* 88, 121–128 (1986).

7. Terstappen, G. C., Functional analysis of native and recombinant ion channels using a high-capacity nonradioactive rubidium efflux assay, *Anal. Biochem.* 272, 149–155 (1999).

8. Hille, B., Ionic channels of excitable membranes, Sinauer Associates, Sunderland, MA (1992).

9. Gill S., Gill R., Wicks D., and Liang D., A Cell-based Rb+- Flux Assay of the Kv1.3 Potassium Channel. *Assay Drug Dev. Technol.* 5 (3), 373–380 (2007).

10. Parihar, A. S., Groebe, D. R., Scott, V. E., *et al.*, Functional analysis of large conductance Ca^{2+} activated K^+ channels: ion flux studies by atomic absorption spectrometry, *Assay Drug Dev. Technol.* 1, 647–654 (2003).

11. McKay, N.G., Kirby, R.W., and Lawson, K., Rubidium efflux as a tool for the pharmacological characterisation of compounds with BK channel opening properties, *Methods Mol Biol.* 491, 267–277 (2008).

12. Karczewski J., Kiss L., Kane S.A., *et al.*, High-throughput analysis of drug binding interactions for the human cardiac channel, Kv1.5., *Biochemical Pharmacology* 77 177–185 (2009).

13. Jow, F., Tseng, E., Maddox, T., *et al.*, Rb$^+$ efflux through functional activation of cardiac KCNQ1/minK channels by the benzodiazepine R-L3 (L-364,373), *Assay Drug Dev. Technol.* 2006 Aug;4(4), 443–450 (2006).

14. Scott, C. W., Wilkins, D. E., Trivedi, S., and Crankshaw, D. J., A medium-throughput functional assay of KCNQ2 potassium channels using rubidium efflux and atomic absorption spectroscopy, *Anal. Biochem.* 319, 251–257 (2003).

15. Wang, K, McIlvain, B., Tseng, E., *et al.*, Validation of an atomic absorption rubidium ion efflux assay for KCNQ/M-channels using the Ion Channel Reader 8000, *Assay Drug Dev. Technol.* 2 (5), 525–534 (2004).

16. Tang, W., Kang, J., Wu, X., *et al.*, Development and evaluation of high throughput functional assay methods for hERG potassium channel, *J. Biomol. Screen.* 6, 325–331 (2001).

17. Murphy, S.M., Palmer, M., Poole, M., *et al.*, Evaluation of functional and binding assays in cells expressing either recombinant or endogenous hERG channel, *J Pharmacol Toxicol Methods.* 54 (1), 42–55 (2006).

18. Sun, H., Liu, X., Xiong, Q., *et al.*, Chronic inhibition of cardiac Kir2.1 and hERG potassium channels by celastrol with dual effects on both ion conductivity and protein trafficking, *Journal of Biological Chemistry* 281, 5877–5884 (2006).

19. Weyermann, A., Vollert, H., Busch, A.E., *et al.*, Inhibitors of ATP-sensitive potassium channels in guinea pig isolated ischemic hearts, *Naunyn Schmiedebergs Arch Pharmacol.* **369** (4), 374–381 (2004).
20. Zhang, J.-H., Chung, T. D. Y., and Oldenburg, K. R., A simple statistical parameter for use in evaluation and validation of high throughput screening assays, *J. Biomol. Screen.* **4**, 67–73 (1999).
21. Vandenberg, J. I., Walker, B. W., and Campbell, T. J., HERK K$^+$ channels: friend and foe, *Trends Pharmacol. Sci.* **22**, 240–246 (2001).
22. Gill, S., Gill, R., Wicks, D., *et al.*, Development of an HTS assay for Na+/K+-ATPase using nonradioactive rubidium ion uptake, *Assay Drug Dev. Technol.* **2** (5), 535–542 (2004).
23. Gill, S., Gill, R., Xie, Y., *et al.*, Development and Validation of HTS flux assay for endogenously expressed chloride channels in a CHO-k1 cell line, *Assay Drug Dev. Technol.* **4** (1), 65–71 (2006).
24. Trivedi, S., Dekermendjian, K., Julien, R., *et al.*, Cellular HTS Assays for Pharmacological Characterization of NaV1.7 Modulators, *Assay Drug Dev. Technol.* **6**, 167–179 (2008).

9

Expanding the Scope of HTMS Methods

Tom G. Holt[1,2], Jun Wang[1], Xun Chen[1], Bernard K. Choi[1],
Neil S. Geoghagen[1], Kristian K. Jensen[1], Maxine Jonas[3],
Qi Luo[1], William A. LaMarr[3], Lorraine Malkowitz[1],
Can C. Ozbal[3], Yusheng Xiong[1], Claude Dufresne[1],
and Ming-Juan Luo[1]
[1]*FAST (Facility for Automation & Screening Technologies), Merck
Research Laboratories, Rahway, NJ, USA*
[2]*now Department of Chemistry, Rutgers University, Piscataway, NJ,
USA*
[3]*BioTrove, Inc., Woburn, MA, USA*

Label-Free Technologies for Drug Discovery   Edited by Matthew Cooper and Lorenz M. Mayr
© 2011 John Wiley & Sons, Ltd

9.1 INTRODUCTION

A label-free enzyme assay based on mass spectrometric quantification of the product of an enzymatic reaction has been developed. The product, cystathionine, a polar dipeptide, was quantified using high throughput mass spectrometry (HTMS). Alternative labeled assays for the enzyme reaction based on colorimetric, fluorescence or radiometric detection lacked either sufficient sensitivity (e.g., measurement of disappearance of substrate when turnover was relatively small and substrate was in excess) or involved cumbersome indirect or coupled assays (e.g., derivatization of analyte to form labeled product). To use the MS assay in a high throughput screening (HTS) environment, RapidFire™ technology was utilized.

RapidFire is a solid phase extraction (SPE) HTMS technology developed for rapid MS analysis (1). It is particularly useful for HTS applications as the typical cycle times are of less than ten seconds per sample. The technology comprises four components: (i) an extremely fast, ultra-low dead volume autosampler for 96- and 384-well microtiter plates; (i) a proprietary SPE cartridge with a about 4 μl bed volume; (iii) a triple quadrupole mass spectrometer typically using electrospray ionization and giving accurate quantitation of subpicomole on-column injections; and (iv) a proprietary data analysis package for rapid peak detection and quantitation using an HTS compatible data file format (Figure 9.1).

The HTMS method was expanded to more relevant *in vivo* assays as the drug discovery project naturally evolved to cell-based secondary assays and animal validation stages. Since the assay was both label-free and based on quantification of the physiologically relevant product of an enzyme reaction, it was possible to utilize the original HTMS method for downstream assays with no further development. Thus, a significant advantage was realized in the applicability of the label-free HTMS method not only for the initial *in vitro* screens but also for cell-based secondary assays and animal validation studies.

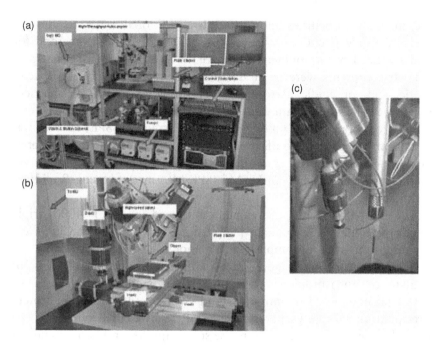

Figure 9.1   (a) The RapidFire instrument with labels indicating the triple quadrupole (QqQ) MS, HPLC pumps, and high throughput autosampler with plate stacker. (b) Close-up of the autosampler highlighting the x/y robotic platform and high speed valves. (c) Close-up of high speed valve showing low dead volume SPE cartridge holder.

Expanding the RapidFire technology to multidimensional "hyphenated" applications is also being explored. A two dimensional HTMS method using size exclusion chromatography (SEC) as the first dimension followed by direct in-line HTMS is reported. This technology was applied to quantitation of a small molecule ligand with affinities for specific proteins in blood.

9.2 DEVELOPMENT OF THE HTMS METHOD FOR UNDERIVATIZED CYSTATHIONINE IN BIOLOGICAL SAMPLES SPANNING *IN VIVO* CELL CULTURE, AND *EX VIVO* ASSAYS

9.2.1 Analytical Method Development

Liquid chromatography MS (LCMS) quantitation of cystathionine via derivatization has been reported by other laboratories (2, 3). To minimize the inherent difficulties introduced by additional steps to form a derivative, it was chosen to develop a quantitative LCMS method for underivatized cystathionine. To prepare the assay sample for mass spectrometry, proteins were precipitated using either trichloroacetic acid, acetic acid, or acidic acetonitrile, depending on the assay matrices employed. The supernatant was then applied to either reversed phase column chromatography (LC) or solid phase extraction (SPE) for removal of salts and nonvolatile buffers prior to quantitative mass spectrometric analysis. To accomplish screening in an HTS environment, the LCMS method was modified to an HTMS (SPE-MS) method using RapidFire technology.

The HTMS method developed employed an API 4000 triple quadrupole mass spectrometer (Applied Biosystems, Foster City, CA). Quantitation was accomplished by monitoring the 223.2 m/e → 134.2 m/e transition (Figure 9.2b) and comparing peak areas of analyte to an isotopically labeled internal standard (DL-[3,3,4,4-^{2}H]cystathionine). The internal standard was added at the protein precipitation sample preparation step. SPE was carried out on a 4 μl cartridge containing a reversed phase solid support, and liquid handling was accomplished using the RapidFire autosampler equipped with three isocratic PU-2080 HPLC pumps (Jasco, Inc., Easton, MD). With HTMS the sample is first applied to the SPE and then the salts and nonvolatile buffers are removed and diverted to "waste" in a wash step of several column volumes. Following the wash step, the analyte is eluted from the cartridge with a sufficiently strong elution mobile phase. Once eluted off the SPE cartridge, the sample passes directly into the mass spectrometer essentially by "direct injection", since in SPE there is negligible chromatographic resolution. One of the challenges of cystathionine HTMS method development was selecting an SPE chemistry that could adequately retain the dipeptide on-column while removing polar buffers and salts. Using a graphitic carbon-based Hypercarb stationary phase chemistry (ThermoFisher, Waltham, MA), the cystathionine was retained by the SPE cartridge for a wash volume of up to seven column volumes, which was sufficient for the analytical method.

The method was applied to 96-well microtiter test plates and showed excellent well-to-well reproducibility with low sample carry over (Figure 9.2d). A calibration curve for cystathionine was also prepared using the *in vitro* enzyme assay buffer matrix (Figure 9.2e). Background and well-to-well carry over remain negligible. The limit of quantitation (LOQ) for the assay was 60 nM, and the linear range was greater than two orders of magnitude (60–10 000 nM).

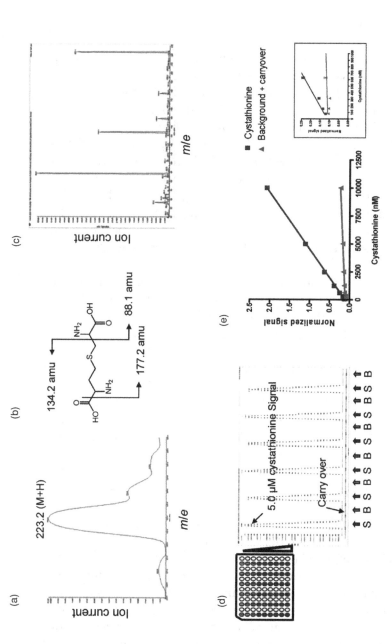

Figure 9.2 HTMS (RapidFire-API 4000) quantitation of cystathionine. (a) Q1 (parent ion) scan of cystathionine. (b) Proposed fragmentation pattern for cystathionine. (c) Q3 (product ion) scan of cystathionine. (d) Representative raw data for cystathionine in a 96-well microtiter plate. Plate map diagram indicates sample titration scheme. Odd-numbered columns of the microtiter plate contained cystathionine samples in twofold serial titration as indicated. Even-numbered columns of the plate contained buffer such that by-row analysis would test carry-over in addition to providing data for calibration curve. Example of raw data (ion current vs. time) showing sample peaks (S) followed by solvent blanks (B). Good well-to-well reproducibility was observed with low carryover. (e) Calibration curve for cystathionine shows LOQ of 60 nM. Run time for the 96-well plate was 12 minutes.

9.2.2 Assay Development

9.2.2.1 In vitro Assay

The *in vitro* enzyme assay was accomplished by incubating enzyme and substrate in assay buffer. After incubation, the reaction mixture was quenched by adding one-sixth volume of 10% formic acid (final 1.7%) containing the DL-[3,3,4,4-^{2}H]cystathionine internal standard. Assay plates were then frozen at $-80\,^\circ$C before shipment to BioTrove (Woburn, MA) for HTMS analysis. Upon receipt, the assay plates were thawed and centrifuged. Only the upper layer (supernatant) of each sample well was sampled in order to prevent clogging of the instrument by particulates. Assay plates were loaded into position using a robot arm (Twister, Caliper LifeSciences, MA). For 96-well microtiter plates, the plate-to-plate cycle time, including time for the robot arm to exchange old plate with a new plate, was 12 minutes.

The MS signal intensities and peak areas for both cystathionine and the DL-[3,3,4,4-^{2}H]cystathionine internal standard in each sample were reported by the RapidFire proprietary data analysis package. Enzyme activity was then reported as the relative amount of cystathionine generated in each sample normalized to the deuterio-cystathionine internal standard. To assess the feasibility of compound screening with the HTMS assay, the effects of DMSO on HTMS detection of cystathionine was tested, since most of the compound samples are provided as DMSO solutions. As shown in Figure 9.3a, the effects of DMSO were negligible at a final assay concentration of 2.5%.

A time course study was then carried out in the presence or absence of a drug candidate. As shown in Figure 9.3b, the enzyme reactions were linear up to 60 minutes with excellent assay statistics ($R^2 > 0.99$). The compound significantly inhibited enzyme activity, as quantified by the reduced production of cystathionine. Z'-factor was calculated in 96-well format with this compound (Figure 9.3c). The Z'-factor scores were typically about 0.8, which was more than adequate for this screening assay (4). A compound titration curve was also generated with this inhibitor (Figure 9.3d). A typical sigmoidal dose response curve was observed. The inhibitory concentration at 50% inhibition (IC_{50}) value for this compound was calculated to be 0.6 mM, consistent with the reported literature (5).

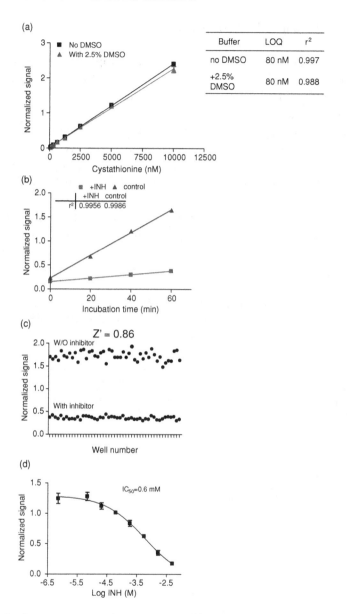

Figure 9.3 *In vitro* assays with HTMS. (a) Calibration curves in *in vitro* enzyme assay matrix with and without 2.5% DMSO. Note no significant effects were observed when assay buffer contains 2.5% DMSO. (b) Incubation time course in the presence and absence of the inhibitor. Data show linear increase in systathionine signal up to 60 minutes. Adequate window can be obtained even at short (<15 min) incubation times. A 60-minute incubation was used for the standard assay. (c) Z' score analysis for a 96-well assay. Enzyme reactions were carried out at the absence or presence of 5 mM of inhibitor, aminooxyacetic acetate (AOA). The Z' for this experiment was 0.86. (d) Dose response curve for the inhibitor AOA.

9.2.2.2 *In Vivo and Ex Vivo Assays*

A significant advantage was realized in the applicability of the label-free HTMS method not only for the initial *in vitro* enzyme assays but also for later validation studies requiring measurements of cystathionine levels in cell-based secondary assays or in animal blood or tissue. With essentially no changes in the analytical method, cystathionine levels were determined in primary rat hepatocytes, mouse liver tissue, and in human serum. The LOQs for these assays were typically higher (80–300 nM), and the linear range was greater than two orders of magnitude (Figure 9.4a).

An example of the cell-based assay is shown in Figure 9.4b. The enzyme activity can be quantified in primary rat hepatocytes with the HTMS assay. When the enzyme inhibitor was titrated in the assay, a typical sigmoidal dose response curve was also observed. IC_{50} value of this compound was calculated to be 3.3 mM, slightly higher than the IC_{50} value determined in the *in vitro* assay (Figure 9.3d). This is expected, since the complexity of the cell-based system often causes a dose dependency right shift in compound potency.

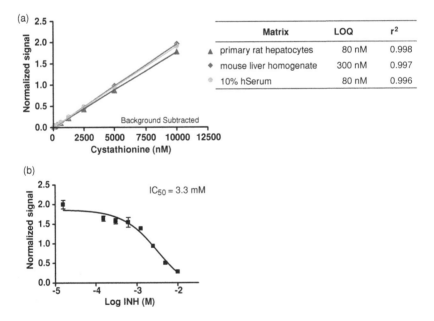

Figure 9.4   (a) Calibration curves for cystathionine for *in vivo* assays. Curves prepared for cell culture assays, liver homogenate, or serum showed little difference. (b) Dose response curve for an inhibitor (aminooxyacetic acetate, AOA) in primary rat hepatocytes. AOA showed comparable dose response curve with slight right shift in IC_{50} in the cell-based assay as compared to the *in vitro* assays.

The label-free HTMS method was used successfully for several screening campaigns of about >120 000 wells with excellent assay statistics. This assay is now considered the gold standard for compound potency determination, and an indispensible tool for supporting medicinal chemistry effort. In addition the assay was useful for rapid analysis of *ex vivo* samples for animal validation studies.

9.3 DEVELOPMENT OF A 2D HTMS METHOD FOR PLASMA-BOUND SMALL MOLECULES

9.3.1 Analytical Method Development

Size exclusion chromatography (SEC) MS is an established analytical tool to investigate specific noncovalent binding of small molecules to macromolecules, such as affinity binding of a ligand to a protein complex (6). Others have expanded this multidimensional methodology to demonstrate screening in an in-line hyphenated setting using SEC directly linked to LCMS. Thus SEC of protein mixture containing ligand is followed by trapping the protein–ligand complex on a reversed phase HPLC column. A weak mobile phase (wash step) is used to remove unbound polar components, which are diverted to "waste." The next step is gradient HPLC, which results both in dissociation of the ligand–protein complex and elution of ligand for MS analysis (7). In one report, in-line SEC-LCMS was used to quantify ligand–protein affinities in serum (8).

An analogous high throughput method was needed to quantify binding of a small molecule ligand to blood proteins. Traditionally, the analytical approach to (i) identify the SEC protein fraction containing the ligand complex and (ii) to quantitate the ligand bound entailed multiple steps. Firstly, the plasma samples were fractionated by SEC (Superose 6 10/300 GL, GE Healthcare Life Sciences, Piscataway, NJ), using a phosphate buffered saline (PBS) mobile phase augmented with 1 mM EDTA. The liquid handling was carried out with Agilent 1100 HPLC pumps (Agilent, Foster City, CA) at ambient temperature and a flow rate of 0.2 ml/min. The resulting fractions were then pooled into a manageable number of samples (typically 96). To prepare the fractions for HTMS, a simple protein precipitation was carried out by adding two volumes acetonitrile containing formic acid (0.1%) to each sample. The supernatant was then applied to RapidFire HTMS.

The HTMS method subsequently developed employed an Agilent 6140 triple quadrupole mass spectrometer (Agilent Technologies, Foster City,

CA). Quantitation was accomplished by monitoring the appropriate parent ion to product ion transition for both P001 and a P001 analogue used as internal standard. The internal standard was added at the acetonitrile protein crash step. Sample supernatants were applied to RapidFire HTMS using a 4 μl C$_4$ cartridge column and PU-2080 HPLC pumps (Jasco, Inc., Easton, MD). The sample containing the P001 analyte was loaded on the C$_4$ column using a relatively weak buffer (20% acetonitrile, 0.09% formic acid, 0.01% trifluoroacetic acid). The column was washed using the same buffer for ten column volumes and then eluted with a strong buffer (80% acetonitrile, 0.09% formic acid, 0.01% trifluoracetic acid). Once eluted off the SPE cartridge, the sample was introduced directly by the mass spectrometer. The method was applied to 96-well microtiter plates and showed excellent well-to-well reproducibility and low sample carry over. The LOQ was 10 nM with a linear range greater than two orders of magnitude (data not shown).

The multistep analytical method was useful, but slow and required the collection of sufficient sample for fraction collection. The development of an in-line method was sought by combining the SEC directly to HTMS, thereby realizing three key advantages: (i) increased first dimension analytical resolution, since there was no need to pool fractions; (ii) lower quantities of sample required due to elimination of fraction collection prior to analysis; and (iii) increased speed and throughput of the method. Thus, the effluent from the SEC instrument was plumbed directly to the inlet of the RapidFire. A syringe pump was employed to add metered amounts of internal standard to the sample stream between the SEC instrument and the HTMS. In addition, a flow splitter was placed after addition of internal standard and upstream of the HTMS (since, in this case, sensitivity was not an issue). This allowed for the option of fraction collection for biochemical analysis of identified fractions.

9.3.2 Application to Small Peptide in Plasma

As part of on-going drug discovery efforts, there was interest in examining the affinity of peptide ligand "P001" with blood proteins. It was decided to develop an HTMS method for P001 and then apply this method to analyse SEC fractions of blood plasma. The aim was to combine the two methods in a hyphenated in-line SEC-HTMS approach. To develop SEC-HTMS methods for P001, firstly P001 was chromatographed over SEC with no plasma present, collected and pooled the SEC fractions; the pooled fractions were then analysed by HTMS. As expected, P001

(a)

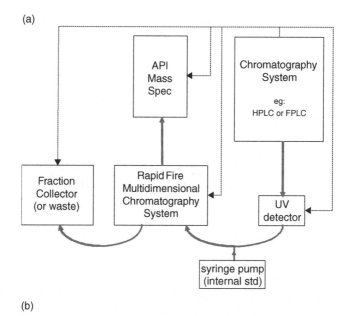

(b)

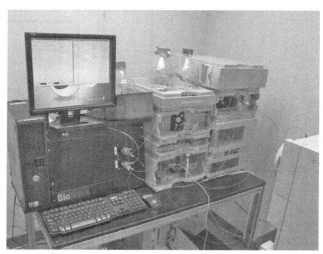

Figure 9.5   (a) Schematic drawing of 2D SEC-HTMS apparatus. (b) Prototype 2D HTMS instrument.

eluted in the final fractions of SEC with all the other small molecule analytes, since P001 was not complexed with protein. Next, an in-line approach was attempted with a prototype instrument combining SEC directly with a RapidFire autosampler (Figure 9.5). This prototype was used to assay again for free P001 in an SEC experiment with no plasma.

(a)   Free P001 (no plasma)

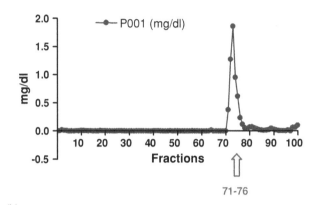

71-76

(b)

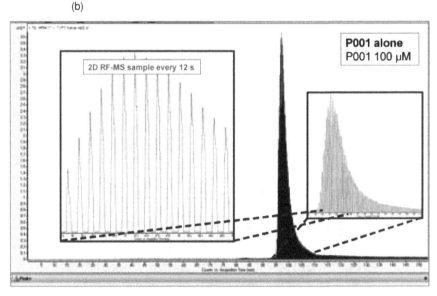

Figure 9.6 (a) HTMS analysis of SEC fractions after SEC of free P001 (no plasma). Unbound P001 elutes at the end of the SEC chromatography, which is expected for unbound small molecules. (b) In-line SEC-HTMS of same run, this time without fractionation.

The 2D SEC-HTMS method resolved P001 with comparable retention time and sensitivity but without the fraction collection step (Figure 9.6). The study was expanded to include P001 spiked into mouse or human plasma. A comparison of the SEC UV chromatograms with both off-line SEC fractionation followed by HTMS and in-line SEC-HTMS showed

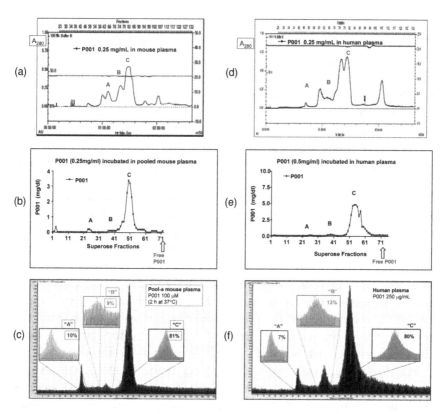

Figure 9.7 SEC, HTMS, and SEC-HTMS results for mouse plasma (a, b, c) and human plasma (d, e, f) spiked with ligand "P001." (a) and (d) SEC UV chromatogram for plasma spiked with P001. (b) and (e) Off-line quantitative HTMS results for P001 for pooled SEC fractions. Note majority of ligand binds to plasma fraction "C." (c) and (f) In-line 2D SEC-HTMS of plasma showing comparable results to off-line experiment, but with higher resolution in first dimension.

good agreement. The results were comparable in identifying the majority the P001 complex with SEC peak "C," and they were comparable in determining the relative amounts of P001 amongst Fractions "A," "B," and "C" (Figure 9.7).

9.4 CONCLUSION

HTMS using RapidFire is a proven methodology for label-free HTS screens. We expanded on this technique and demonstrated that HTMS can be used as a universal method for a particular target as the drug discovery project evolves from broad-based *in vitro* screening assays to cell-based secondary assays and, ultimately, animal validation studies. Using cystathionine as an example, some of the analytical challenges of the technique were demonstrated, such as retention of a polar dipeptide by SPE or obtaining an adequate LOQ and linear range. All of these challenges were met resulting in a robust analytical method and a robust overall assay. Other challenges of HTMS are integration of an extremely fast autosampler with the mass spectrometer and having adequate software for peak detection and quantitation. These challenges were addressed in this case by using the commercially available RapidFire technology. The advantages realized in the cystathionine study were threefold: (i) a label-free approach, with all the advantages of assaying the actual product and not a labeled analog; (ii) a rapid approach that is compatible with HTS for screening densities of up to 384 wells per plate; and (iii) one single analytical method for all stages in the drug discovery project, from initial screening to cell-based screens and ultimately animal validation studies. This third point, the broad applicability of the method to various matrices, may also prove useful in the future for quantitative biomarker analysis in large populations, where the speed and relative per-well cost of the technique is important.

HTMS methods utilizing LCMS, rather than SEC-MS, may also be applicable to cystathionine analysis, albeit at a somewhat slower well-to-well rate of analysis (9). In the case of the cystathionine assay, a potential advantage of a method utilizing an LC column would be the chromatographic resolution and quantitation of both cystathionine and the more polar substrate, homocysteine. In our laboratory, homocysteine was not retained on the SPE cartridge, but with an LC column of sufficient length, the two analytes could be resolved (data not shown). However, LCMS methods allowing for chromatographic separation increase analysis time and require multiplexing to approach speeds required for HTS. In cases where SPE provides sufficient retention of analytes while nonvolatile buffers and salts are removed, RapidFire HTMS is advantageous because of its unparalleled speed while still being capable of quantifying multiple analytes in a single run. RapidFire HTMS provides the only proven approach with well-to-well sampling times of about 12 seconds. The RapidFire autosampler is unique in its speed and simplicity (obviating the need for multiplexing), and the data analysis software greatly simplifies the analysis by providing data files per plate rather than per sample.

Finally, the HTMS methodology was expanded by linking it directly to SEC in a multidimensional approach. The example here was a ligand of interest to drug discovery. Quantitation of the ligand bound to specific fractions of proteins as separated by SEC was demonstrated. Carrying out the experiment in-line as a contiguous technique resulted in the three following advantages: (i) removing the need to collect and pool fractions, thus giving higher analytical resolution in the SEC first dimension; (ii) offering the ability to use smaller sample size, since there was no need to collect fractions; and (ii) providing a rapid, high throughput method. For future screening, the increase in speed and decrease in sample size should also result in a lower per-well cost of analysis. Cost and time savings become increasingly important in screening for the ligand–protein complex in large cohort studies.

REFERENCES

1. C. C. Ozbal, W.A. LaMarr, J.R. Linton, et al., Assay Drug Dev. Technol. 2, 373 (2004).
2. W. Lu, E. Kimball, and J. D. Rabinowitz, J. Am. Soc. Mass Spectrom. 17, 37 (2006).
3. K. Sugahara, J. Ohta, M. Takemura, and H. Kodama, J. Chromatogr., Biomed. Appl. 579, 318 (1992).
4. J. Zhang, T. Chung, and K. Oldenburg, J Biomol Screen 4, 67 (1999).
5. A. Amadasi, M. Bertoldi, R. Contestabile, et al., Curr. Med. Chem. 14, 1291 (2007).
6. A. R. de Boer, H. Lingeman, W. M. A. Niessen, and H. Irth, Trends Anal. Chem. 26, 867 (2007).
7. D. A. Annis, J. Athanasopoulos, P.J. Curran, et al., Int. J. Mass Spectrom. 238, 77 (2004).
8. K. F. Blom, B. S. Larsen, and C. N. McEwen, J. Comb. Chem. 1, 82 (1999).
9. T. P. Roddy, C.R. Horvath, S.J. Stout, et al., Anal. Chem. 79, 8207 (2007).

10

A Novel Multiplex SPR Array for Rapid Screening and Affinity Determination of Monoclonal Antibodies: The ProteOn XPR36 Label Free System: Kinetic Screening of Monoclonal Antibodies

Vered Bronner, Oded Nahshol, and Tsafrir Bravman
Bio-Rad Laboratories, Inc., Haifa, Israel

Label-Free Technologies for Drug Discovery   Edited by Matthew Cooper and Lorenz M. Mayr
© 2011 John Wiley & Sons, Ltd

10.1 INTRODUCTION

Development of new monoclonal antibody (mAb) diagnostics and therapeutics requires the production and purification of monoclonal antibodies with very high affinity for the intended ligands, as well as very high specificity and low cross-reactivity. However, current methods for screening potential mAb candidates are slow, usually requiring purification of the antibody from the monoclonal supernatants before screening can occur, and sometimes can require time consuming and laborious preparation of labeled ligands.

Surface Plasmon Resonance (SPR) optical biosensing is a technique that requires neither radiochemical nor fluorescent labels to provide real-time data on the affinity, specificity and kinetics of protein interactions. It can detect picomolar affinity levels of proteins and other molecules as small as a few hundred Daltons (1). Until recently, many SPR experiments for the determination of kinetic rate constants could only be run sequentially. Following the immobilization of a ligand on the sensor surface, a single concentration of analyte was flowed over the ligand and the corresponding response data was measured. The surface was then regenerated (analyte removed) to prepare the ligand for the next concentration of analyte. This sequence was repeated until a full analyte concentration series was measured (2, 3). Recently, however, several biosensors have been introduced to increase sample throughput with different approaches for sample delivery (4–6). These systems are capable of screening large numbers of samples in many areas, including drug discovery (7).

One approach utilizes the Bio-Rad ProteOn^{TM} XPR 36 protein interaction array system (Bio-Rad Laboratories, Hercules, USA), and its unique One-shot Kinetics^{TM} approach (8). This system integrates a unique 6×6 interaction array for the analysis of up to six ligands with up to six analytes, producing 36 data points in a single experiment. Multiplexing improves and expands the capabilities of traditional technology and workflow by enabling multiple quantitative protein binding experiments in parallel. Because multiple conditions can be tested in parallel, comprehensive kinetic analysis of an analyte concentration series can be handled in one experiment. This one-shot parallel approach generates a complete kinetic profile of a biomolecular interaction, without the need for regeneration, in one experiment, using a single sensor chip.

One important application of this multiplex, one-shot kinetics approach is hybridoma screening. This system can screen 250 supernatants and provide final results in just 17 hours, much faster than traditional methods that require purification of the mAbs from the supernatants before screening. Demonstrated here, in two separate experiments, are the efficient and rapid screening, ranking, and kinetic binding analysis of about 250 monoclonal antibody supernatants against each of two human antigens, human interleukin 12 and a hemoglobin variant. These proteins play important roles in both diagnostic and therapeutic applications.

10.2 OPTIMIZED ASSAY CONFIGURATION

The kinetic binding and affinity constants were determined for hundreds of monoclonal supernatants raised against two antigens: interleukin 12 and a hemoglobin variant. The assay configuration was optimized for rapid and efficient binding kinetic analysis, exploiting the parallel data collection mode of the ProteOn XPR36. The assay configuration was as follows (Figure 10.1):

1. Anti-mouse IgG (whole molecule) was immobilized covalently on six channels using amine coupling chemistry in the horizontal orientation.
2. Six different monoclonal supernatants containing mouse IgG antibodies against one of the two antigens were captured by the immobilized anti-mouse IgG antibodies in the vertical orientation.
3. Five concentrations of IL-12 and four concentrations of the hemoglobin variant were injected simultaneously in the horizontal orientation. Running buffer was injected in the sixth channel as a reference to correct for the decay of the monoclonal supernatant antibody from the anti-mouse IgG capture antibody.
4. A regeneration step was performed to remove the captured antibodies, allowing the capturing of six different additional supernatant antibodies.

10.3 SELECTION OF THE OPTIMAL CAPTURE AGENT

The first step before the binding kinetics analysis of the IL-12 and hemoglobin variant monoclonal supernatants was to characterize and determine the best capture agent for the mouse monoclonal antibodies. Using the ProteOn XPR36 system, up to six different capture agents can be tested in parallel by immobilizing them in six different channels

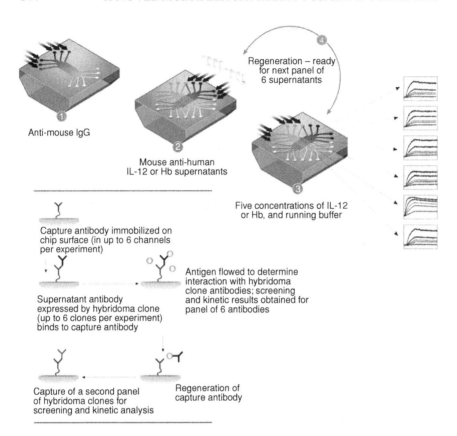

Figure 10.1 The workflow for the kinetic analysis of antibodies supernatants. The steps are: (1) Anti-mouse IgG is covalently immobilized in six horizontal channels. (2) Six different monoclonal supernatants are injected in the vertical channels. (3) Different concentrations of the antigen and running buffer are injected in the six horizontal channels, and kinetic data is collected. (4) The antigen/monoclonal antibody complex is stripped from the sensor chip, which is regenerated to allow the capture of six new supernatant antibodies. The inset illustrates the molecular events occurring at the surface of the sensor chip, from binding to regeneration of the capture antibody. Reprinted from [8] with permission from Elsevier.

and testing them simultaneously and independently. The optimal capture agent should meet several criteria: the ability to bind to the sensor chip in high density; the capability to capture a sufficient amount of the supernatant antibodies to produce acceptable analyte signal levels; the ability to form highly stable complexes with the target monoclonal antibody; preservation of the activity of the target monoclonal antibody after capture; and the stability to withstand multiple regeneration cycles without significant loss of capture antibody from the sensor chip surface.

The capture agents evaluated were: Anti-mouse IgG whole molecule; protein A/G; anti-mouse IgG Fc specific; and anti-mouse Ig. These four proteins were immobilized in parallel in four different channels using the same conditions. The three antibodies anti-mouse IgG whole molecule, anti-mouse IgG Fc specific and anti-mouse Ig were immobilized to about 9800, 9100 and 8850 RU (response units), respectively, while protein A/G was immobilized up to 5300 RU. This level of immobilization is sufficient to capture a sufficient quantity of the supernatant antibodies to produce statistically significant analyte signal with any of the four tested agents.

Six different, randomly selected mouse anti supernatants raised against the hemoglobin variant were then injected simultaneously into the sensor chip containing the capture agents, and the amount of each monoclonal antibody captured by each of the four capture agents was determined, along with the stability of each capture agent/monoclonal antibody complex. Figure 10.2a shows a single supernatant out of the six tested. It can be seen that protein A/G could capture the most antibody from the supernatants (about 4000 RU) compared to the antibody capture agents (about 800 RU). However, dissociation of the captured monoclonal antibody from the protein A/G capture agent after injection of the supernatant is terminated at 360 seconds (Figure 10.2a) and is relatively fast, compared to other capture proteins tested, as shown by the exponential decline in RU. Since the antigen injection is the next step, the antigen–antibody signal would have an exponential decay caused by

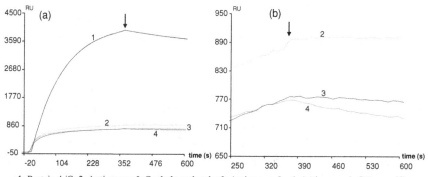

1: Protein A/G; 2: Anti-mouse IgG whole molecule; 3: Anti-mouse Ig; 4: Anti-mouse IgG Fc specific.

Figure 10.2 Efficiency of the capture agents. (a) The binding signals from one member of a randomly chosen set of six supernatants, by the four different capturing agents. (b) The dissociation phase of the supernatant antibody from the three antibody capturing agents. Arrows indicate the start of the dissociation phase. Reprinted from [8] with permission from Elsevier.

the dissociation of the antibody from the capturing agent, which com-plicates the binding analysis of the antigen. A much slower dissociation would be more optimal for obtaining accurate measurement of kinetics of binding of the monoclonal antibodies in the supernatants. Therefore, it was decided not to use protein A/G as a capture agent.

Of the three antibodies tested as capture agents, anti-mouse IgG Fc specific also had a faster dissociation of the capture agent/monoclonal antibody complex compared to the other two (Figure 10.2b), making the IgG Fc specific antibody a suboptimal capture agent as well. Both anti-mouse IgG whole molecule and anti-mouse Ig showed similar slow dissociation rates. These observations were also validated by determin-ing the dissociation rate constants of the capturing agent – supernatant antibody complex. The values for anti-mouse IgG whole molecule; pro-tein A/G; anti-mouse IgG Fc specific and anti-mouse Ig were $<10^{-6}$, 3.0×10^{-4}, 2.1×10^{-4} and 5.3×10^{-5} sec^{-1}, respectively. These results demonstrate that the anti-mouse IgG whole molecule can form the most stable complex.

Another crucial parameter is preservation of the captured antibody activity for antigen binding. The anti-mouse Fc specific antibody was tested as a capture agent, because it was hypothesized that the Fab portion of the monoclonal supernatant antibody would remain free to bind the antigen. The signal levels (at the end of injection) of the antigen interacting with the antibodies that were captured by the four different capturing agents were measured. These signal levels were nor-malized according to the amount of captured antibody. The normal-ized values of the signal levels were all similar (about 10% of the expected maximal signal, R_{max}, for this specific injection length), sug-gesting that all supernatant antibodies maintained similar activity for antigen binding.

The last important parameter relating to selecting the capture pro-tein is the stability of the capture agent toward numerous regenera-tion treatments. The ability of each capture agent to recapture a se-lected monoclonal antibody supernatant after 20 and 40 regeneration cycles was tested (Figure 10.3). Specifically, the selected antibody su-pernatant was captured followed by 20 regeneration injections. Then, it was recaptured again and an additional 20 regeneration injections were performed. Finally, the selected antibody supernatant was cap-tured again after overall 40 regeneration cycles. Since the signals of the antibody supernatant capturing reached the same level it was con-cluded that there is no observable loss of capture capability after 20 and even 40 regeneration cycles (the number required to complete

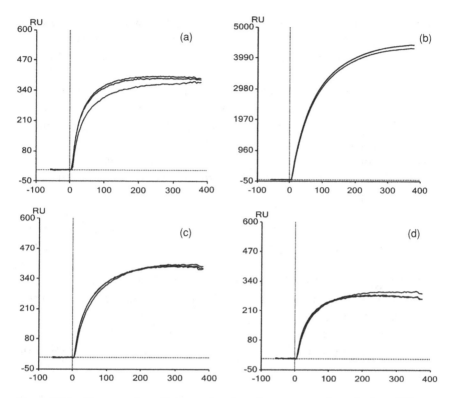

Figure 10.3 Regeneration efficiency of a selected supernatant from the four different capturing agents after 0, 20 and 40 regenerations cycles. Anti-mouse IgG whole molecule (a), protein A/G (b), anti-mouse IgG Fc specific (c) and anti-mouse Ig (d). Reprinted from [8] with permission from Elsevier.

the screening of about 250 supernatants) for all the four capturing agents tested.

Based on these results, anti-mouse IgG whole molecule was chosen as the capture agent for the hybridoma screening experiments. Different supernatants may exhibit different binding characteristics to different capture agents, and these optimization experiments were performed in order to select the best capture agent for use in the screening of a large number of supernatants.

10.4 KINETIC ANALYSIS OF 192 HUMAN ANTI-IL-12 SUPERNATANTS

The kinetic analysis of all mouse anti-human IL-12 supernatants was performed by first capturing the mouse anti-human IL-12 antibodies from the supernatants (using the anti-mouse IgG whole molecule capture agent) and then monitoring and analyzing the interaction between these anti-IL-12 antibodies and different concentrations of IL-12 antigen.

Anti-mouse IgG whole molecule was immobilized in the horizontal orientation in all six channels of a GLM sensor chip, to a level of about 9800 RU. This step was performed only once for the entire experiment, which consisted of 42 cycles, each cycle providing the full determination of the binding constants of six different monoclonal supernatants raised against human IL-12. The experimental protocol consisted of the following steps

1. Capturing six different supernatant mouse anti human IL-12 monoclonal antibodies in parallel, in the vertical orientation of the sensor chip.
2. Antigen (IL-12) injection in the horizontal orientation, using five different concentrations in five channels and running buffer in the sixth channel.
3. Regeneration to remove the anti-human IL-12 antibody/IL-12 antigen complex from the IgG capture agent, followed by injection of another panel of six supernatants.

This assay configuration utilized two types of referencing required for appropriate data processing and analysis. The first reference, horizontal interspots, was used to correct bulk effects and nonspecific binding of the antigen to the sensor chip. Horizontal interspots contain only the anti-mouse capture agent (no bound monoclonal antibody) and any antigen (IL-12) which bound nonspecifically (Figure 10.4). During reference subtraction, data collected from the horizontal interspots were subtracted from the kinetic profile data. Vertical interspots were used to determine the amount of monoclonal supernatant antibodies being captured by the anti-mouse IgG, providing useful information about expression levels of the IL-12 antibodies in the various supernatants.

A second reference was used to correct for the exponential drift stemming from the decay of the anti-mouse IgG capture antibody/mouse anti-human IL-12 antibody complex. Although the capture agent was chosen to minimize such decay, the subtraction of this decay from the kinetic data can ensure an even more accurate reflection of the antigen–antibody binding kinetics. This correction was done by subtracting the signal of the running buffer injected in the sixth channel from the antigen signals obtained from each of the five channels. It should be noted that

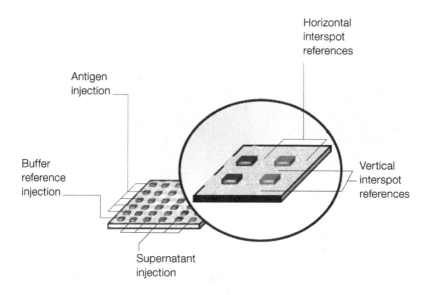

Figure 10.4 Interspot references are located in the horizontal and vertical channel flow path of the sensor chip, immediately before and after each reaction spot. Reprinted from [8] with permission from Elsevier.

this correction cannot account for the change in surface capacity during the decay (which might impact the association phase) but it provides a means to eliminate the nonlinear drift, thereby facilitating data analysis. Since the decay is not linear, the reference buffer injection must be performed at the same time with the antigen injection. This correction is made possible by the parallel mode of data collection enabled by the ProteOn XPR36 system (8).

The output of a single cycle using the one-shot kinetic approach included the determination of six sets of association and dissociation rate constants, from which the affinity constants could also be derived (Figure 10.5a). This parallel mode of operation allows the complete determination of the kinetic constants after a single monoclonal antibody capturing step. Since five antigen concentrations interact simultaneously with the captured antibody, there is no need to recapture the same supernatant. Moreover, the five different antigen concentrations interact with the same level of captured antibody allowing a single global R_{max} calculation, making the data analysis more thorough.

The binding curves obtained from the interaction between the different concentrations of human IL-12 antigen and each mouse anti-human

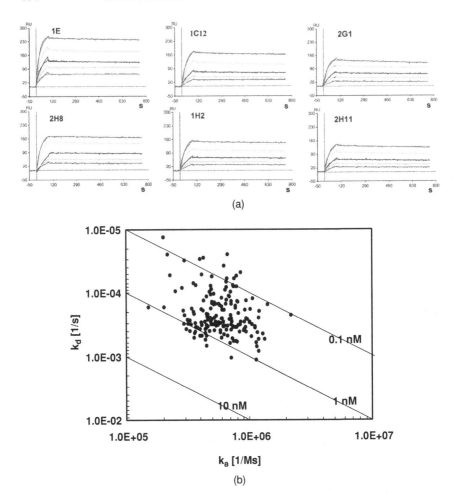

Figure 10.5 (a) One-shot kinetics results of human IL-12 antigen (50, 25, 12.25, 6.25 and 3.12 nM) interacting with six different mouse anti-human IL-12 hybridoma supernatants. All the binding responses were generated in a single injection using the one-shot kinetics approach, and they are grouped so that each plot contains a single supernatant interacting with the five antigen concentrations. (b) The kinetic binding constants were plotted on a k_a versus k_d plot for the interactions of the different anti-human IL-12 supernatants and human IL-12 antigen. Data points along the same diagonal have identical binding affinities. Reprinted from [8] with permission from Elsevier.

IL-12 monoclonal supernatant were all fitted using the Langmuir model describing a 1:1 binding stoichiometry. For each supernatant antibody interacting with the five antigen concentrations, a single global k_a, k_d and R_{max} were fitted.

All 192 anti-human IL-12 monoclonal supernatants were analysed using a single chip. The kinetic binding constants and the affinity constants (from $K_D = k_d/k_a$) were determined and plotted in a k_a versus k_d graph (Figure 10.5b). Most supernatants have affinity constants between 0.1 and 1 nM and a few very high affinity candidates have affinity constants below 0.1 nM. Each cycle, which included the capture of six mouse anti-human IL-12 monoclonal antibodies, interaction with the antigen, followed by regeneration of the capture surface, could be completed in about 20 minutes. Thus, the entire experiment was completed in about 14 hours (including assay set up, instrument and data analysis time), yielding the kinetic binding constants (k_a and k_d) of all 192 supernatants.

10.5 KINETIC ANALYSIS OF 243 HUMAN HEMOGLOBIN SUPERNATANTS

In a second experiment, the ProteOn XPR36 system was used to screen a large number of monoclonal supernatants in order to identify antibodies having significantly high affinity for the hemoglobin variant. For this purpose, four different concentrations of the hemoglobin variant antigen were used to determine the kinetic binding parameters. The HbA0 antigen was tested at a single concentration (similar to the highest concentration of the hemoglobin variant being studied) to verify that its' affinity was indeed much lower for each monoclonal antibody than that for the hemoglobin variant. Running buffer was injected in the sixth channel to correct for decay of the capture antibody/anti-hemoglobin variant antibody complex (Section 10.4). All six samples (four concentrations of the hemoglobin variant, HbA0 and running buffer) were injected in parallel using the one-shot kinetics approach. Figure 10.6a shows a representative output of six captured supernatant antibodies interacting with the four concentrations of the hemoglobin variant. No binding signals were observed for the HbA0 variant.

In this manner, all the binding constants of all 243 supernatants were determined in a total overall tome of about 17 hours, which included assay set up, instrument time and data analysis time. The kinetic parameters were plotted in a k_a versus k_d plot (Figure 10.6b). After screening and kinetic analysis, most supernatants against the hemoglobin variant showed affinity constants ($K_D = k_d/k_a$) between 1 and 10 nM, while a small number had very high affinities, with affinity constants below 1 nM. None of the supernatants showed any significant binding to the HbA0 hemoglobin. Many negative clones that produced no signal upon

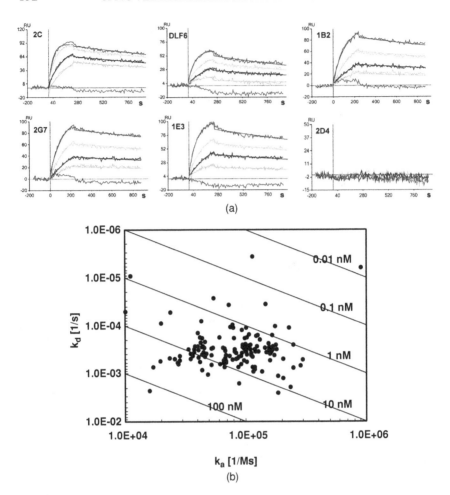

Figure 10.6 (a) One-shot kinetics results of a human hemoglobin variant (100, 50, 25 and 12.25 nM) interacting with six different mouse anti-human supernatants to the same variant. All the binding responses were generated in a single injection using the one-shot kinetics approach and are grouped so that each plot contains a single supernatant interacting with the four hemoglobin variant concentrations and the single HbA0 concentration (100 nM, the lowest curve on all graphs). (b) The kinetic binding constants were plotted on a k_a versus k_d plot for the interactions of the different anti-human hemoglobin variant supernatants and the hemoglobin variant antigen. Data points along the same diagonal have identical binding affinities. Reprinted from [8] with permission from Elsevier.

antigen injection were also found. Antibodies from these clones were captured efficiently by the capturing agent but no antigen binding was observed. Out of the 243 clones tested, 152 were positive and their binding kinetics could be determined.

10.6 CONCLUSIONS

Two relatively large sets of hundreds of monoclonal antibodies to two different antigens of potential clinical significance (IL-12 and a human hemoglobin variant) were screened and their kinetic binding constants and affinities determined. Interleukin 12 and the more recently discovered IL-23 and IL-27 constitute a unique family of cytokines which regulate cell-mediated immune responses, and they may have a central role in the development and progression of cell mediated autoimmune diseases. Therefore, pharmacologically targeting cytokines of the IL-12 family would be useful in the modulation of several autoimmune diseases (9). The hemoglobin variant analysed in this study is of interest for diagnostic applications. High affinity, highly specific monoclonal antibodies for both of these antigens could, therefore, be valuable therapeutic and/or diagnostic tools.

The multiplex advantage of the ProteOn XPR36 protein interaction array system enables the rapid screening of large numbers of monoclonal antibody supernatants to accurately identify high affinity, high specificity antibodies for antigens of interest. The kinetic analyses can be performed without the need for antibody purification. Data collection was performed in cycles of six different supernatants each, and the binding kinetic constants of the six supernatants in each cycle were determined in parallel. The parallel analysis mode enables correction for the drift (but not for the change in surface capacity) caused by the decay of the capture antibody/supernatant antibody complex from the anti-mouse IgG capturing agent, improving the accuracy of the analysis. Most importantly, the kinetic analysis of 192 monoclonal antibody supernatants raised against IL-12 and 243 supernatants raised against a hemoglobin variant could be completed in only 14 and 17 hours of instrument time, respectively.

Traditional screening methods for monoclonal antibodies can be slow and inaccurate. A method that can distinguish between low antibody concentration and low affinity for the antigen is essential. There are several SPR platforms available now that provide high throughput capabilities. These can be used for screening and affinity ranking of hundreds of antibodies during the development of therapeutic antibodies within a relatively short time (4, 6). The primary advantage of the ProteOn XPR36, however, is that it allows the full kinetic determination of up to six different antibodies using six different antigen concentrations in parallel in a single run (4, 8). This makes the ProteOn XPR36 array system a valuable tool for rapid, high throughput screening and selection of candidate antibodies for the development of diagnostic and therapeutic applications.

REFERENCES

1. D.G. Myszka, *Current Opinion in Biotechnology* **8**, 50 (1997).
2. G.A. Canziani, S. Klakamp, and D.G. Myszka, *Anal. Biochem.* **325**, 301 (2004).
3. P. LinksSäfsten, S.L. Klakamp, A.W. Drake, *et al. Anal. Biochem.* **353**, 181 (2006).
4. R.L. Rich and D.G. Myszka, *Anal. Biochem.* **361**, 1 (2007).
5. Y. Abdiche, D. Malashock, A. Pinkerton, and J. Pons, *Anal. Biochem.* **377**, 209 (2008).
6. M.A. Cooper, *Drug Discov. Today* **11**, 1061 (2006).
7. M.A. Cooper, *Nat. Rev. Drug Discov.* **1**, 515 (2002).
8. T. Bravman, V. Bronner, K. Lavie, *et al. Anal. Biochem.* **358**, 281 (2006).
9. B.Y. Kang and T.S. Kim, *Curr. Med. Chem.* **13**, 1149 (2006).

11

Biophysics/Label-Free Assays in Hit Discovery and Verification

Johannes Ottl

Novartis Institute for BioMedical Research, Centre for Proteomic Chemistry, Basel, Switzerland

Label-Free Technologies for Drug Discovery Edited by Matthew Cooper and Lorenz M. Mayr
© 2011 John Wiley & Sons, Ltd

11.1 INTRODUCTION

Drug discovery has seen dramatic changes over the past decade, especially in the early drug research and discovery process. To keep pace with the growing demand to supply new molecular drug entities, high throughput screening (HTS) has become one of the main methods for generating leads for drug discovery (1). The capabilities, capacity and throughput of screening have been growing steadily for the last two decades. In particular, the development and utilization of miniaturized, homogeneous assay technologies and various signal detection methodologies has made possible the screening of hundreds of thousands, and even millions, of samples in a relatively short time. Despite these advances in drug discovery, there still remains a continuous fight against bottlenecks and high attrition rate. Although HTS and the discovery of high numbers of potential new leads were key focus areas over the last decade, it has become apparent that the later stages of the drug discovery pipeline could not cope efficiently with the pertinent question of how to identify and advance the few truly good drug candidates from a vast set of possible ones. Identification and qualification of target binding, moreover distinguishing specific from nonspecific action, and ultimately resolving the mode-of-action, are crucial technology necessities for lead finding. Biophysics, with its broad range of applications, has become a powerful tool to solve some of these fundamental needs for pharmaceutical lead and drug discovery research.

11.2 WHY BIOPHYSICS?

Biophysics / label-free technologies have evolved during the past few years as powerful processes that can be utilized to systematically validate and investigate the binding of hits and leads to their respective targets (2–4). Compared with the more classical assay technologies, a biophysical readout often is more direct, relying on parameters which are naturally intrinsic to the target. This offers several advantages that will efficiently complement existing assay technologies in the coming years. During the last few years, methods were evolving which were already being used in productive screening as orthogonal or secondary readout. Some of these assays do have suitability for high or medium throughput screening. Therefore, the pharmaceutical industry has started to build up a biophysics technology toolkit for its lead finding research; even if it may appear to be premature to place this novel technology field in an industrialized drug discovery environment.

Although the application of biophysics in an academic environment is reasonably well established, modern pharmaceutical lead discovery presents different scientific challenges that are not yet addressed as adequately as with classical assay technologies. The key requirements are more efficient and robust tools in identifying true and specific target binders out of very large numbers of compound candidates, which is currently a lengthy and resource intensive endeavor.

The vision for biophysics is to understand the biophysical mechanisms of binding and activity for screening hits in a timely manner, to advance hits in order to generate meaningful lead candidates more efficiently, and certainly to minimize wasted resources on false positives; in summary: to identify and discard "bad compounds" early.

Another opportunity for biophysics is to confirm and characterize weaker hits and singletons and in the process to gain novel capabilities that will complement the known assay technologies with predictive tools for drug discovery, that is to:

- Help establish structure–activity relationship (SAR).
- Gain deeper understanding of compound mode-of action (e.g., mode of binding, kinetics, thermodynamics).
- Cross-compare and validate candidates with other assays (K_D versus biochemical and cellular EC_{50}).

Despite all scientific hope and excitement, it must be stressed that today most biophysical methods are still difficult, resource intensive, and, yet, quite low throughput! Secondly, biophysics is complementing, and by no means replacing, other existing and well established assays and methods!

11.2.1 Quests of Lead Discovery Program Teams for Biophysics

Biophysics can obviously be applied in a variety of lead and drug discovery stages for a variety of questions. During the very early target identification and validation process, before actual hit identification can be started, there is a need to qualify and quantify interactions of functionally not yet well characterized proteins in order to prove their feasibility for lead finding.

In the hit identification phase, activity assays are sometimes incapable of characterizing target–protein interactions or these assays are simply not turn-key. For example, there can be a need to run a target binder screen, potentially in order to identify tool compounds for establishing or validating HTS activity assays.

Once hits have been identified by any means, project teams are eager to move forward as efficiently as possible with the first good meaningful candidates to prove their hypothesis. Especially when regarding large numbers of hits – for example, from HTS – verification is the key task of biophysics. Often enough target proteins are prone to artifacts and it is important to get to the true hits and rule out "promiscuous" actives. The main goal is to verify that hits are actually binding specifically to the target and not acting by simply deactivating nonspecifically any of the assay interaction partners.

In later stages, the stoichiometry of compound binding, their affinity ranking and K_D are crucial requirements. Recently, even the requests for systematic detailed quantification of binding kinetics, mode-of-action, and thermodynamic properties of compound classes are becoming customary.

11.3 BIOPHYSICS / LABEL-FREE TOOLBOX

Biophysical methods are becoming an important tool for validating molecular interactions and determining kinetic and structural parameters for molecular recognition by protein targets. A collection of long standing, gold standard methods is rapidly being augmented by novel, higher throughput techniques, presenting both an extensive, but also confusing, landscape of tools. The various technologies offer very diverse information content and totally different needs for resource (sample requirement, achievable throughput, level of complexity, etc.). Taking into account that methods should be suitable and efficient for early lead discovery

Table 11.1 Biophysics toolbox.

Technology	Type of data / information
DLS	Compound / protein aggregation / insolubility
MS	"yes/no" binding; covalent?; activity assay
SPR, RWG, BLI, NMR	"yes/no" binding; K_D
DSF/DSLS/DSC/CD	stability of protein "folding" ($\Delta T_{folding}$)
SPR	stoichiometry, nonpromiscuous binding, K_D, k_{on}, k_{off}
ITC	stoichiometry, ΔH, ΔS
X-ray, NMR, CD	3D structure and dynamics

BLI: Biolayer Interferometry (aka "Fortebio"); CD: Circular Dichroism; DSC: Differential Scanning Calorimetry; DSF: Differential Scanning Fluorimetry (aka "Thermofluor"); DSLS: Differential Static Light Scattering (aka "Stargazer"); ITC: Isothermal Titration Calorimetry; MS: Mass Spectrometry; NMR: Nuclear Magnetic Resonance; RWG: Resonant Waveguide Grating (for example Epic^{TM}, SRU Bind^{TM}); SPR: Surface Plasmon Resonance (aka "Biacore").

and even higher sample numbers, few appropriate biophysics tools are remaining.

Very recently, for the needs at Novartis for low molecular weight compound lead finding, such a custom toolbox has started to be developed, implemented, and adapted. Table 11.1 lists our view on the currently available biophysics tools and key words for their main information content.

11.4 WHICH BIOPHYSICAL MEASUREMENT AT WHICH STAGE OF A DRUG DISCOVERY PROJECT FLOWCHART?

It is of great importance that the right biophysics tools are placed at a suitable place in a drug discovery assay project flowchart. Obviously, other approaches need to be available and used in addition to biochemical and cellular activity assays, as well as compound quality control! Figure 11.1 places the biophysics tools and the key technology requirements inside an exemplified lead discovery project flowchart.

11.4.1 Hit Finding

For very specific hit finding efforts – such as the fragment-based screening (FBS) – high sensitivity for identification of even very weak binding fragments is mandatory. Nuclear Magnetic Resonance (NMR), X-ray, as well as Surface Plasmon Resonance (SPR) techniques fulfill those

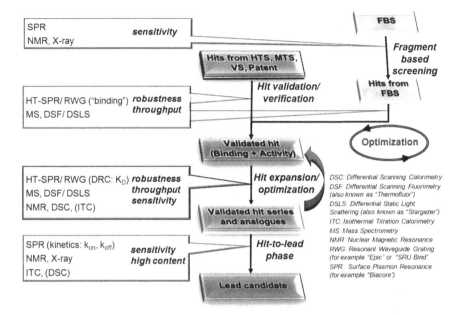

Figure 11.1   Biophysics technology examples in a drug discovery project flowchart.

requirements for screening typically carefully selected smaller libraries at very high compound concentration (5, 6).

11.4.2 Hit Validation

Hit validation requires different biophysics needs. Typically, larger hit sets derived from high throughput screening (HTS), medium throughput screening (MTS), virtual screening (VS) or patent busting approaches have to be profiled. Those compound sets are typically largely unclassified and often contain a variety of nonproductive or artifactual compounds, which serve to not only falsify assay results but which can also harm following experiments. Vital requirement of the methods in this phase are certainly robustness and a decent throughput, both of which are often mandatory due to the high number of hits.

In our experience and known from literature, dynamic and static light scattering are useful tools for annotation of even larger compound sets regarding eventual insolubility and aggregation (7). Thermal protein unfolding, denaturation or aggregation assays assess whether assay additives or actually the test compounds cause modulated target unfolding (8, 9). Differential Static Light Scattering (DSLS, aka "Stargazer") and

Differential Scanning Fluorimetry (DSF, aka "Thermofluor") are microtiter plate-based assays, easy to set up and run in order to quickly profile and cherry-pick hit compounds that eventually stabilize the target protein folding. It is important to note, however, that this assay concept should be regarded more as an opportunistic approach to move forward the most prominent hits rather than a go/no go decision for the fate of compounds.

SPR and Resonance Waveguide Grating (RWG, for example Epic™ or SRU Bind™) techniques today enable medium to even high throughput characterization of compound binding on protein targets (4, 10). The RWG techniques especially offer high suitability in this phase. The applications are still rather novel, but very robust and highly scalable in throughput. SPR additionally yields information about binding kinetics in real time, which are valuable data typically needed in later stages to qualify more advanced hit classes (11–13).

Mass Spectrometry (MS) helps to identify whether or not compounds bind reversibly or irreversibly, and often serves as a generic activity assay detection set-up (14).

11.4.3 Hit Expansion

Once activity and target binding of hits are verified, they can be regarded as "validated hits" and the iterative hit expansion and optimization process starts. At this phase, the vital technology requirements are not only assay robustness and throughput, but also sensitivity and high data content.

Besides RWG – offering sufficient throughput – SPR can now bring in its core strengths with real time binding information to resolve binding kinetics. Most SPR systems additionally offer multiplexing to investigate the binding on more than one target protein in parallel during the same experiment.

Nuclear Magnetic Resonance (NMR) is a highly versatile technology to identify and characterize a variety of binding events (15, 16). It is performed free in solution and just this fact means that NMR often serves as complementary technology to further strengthen binding information derived from technologies working with immobilized targets (SPR, RWG, etc.)

Downstream of the drug discovery project flowchart (Figure 11.1), binding affinity, real stoichiometry, and, ultimately, thermodynamic parameters can be quantified free in solution with isothermal titration calorimetry (ITC), certainly at the cost of relative low throughput and comparably high protein amounts (17).

11.5 EXAMPLES OF HIGHER THROUGHPUT BIOPHYSICS APPLIED IN HIT AND LEAD FINDING

Although a variety of biophysics technologies can be applied in hit and lead finding, described here, in an exemplified and focused manner, are a few of those typically utilized to better qualify to investigate HTS hit lists in the hit validation phase.

11.5.1 Compound Aggregation Artifacts

For typical HTS libraries, the compound aggregation phenomenon has been published as a serious screening artifact, causing false positive hits (7). In fact, experience in the past years has shown that this kind of artifact alone can fool project teams with fruitless hit compounds that in the end prove to be nonproductive. To address this issue, we and others have started to systematically annotate hit lists regarding these phenomena.

Aggregation and solubility of low molecular weight organic compounds is sharply assay and buffer dependant: for example, the aggregation of tetraiodophenolphthalein – a well known aggregator (7) – shows aggregation starting at 0.5 or 50 micromolar, which depends on the actual buffer conditions.

Such "promiscuous" compounds, which are frequently active in HTS assays, are often linked with the compound aggregation phenomena. In an internal study, it has been found that a normal screening library contains 17% aggregating or insoluble compounds under standard screening conditions (10 micromolar compound, PBS buffer, 0.005% Tween20, 2% DMSO).

A "frequent hitter" compound library set – assembled with the knowledge of >25 biochemical HTS studies – yielded 57% aggregating or insoluble compounds under the same screening conditions. The aggregation phenomenon is complex; some compounds appear as large particle aggregates (precipitates), others have particle sizes distributing from colloidal aggregates to visible precipitates.

Compound aggregation is, *per se*, not yet a problem because it has to be evaluated with respect to the compound's activity for the given target! For example, staurosporine, a well known and characterized true kinase inhibitor and binder, often shows kinase inhibition in the low nanomolar activity range. On the other hand, this compound class could be defined as "promiscuous" in assays for targets like protein–protein interactions, displaying activities in the single to double digit micromolar range, which is the same concentration range where aggregation of such staurosporine-like compounds are experienced. In other words, staurosporine is certainly a true and productive kinase inhibitor, but also a weak "promiscuous", nonproductive inhibitor for some protein–protein interaction targets.

11.5.2 Direct Binding of Compounds on Proteins: High Throughput is Still Challenging!

Early in the lead discovery phase, it is already of very high importance to assay for the actual binding of hit compounds to their respective target. Classically, this type of information can be derived from long standing methods like enzymology or radiometric filter binding assays. In the last few years, label-free detection systems have been developed for this purpose, and such assays have emerged as a new detection paradigm in HTS and related applications (2–4). These include the development of evanescent wave technologies and interferometry; a few have even been adapted to allow the detection of binding at the surface of microtiter plates, such as Corning's Epic^{TM} system, the Bind^{TM} system from SRU. In comparison, Fortèbio's Octet^{TM} system detects binding events via protein immobilized on a sensor tip dipping into microtiter plates containing the test compound (10). Consequently, HTS-compatible techniques are evolving to measure direct binding events on immobilized molecules, typically the target proteins, for example via changes in refractive index.

For productive results, the requirements are good protein immobilization strategies and high quality protein. Binding of ligands (compounds) is often measured as mass signature on immobilized targets (proteins). Over the last decade, technologies have been applied and optimized to investigate binding events of relative large binding partners on typically surface immobilized ligands (e.g., protein–protein or antigen–antibody interaction). Currently, technologies are now being used to screen for binding of low molecular weight test compounds (molecular weight <400 Da) on large targets (e.g., protein with a molecular weight >60 000 Da).

Depending on the assay set-up, the detection of direct compound binding is more or less straightforward. A considerable challenge of low molecular weight compound binding is the necessity for assay sensitivity. In label-free terms, the sensitivity of the assay should detect, for example, the binding of a 400 Dalton compound on a 60 000 Dalton protein in a 1:1 binding event, which yields only 0.66% of mass increase at saturation of binding. This challenge is further complicated by the fact that any slight change in the state of the assay components and the commencement of aggregating or insoluble compounds can significantly falsify true binding signals. Therefore, proper controls and correction experiments are mandatory.

11.5.2.1 Feasibility Study for HTS Hit List Follow Up: Two Examples for "SPR-like" Technologies

Binding studies have been run with a "mimicked" nuclear receptor HTS hit list containing 690 well qualified compounds. The set contained true and active binders, false positives, known artifact compounds from HTS ("challenge compounds"), and inactive nonbinders. From the biophysics data, the wish was to group the hit list into:

- Target binder (256 in test set).
- Nonbinder (227 in test set).
- Challenge compounds (207 in test set).

Binding was tested with two quite different assay systems, the Corning Epic™ RWG system and the GE Healthcare Biacore A100C SPR module, both designed to investigate binding at higher throughput.

Epic™ Assay Study
The Epic™ system has a much higher throughput; therefore, full dose response has been run for all the compounds (0.13–17 micromolar). This RWG system is microtiter plate based and one prominent advantage is that each data point is obtained in its individual microtiter plate well. Potential cross-contamination between compounds as in a flow system is thereby fully avoided, albeit at the cost of relative high protein consumption. The total protein consumption was roughly 6 mg for all 690 compounds tested in full dose response.

A100™ assay
Due to the A100's comparably lower throughput, the compounds have only been tested at a single concentration (five micromolar). Due to

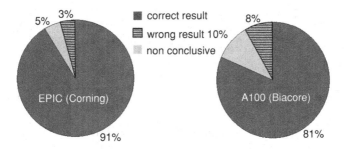

Figure 11.2 Predictability of binding assay outcome: Epic™ versus A100™.

the comparably higher sensitivity of this SPR system, it was expected still to be able to detect hit compounds efficiently. The presence of the many "promiscuous" compounds from the "challenge library" did lead to a loss of binding efficiency for regularly injected control compounds (about –30% in 24 h). Binding experiments were performed in parallel with two nontarget related control proteins. This significantly helped in qualifying compounds as selective target or "promiscuous" binder compounds. Total protein consumption was very low; in total 0.05 mg target protein was necessary for the whole assay.

As can be seen in Figure 11.2 the results of both approaches appear quite promising. Both delivered an accuracy of >80% for the predicted binding result.

11.5.3 Affinity MS Screening: Qualitative and Quantitative Screening Free in Solution

Mass spectrometry enables generic direct and selective label-free detection of the involved assay components free in solution. The main application next to classical analytics is the so-called "functional activity MS" measuring the outcome of an enzymatic transformation, for example, the formation of a product (18, 19). Although MS offers very versatile application, here the focus is on binding assay applications.

Direct compound binding assays, for example, SPR and RWG as described above, are becoming increasingly important as tools to assay the binding of low molecular weight compounds on targets. However, these technologies require immobilization of one of the binding partners on a sensor chip surface in our application; it is typically the target protein.

Even if a variety of good immobilization strategies offers versatility in assay design, it must not be forgotten that ligand immobilization

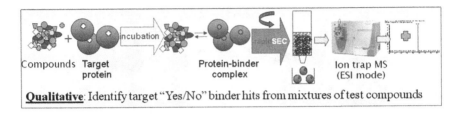

Qualitative: Identify target "Yes/No" binder hits from mixtures of test compounds

Figure 11.3 Affinity MS screening assay set-up.

can significantly influence the activity and binding properties of a target protein. Therefore, mass spectrometry is being used as an alternative binding assay set-up for projects where we experience problems with protein immobilization or issues with large target protein size are faced.

In the affinity MS screening set-up, the target protein of interest is incubated with test compounds (Figure 11.3) (14). The protein/compound complex is then separated from unbound compounds with a microtiter plate-based chromatographic separation step. Even in the presence of the protein or other MS signals, the bound compounds can be identified by focusing on the m/z signals from the known cocktail of test compounds with LC/MS.

There are alternative approaches that use a size exclusion ultrafiltration step, such that the protein–ligand complex remains trapped in the filter plate rather than flowing through (20), as occurs with size exclusion chromatography (21). This screening method has been extended to allow screening of integral membrane proteins such as GPCRs (22). The major advantage of these methods is the obvious ease of set-up, even in such cases as the absence of functional activity of the target, for example, for orphan or new genomic targets.

Affinity selection MS, in conjunction with a known reporter, can give additional valuable information (Figure 11.4). This information

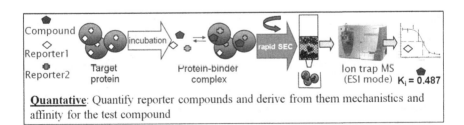

Quantative: Quantify reporter compounds and derive from them mechanistics and affinity for the test compound

Figure 11.4 Affinity MS screening assay set-up using a reporter molecule for affinity determination.

may include not only the confirmation of compound binding to the target, but also its affinity ranking and the mode-of-action about the binding site (displacement of known binder/reporter). These data are gleaned by quantifying the reporter bound to the protein and eluted as protein–binder complex. MS/MS detection makes this method very selective for the detection of the reporter, independent of the ionization of the actual test compounds.

11.6 CONCLUSION

Our goal is to apply biophysics technologies in order to systematically annotate large numbers of hit compounds with data that help in their selection and promotion towards lead candidature. Key biophysical information at this stage is encompassed in data that disclose comprehensive details concerning the binding of the candidate compounds to the actual target. Cumulative data are, therefore, a combined effort from several technologies that complement each other. Conflicting data can be resolved by applying orthogonal methods on a case-by-case basis, for example, binding by NMR and SPR.

Our strategy is to deliver a solid experimental data package, containing several information layers for the compound:

- Activity in the parent assay (EC_{50}), orthogonal assay readout and including selectivity or toxicity.
- Integrity, purity, and annotation about aggregation/insolubility in the respective assay system.
- Target binding, binding stoichiometry, and, ultimately, affinity (K_D) or potency ranking.

This data package enables project teams to prioritize their downstream biological and chemical efforts. At this stage, the application of biophysics is utilized to annotate a select number of compounds with binding properties such as kinetics and, eventually, thermodynamics. Naturally, the chosen strategy of biophysics is obviously target dependent. The actual mode of action and binding plays a very significant role, often only resolved by crystallization of the compound/target complex.

Altogether, biophysics in pharmaceutical hit and lead discovery plays an increasingly important role. However, it must be stated that this is still a quite novel field for most, if not all, biophysics technologies. As a whole, to progress from dealing with a few dozen well characterized, freshly dissolved, and soluble compounds towards hundreds or thousands of uncharacterized compound archive solutions of potentially insoluble compounds is still a major challenge! However, the technologies, methods, and processes are developing, causing technology providers and the pharmaceutical industry to move up the learning curve. And, in response, biophysics has contributed considerably to strengthen the quality lead candidature in drug discovery.

11.7 OUTLOOK

The clear need is seen for applying a solid mix of complementing technologies that are carefully selected from the biophysics toolbox, tailored according to the individual information needed. In addition to these available methods, there is an obvious requirement to further develop novel methods and technologies to keep pace with the changing challenges in the lead discovery field. One crucial challenge is the lack of sufficiently sensitive analytical tools to probe the real time relationship between structural change and molecular function or behavior. Obviously, NMR is capable of investigating this, but at the cost of comparably high protein consumption, low throughput, and an eventual need for protein labeling.

The dual polarization interferometry (DPI) technology from Farfield's AnaLight® measures optical interference patterns caused by changes in the structure and/or mass of immobilized molecules. Thus, DPI gives insights into the structural changes taking place in molecular systems as they function and interact (23, 24). In the future, it is a very promising technology that could answer some of the necessary questions.

The necessity of target immobilization for many of the above mentioned technologies (SPR, RWG, BLI and also DPI,) can significantly limit their application. In response to this conundrum, free solution, label-free molecular interactions were recently investigated with back-scattering interferometry (BSI) in an optical train composed of a helium–neon laser, a microfluidic channel, and a position sensor in a miniaturized format (25). Molecular binding interactions between proteins as well as small molecules and protein could be monitored without labeling or immobilizing any of the interaction partners.

Technologies like these will certainly augment the available biophysics toolkit to strengthen its application in lead discovery. It is apparent that biophysics is rapidly developing and its technology field is becoming broader. Thus, in the early lead discovery phases, the support of novel technologies and applications in biophysics to aid in understanding better the mechanisms of activity for low molecular weight drug candidates is expected.

REFERENCES

1. R. Macarron, *Drug Discov. Today* **11**, 277 (2006).
2. M.A. Cooper, *Anal Bioanal Chem.* **377**, 834–842 (2003).
3. A. K. Shiau, M. E. Massari, and C. C. Ozbal, *Combinatorial Chemistry & High Throughput Screening* **11** (3), 231–237 (2008).
4. B. T. Cunningham and L. G Laing, *Expert Opinion on Drug Discovery* **3** (8), 891–901 (2008).
5. R. A. Carr, M. Congreve, C. W. Murray, and D. C. Rees, *Drug Discov. Today* **10**, 987–992 (2005).
6. D. A. Erlanson, R. S. McDowell, and T. O'Brien, *J Med. Chem.* **47**, 3463–3482 (2004).
7. B. K. Shoichet, *Drug Discov. Today* **11**, 607–615 (2006).
8. M. Vedadi, F. H. Niesen, A. Allali-Hassani, *et al. PNAS*, **103** (43), 15835–15840 (2006).
9. G. A. Senisterra and P. J. Finerty, Jr., *Mol. BioSyst.* **5**, 217–223 (2009).
10. M. A. Cooper, *Nature Reviews Drug Discovery* **1** (7), 515–528 (2002).
11. R. L. Rich and D. G. Myszka, *Analytical Biochemistry* **361** (1), 1–6 (2007).
12. S. Löfas, *ASSAY and Drug Development Technologies* **2**, 4, 408–415 (2004).
13. D. G. Myszka and R. L. Rich, *PSTT* **3**, 9, 310–317 (2000).
14. H. Zehender and L. M. Mayr, *Current Opinion in Chemical Biology* **11** (5), 511–517 (2007).
15. A. L. Skinner and J. S. Laurence, *Journal of Pharmaceutical Sciences* **97** (11), 4670–4695 (2008).
16. J. Klages, M. Coles, and H. Kessler, *Analyst (Cambridge, UK)* **132** (7), 693–705 (2007).
17. U. Rester, *Current Opinion in Drug Discovery & Development* **11** (4), 559–568 (2008).
18. C. C. Ozbal, W. A. LaMarr, J. R. Linton, *et al. Assay Drug Dev. Technol.* **2**, 373 (2004).
19. T. P. Roddy, C. R. Horvath, S. J. Stout, *et al. Anal. Chem.*, **79**, 8207 (2007).
20. K.M. Comess, M.E. Schurdak, M.J. Voorbach, *et al. J Biomol Screen.* **11**, 743 (2006).
21. D. A. Annis, N. Nazef, C.-C. Chuang, *et al. J. Am. Chem. Soc.* **126**, 15495 (2004).
22. C. E. Whitehurst, N. Nazeef, D. E. Annis, *et al. J. Biomol. Screen.* **11**, 194 (2006).
23. G. Cross, A. Reeves, S. Brand, *et al. Biosen. Bioelectron.* **19**, 383 (2003).
24. M. Swann, L. Peel, S. Carrington, and N. Freeman, *Anal. Biochem.* **329**, 190 (2004).
25. D. J. Bornhop, J. C. Latham, A. Kussrow, *et al. Science* **317**, 1732 (2007).

12

Harnessing Optical Label-Free on Microtiter Plates for Lead Finding: From Binding to Phenotypes

Julio Martin

GlaxoSmithKline, Centro de Investigacion Basica, Tres Cantos, Spain

Label-Free Technologies for Drug Discovery   Edited by Matthew Cooper and Lorenz M. Mayr
© 2011 John Wiley & Sons, Ltd

12.1 INTRODUCTION

Now that the productivity of pharmaceutical Research and Development is under scrutiny and in question, all those involved are interrogating themselves about causes of failure and ways of improvement. In the context of early drug discovery, there are at least three points of intervention that may have hampered the success: (i) limited access to tractable therapeutic targets and exploitation of chemical-genomics; (ii) poor predictability of the therapeutic action of chemical compounds in biological assays; and (iii) inadequate selection of candidate molecules that fulfil the right biological and physicochemical profile of a drug.

12.1.1 What's Limiting the Development of Chemical-Genomics?

With the explosion of genomics in the 1990s, it was expected that an abundant supply of new targets that might serve as candidates for pharmaceutical intervention and be used in high throughput drug screening assays would be generated. Currently, marketed drugs are directed against some 500 therapeutic targets, leaving the prospect that about 90% of all drug targets remain to be exploited. An estimation following the genome sequencing points out that only 20% of gene products are known, and 40% of human genes have molecular function unknown (1). Conceptually, the conventional approach includes the following sequence of events: precise definition of a few selected targets, formal biological validation of a few of these, and drug screening against this subset performed *in vitro*. By contrast, the genomics-based approach, recently referred to as chemical-genomics (or chemogenomics or chemical proteomics), can be summarized as follows: genome-wide definition of many targets, high throughput drug screening for most of them, and complete biological validation of a few targets using compounds found formerly. In a broader sense, chemical-genomics can also be extended to the study of the genomic or proteomic response of whole cells or organisms to novel chemical compounds. One of the obvious advantages of the chemical-genomics approach is the fact that many more protein structures can be used to challenge libraries of compounds, further increasing the probability of finding relevant molecules. However, the chemical-genomics approach introduces a new difficulty: the rapid definition of automated drug screening assays for such large numbers of proteins.

Targets of almost all drugs on the market today are the proteins produced by genes. In their drug discovery programs, pharma-certified companies generally screen large numbers of compounds to determine if they modulate the function of the target protein. Therefore, this approach requires that the function of the protein is understood and can be experimentally assayed, which, in some cases, represents a significant roadblock to exploit a potentially relevant target. Protein targets can be classified into classes according to their function, and hence generic screening methodologies can be developed for each class. Even so, specific probes, reagents and engineered cells have to be designed and produced on an *ad hoc* basis. In the end, assay development may demand excessive allocation of resources (i.e., time, money, and people) prior to and at risk of not knowing the actual tractability of the target.

But the question still remains: how to exploit those genes and their proteins that have therapeutic potential as drug targets, and whose specific function has not been identified or cannot be measured? Or, in other words: how can we go from gene or target to screen bypassing the function as an obligatory preliminary step in the screening process?

The universal principle of the action of drugs is the binding to their target.

"Corpora non agunt nisi fixate" *("A drug will not work unless it is bound")*
—Paul Ehrlich (1854–1915)

So one solution resides in screening methodologies that can directly determine the binding of a compound to a given protein, which is a highly predictive feature of a relevant biological interaction.

12.1.2 Why are Biological Assays of the Therapeutic Relevance of a Compound Not Equally Predictable?

Some screening assays may not be predictable of compound activity in a more disease-relevant scenario. Current detection systems used in screening and early drug discovery are predominantly based on physicochemical principles that are not generally intrinsic to the nature of the biological system tested. Extrinsic labels and artificial biology (e.g., overexpression of proteins, chimeras, artificial coupling of signaling and reporting systems) have to be engineered in order to probe the activity of the target. As a result, assay development will be hampered in many cases, and always complicated. The biological texture of the target is altered more or less significantly, and no longer resembles all features of a native environment. The outcome of the assays may thus be misinterpreted and mislead the judgment on the biological relevance of an effect caused by a particular compound.

> *"The prismatic qualities of the assay distort our view in obscure ways and degrees"*
>
> —(James W. Black)

No matter how complex an assay can be designed, it will always be a reductionist approach by nature. The argument around the biological, physiological or therapeutic relevance of a particular assay is a quite common argument of discussion in the day-to-day activities of a lead discovery team. Relevance should better be linked to predictability, rather than to complexity of performance. As aforementioned, binding of the drug to the target is a simple but primary and relevant event to the therapeutic action. Likewise, testing the activity of compounds in primary or native living cells that have not been manipulated and only express endogenous receptors naturally coupled *a priori* will be a more relevant surrogate of the disease environment. Moreover, measuring these responses in real time and nondestructively will be priceless to drug discovery.

12.1.3 Compounds Hitting an Assay are not Always Genuine and Tractable Hits of the Target

All assays are prone to interference that can mislead decisions on the triage of compounds. Setting aside nuisance compounds interfering with the assay detection system, there are mechanisms for promiscuity that are general; for instance, compounds that nonspecifically bind to protein matrixes or form macromolecular aggregates that can seclude target proteins. The early identification and flagging out of such compounds alleviates future attrition rate, waste of resources and false expectations. Label-free assays can be exploited as an orthogonal approach to confirm genuine responses of compounds, particularly for those primary screens which (a) are very cheap to run, (b) have low false negative rate, and (c) have a significant rate of false positives.

Plate-based label-free biosensors coupled to optical detection are compatible with current screening technologies and infrastructure. They constitute a versatile platform that can accommodate a broad range of applications and fit within drug discovery research in order to fill the gaps described above. This chapter describes the basic principles of this technology, the state of the art for applications in early drug discovery, as well as some of the challenges that will have to be faced.

12.2 VALUE PROPOSITION AND ADVANTAGES OF LABEL-FREE METHODOLOGIES

Since the first introduction of Surface Plasmon Resonance (SPR) sensors in the early 1990s, a variety of different label-free methodologies have been developed and adapted for use in basic research (2, 3). Nevertheless, and in contrast with the large variety of labeled methods, there are still relatively few methods that allow detection of molecular and cellular interactions without labels. Amongst the main advantages of label-free detection, it is worth highlighting:

- Biological relevance of native systems: label-free removes the experimental uncertainty stemming from the effect of introducing an exogenous label on the specimen of study (e.g., engineered cells that overexpress receptors, chimeras or artificial pathways, conformational restrictions, steric hindrance in ligands and proteins, etc.). Thus, there is a closer resemblance to native ligands, substrates, proteins and cells.
- Systematic and generic approach to assay development and screening: this may be translated into faster turnaround times, less demand of resources, lower cost, and higher tractability of reluctant targets.

- Nondestructive and direct monitoring: the events occurring on the species of interest are studied in real time without further alteration of their properties. On- and off-kinetics and receptor desensitization can be measured. There is the prospect of re-usage of cells and proteins in sequential experiments.

The sensitivity, specificity and throughput of a biosensor system will determine its usefulness. Biosensors embedded in a flow chamber are constrained by the limit for parallel flow and time to re-establish initial conditions after each experiment. In contrast, systems based on simple and disposable assay vessels (such as microtiter well plates) can provide an unsurpassed processing capacity. Nowadays, there are at least two distinct technology platforms compatible with assays running in microtiter well plates and high throughput mode. They essentially differ in the biophysical principle of detection, namely electrical impedance or index of refraction. The fundamental advantage of the latter is that a direct electrical connection between the excitation source, the detection transducer, and the transducer surface (i.e., the sensor) is not required. Consequently, design and fabrication of sensors exposed to liquid samples becomes advantageously simplified and versatile. Moreover, optical biosensors and corresponding detectors can be designed to allow the measure of images with resolution of a few microns (e.g., an area as small as $1\,cm^2$ can be used to perform several hundred parallel determinations). In all, the main advantages of optical label-free platforms based on refractive index changes over electrical impedance platforms are:

- Versatility of biological applications: from direct binding of low molecular weight compounds to phenotypic cellular assays
- Miniaturization: lower costs of sensor, reduced consumption of reagents and higher throughput.
  - Design and fabrication of sensor surface and detection is insensitive to assay density and array format.
  - Inexpensive plastic material. One time use before disposal.
- Resolution.
  - Prospect of measuring species spotted on locations separated by only a few microns.
  - Individual cells can be monitored, instead of average detection of confluent cells.

In summary, optical biosensors on microplates fulfill most, if not all, of the requirements for its adoption as a label-free, any target drug discovery platform:

- amenable to high throughput, that is able to rapidly, robustly, and inexpensively assess hundreds or thousands of compounds in a single independent experiment;
- sensitive to detect binding of small molecular weight compounds (200–600 Da), formation of macromolecular complexes, and phenotypic changes in cells;
- not based on specific probes and labeling;
- not based on the function of the target;
- amenable to massive and parallel assay development.

12.3 DETECTION PRINCIPLE OF AN OPTICAL LABEL-FREE RESONANT GRATING SENSOR

Rather than detecting mass directly, all optical biosensors rely on the dielectric permittivity of detected substances to produce a measurable signal that correlates with the index of refraction. By far, surface plasmon resonance (SPR) has been the most widely adopted optical label-free methodology in basic research. Despite the fact that surface plasmon resonance has been used in high density sample arrays avoiding flow chambers and microfluidics, it has not been exploited as a high throughput platform in microtiter plates. Recently, biolayer interferometry, another optical label-free technology, has been developed for detecting biomolecular interactions (e.g., binding of small compounds to proteins) in 96-well sample plates (4). However, no cellular applications have been described yet.

In 2001, a novel class of optical biosensor was introduced ready for use in drug discovery applications, with the first commercial product being launched in 2004 (5). These sensors exploit the unique properties of optical devices known as "photonic crystals", which are structures incorporating at least two different dielectric materials with a periodically repeating structure. In this technology, a nanostructured subwavelength optical grating is used as the binding surface. This novel kind of surface hologram reflects only one single infrared color when illuminated with white or broadband light. The nature of the physical phenomenon taking

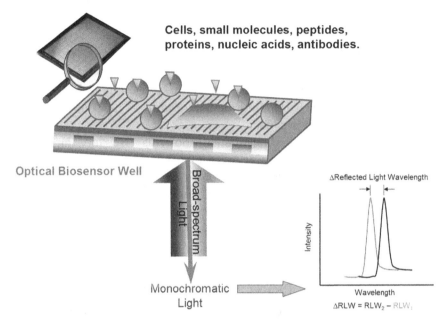

Figure 12.1   Signal Generation on an Optical Resonance Grating Biosensor. The figure depicts the detection principle of these optical biosensors. The biosensor is incorporated into standard microplate formats, i.e. 96-, 384- and 1536-well formats, for drug discovery applications. The Reflected Light Wavelength (RLW) varies depending on the local index of refraction of material bound at the sensor surface. The magnitude of RLW red shift is proportional to the mass increase of material bound to, or within about, 150 nm of the sensor surface. The biosensor provides very sensitive measurements of changes in binding or adherence of cells or proteins in response to ligand additions in the proximity of the biosensor surface. Reprinted with permission from Russell Publishing. Copyright 2008.

place when light enters and interacts with the sensor may differ from one sensor to another depending upon the peculiar properties of each grating and mode of illumination. At least two different mechanisms have been described in the literature, that is, Guided Mode Resonance (a total reflection at a single wavelength based on the energy field created at the site of binding) and Waveguide Resonance (a waveguide traveling through the grating before reflecting back at a single wavelength).

From the user's standpoint, regardless of what the intimate mechanisms of interaction between light and subwavelength grating are, the detection principle is identical: illumination with broadband light and reflection of monochromatic light whose wavelength is characteristic of the index of refraction in the sample of analysis (Figure 12.1). The optical biosensors provide very sensitive measurements of changes in binding or adherence of cells or proteins in response to ligand additions in the proximity of the biosensor surface. When compounds or biological material (e.g., DNA, protein, peptides, antibodies, cells, viruses, etc.) are attached to the surface, the reflected wavelength (i.e., color) is shifted to the red due to change of the optical path of light that is coupled into the grating. This shift of wavelength is a measure of the change in the refractive index occurring in the proximities of the sensor (about 150–200 nm). Strikingly, there is a directly proportional relationship between wavelength shift and increase of mass over a large dynamic range. This feature allows quantification of net increase of mass as a result of a direct binding event, hence estimation of stoichiometry. Sensitivity is determined by the pairing formed by the sensor and the detecting light spectrometer. The current platforms are able to detect mass changes in the range of a few picograms per mm^2, which corresponds to a limit of detection around one picometer wavelength shift. Detection devices have been developed that can either average the area of individual wells in the plate or scan each sample to obtain images at low microns resolution, the latter thus offering an unrestricted reading array to obtain images of mass distribution (6). This kind of sensor hologram can be inexpensively mass produced from plastic using an embossing process, and can be incorporated into standard microtiter plate formats (i.e., 96-, 384- and 1536-well) or microarray slides, so high throughput screening assays can be performed using conventional liquid handling and robotics for automated operations.

One important component of the sensor is the chemical nature of the surface on which the specimen is bound or adhered. The range of sensor plates described so far in the literature and commercially available is broad and allows a variety of common biological applications to be covered, such as imines chemistry for attachment of proteins through lysines, streptavidin coating for the capture of biotinylated proteins or ligands, polycationic surfaces or extracellular matrix proteins (i.e., fibronectin, collagen, etc.) for the adherence of cells.

12.4 BIOLOGICAL APPLICATIONS OF OPTICAL LABEL-FREE IN LEAD DISCOVERY

Optical label-free based on resonant grating sensors is still an incipient platform. Nevertheless, and because of its universal principle of detection and amenability to high throughput, it has already been explored as a general purpose methodology to facilitate a broad range of assays in drug discovery.

12.4.1 Direct Binding of Compound Libraries to Protein Targets

HTS (High throughput screening), compound profiling or hit validation
Optical label-free is challenged as a high throughput and cost effective alternative to experimentation on compound binding carried out by SPR. Three main factors control the magnitude of the response for a given compound–protein–sensor system: binding thermodynamics (i.e., K_D, k_{on}, k_{off}, ligand concentration, stoichiometry, molecular weight), protein loading (i.e., coating capacity of the sensor, binding sites available, conformational homogeneity, protein functionality) and sensor sensitivity (i.e., limit of detection, dynamic range). Current sensors have demonstrated ability to detect binding of compounds as small as 200 Da to proteins of about 30 kDa or a compound of 350 Da binding to a protein as large as 130 kDa (Figure 12.2a). In principle, larger proteins will expose less binding sites per sensor area unit than a smaller protein. The magnitude of the signals is usually small, thus controlling experimental noise on refractive index is critical. Special attention has to be paid to DMSO mismatches from compound libraries, temperature shifts produced by air draughts, bulk effects caused by volume addition, and mixture of buffers with different salt concentrations.

One important caveat in optical label-free is the signal coming from chemical compounds in the absence of any target protein. Compounds with avidity to the sensor chemical matrix or colloidal and aggregating compounds can be detected. Users should have heightened awareness to these compound behaviors and their most appropriate interpretations. Examination of stoichiometry, time course, concentration response curves, use of reference surfaces, and competition experiments will help the users to tell apart genuine specific binding and signals owing to the intrinsic physicochemical properties of a problematic compound in aqueous solution. The detection of their absorbent behavior can also be used to advantage. Some compounds form small aggregates that can generically interact with proteins or other components of a screening assay, appearing as promiscuous or frequent hits (7). Optical label-free has the prospect to identify these behaviors and assist the triage of effective hits.

Grating-based sensors in microtiter plates have been efficiently used for fragment-based screening, screening of focused libraries and HTS of

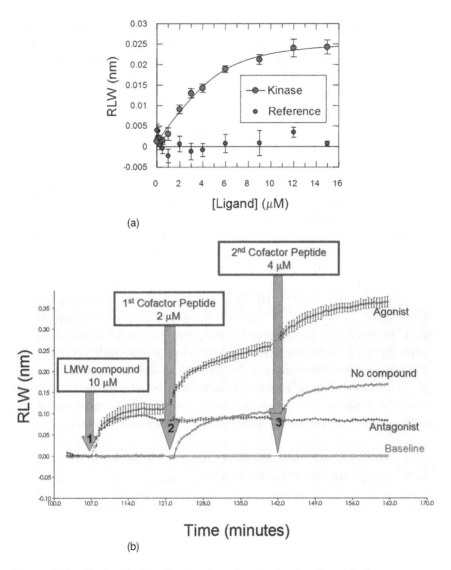

Figure 12.2 Biochemical applications based on monitoring direct binding to a target biomolecule immobilised on the sensor. (a) A low molecular weight compound (365 Da) is bound to its specific kinase target (130 000 Da) (upper curve), but not to a reference surface of bare sensor (lower line); the curve is fitted to a single site equilibrium binding equation with 1:1 stoichiometry. (b) Sensor coated with a nuclear receptor (25 000 Da) is challenged with either an agonist or an antagonist ligand (MW <400 Da) (arrow 1); the ability of the nuclear receptor to recruit a co-activating peptide (3000 Da) turns out to be enhanced by the agonist but abrogated by the antagonist (arrows 2 and 3). Reprinted with permission from Russell Publishing. Copyright 2008.

diversity libraries (8, 9). Despite using a static liquid vessel, K_D, k_{on} and k_{off} rates, as well as binding stoichiometry, have been determined, hence proving to be a valuable tool not only for hit identification, but also for validation and profiling of hits.

12.4.2 Functional Biochemical Assays

Multicomponent complex enzymes (e.g. proteases, kinases)
Biochemical assays have been configured looking at: (a) the ability of a target protein to recruit other biomolecules to form a functional multicomponent complex (e.g., DNA-interacting protein with oligonucleotides, protein ligand with its protein receptor, co-activating peptide with its nuclear receptor, etc.) (9, 10); and (b) the enzyme activity of a target on an immobilized substrate (e.g., protease cleaving its substrate, kinase phosphorylating a substrate that is subsequently recognized by a specific antibody, etc.) (11). The fact that the detection is not destructive allows assay multiplexing. Figure 12.2b illustrates a case in which the direct binding of a compound to a nuclear receptor and its effect on a recruitment assay are sequentially monitored in the same well. Screening of antibodies can be efficiently run following a similar sequential strategy. Titer of antibody can be estimated from the amount captured by a matrix of a secondary antibody and antibody affinity from the subsequent binding to the corresponding antigen on the same assay well.

12.4.3 Cellular Phenotypic Assays

GPCRs (G-protein coupled receptors), RTKs (receptor tyrosine kinases), ion channels, and so on
The applications above described are based on the measurement of wavelength shift responses as a result of a net increase of mass in the immediacies of the sensor. Cells can also be attached to the surface of the sensor and produce a concomitant change of local refraction index that is also measurable. Optical refraction label-free has emerged as a practical alternative to electrical impedance for cell-based assays (12, 13, 14). Notably, cells need to establish an intimate contact and adherence with the sensor in order to be detected. Suspension cells that merely settle down on the sensor surface may not give a response, possibly because the aqueous layer is not excluded within the 100–200 nm detectable distance. Cell duplication, cell growth, cell motility, cell differentiation, and

cell detachment are events taking place within this distance, thus prone to be monitored as a sheer net mass change. However, recruitment of cells, viruses, bacteria, and large protein complexes may occur far from this distance and remain somewhat invisible. Likewise, it should be expected that the cell layer deployed on the sensor does not contain enough protein receptor molecules exposed per sensor area unit to allow efficacious detection of direct binding of small compounds and ligands. Yet, resonant grating sensors have proven to be able to detect changes in the attached cells in response to this kind of external stimuli. How is this possible? The precise molecular mechanisms involved in the transduction of the biological cell response into an optical sensor signal remain to be unveiled. Cytoskeleton rearrangement is a common biological response downstream of many receptor signaling pathways and has been proposed as a possible end-point for impedance label-free detection. Change in adhesion properties of a cell to its matrix could also be hypothesized. Overall vectorial redistribution of mass within the cells as a consequence of protein trafficking has been proposed as the ultimate phenotypic change observable. Mathematical models have been developed for this vertical or horizontal dynamic redistribution of mass in order to explain the distinct temporal signatures observed upon receptor activation (15). In addition to cytoskeleton rearrangement and recruitment of cells, microorganism and proteins, other cellular events that can induce mass redistribution are endocytosis, receptor internalization, exocytosis, apoptosis, cellular communication, and ligand-driven activation of cellular receptors (e.g., G-protein coupled receptors, receptor tyrosine receptors, nuclear receptor) and ion channels. Therefore, there is a plethora of potential cellular applications.

GPCRs constitute the most abundant target class for current drug therapeutics and still attract a significant part of the drug discovery efforts in the pharmaceutical industry. Both native cells expressing endogenous GPCRs and cells overexpressing one particular receptor have been monitored by optical grating sensors in response to stimuli by specific ligands. RTKs and ion channels have also been shown as amenable to this technology. Strikingly, distinct temporal fingerprints are exhibited that seem to be characteristic of the particular receptor coupling pathways triggered by each ligand on a determined cellular background. In particular, Figure 12.3 illustrates examples of the kinetic profile observed in HEK MSRII (human embryonic kidney cells stably expressing the macrophage scavenger receptor class II) cells upon selective activation of each G-protein coupling signaling mechanism. Other different cellular backgrounds may exhibit a different kinetic profile for the

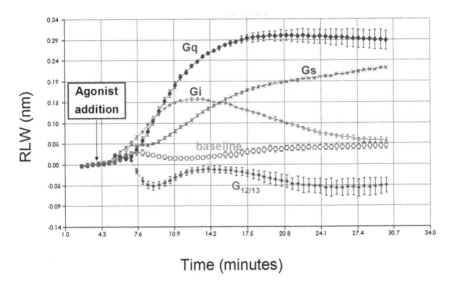

Time (minutes)

Figure 12.3 Kinetic profile of cells in response to selective activation of endogenous G-protein coupled receptors (GPCRs). HEK MSRII cells expressing endogenous receptors are challenged with a series of agonists exhibiting functional selectivity for G-protein coupling pathways. Reprinted with permission from Russell Publishing. Copyright 2008.

same G-protein coupling mechanism. Although each particular GPCR usually posseses a preference for one G-protein coupling type, it is not uncommon that one GPCR can activate more than one pathway depending upon the agonist molecule and the cell type. This phenomenon has been named as agonist trafficking, ligand-biased agonism or functional selectivity (16). Optical label-free allows the possibility of studying agonist trafficking in any cellular background, including native primary cells, without additional experimental complications other than cell handling. The key is having a strategy and tools to deconvolute the combination of signatures (e.g., gene knock-outs, knocking down receptors or pathways with siRNA, specific antagonists and agonists, selective pathway blockages, etc.). Deciphering the signature encrypted in a temporal response may be the Rosetta stone of cellular label-free.

Taking advantage of the nondestructive nature of this technology, valuable primary cell lines derived from rat brain have been subjected to sequential challenges of GPCR ligands with negligible alteration of the magnitude and profile of the response. In the context of maximizing the usage of precious cells, a high performance reader may employ less than one thousand cells per well. Moreover, a scanner with high spatial resolution can monitor responses from individual cells.

The magnitude of the shift of the reflected light wavelength for cellular responses is usually far above the limit of detection. The optimization of the experimental design is focused on sensor coating (e.g., use of proteins from extracellular matrix or polycations, concentrations, coating time, etc.), cell health and handling (e.g., confluency, passages, seeding density and time, cell starvation, etc.) and compound addition (e.g., effect of DMSO on cell biology, dilution and mixing procedure, etc.). Grating sensors have been efficiently used for the identification of GPCRs agonists and antagonists by screening of compounds libraries of about 100 000 compounds.

12.5 CURRENT AND FUTURE CHALLENGES

Optical label-free in microtiter plates is still an incipient methodology awaiting a definitive and extensive adoption by the scientific community as a routine platform. Limited know-how has been spread out so far. As for any other technology, users should have heightened awareness to some technical tips and caveats that will need to be challenged.

- **Development of new alternative surface chemistries.** Proteins and cells need to be efficiently immobilized in an effective and healthy state or conformation that preserves the functionality of the biological species and reduces the usage of material. For instance, imine chemistry is random, thus heterogeneous, and cannot guarantee success for all proteins. Oriented attachment is desirable.
- **Fluidics and thermodynamics.** Systems where the target is not free in solution can be rate-limited by mass transport, rather than by on- and off-rates. In the absence of mixing, mass transport limitation may increase. For an accessible, low density surface with slow binding, kinetic constants can be measured without flow. In a static well, depletion of ligand occurs by binding to the target. Hence, the tight binding lower limit for K_D is much higher for plate systems than for flow systems. Off-line washing may not be required if a competing agent is used. The large volume of the well gives effective dissipation of displaced ligand, provided that the on-rate of the competing ligand is high.
- **Deciphering the signature of the cellular responses.** The lack of efficient strategies to deconvolute the complexity of the behavior of a

cell in response to a receptor ligand can hamper the tremendous potential of this technology. Biological (e.g., knocking down receptors or pathways with siRNA) and chemical (e.g., specific antagonists, agonists and pathway blockages) tools are required to ascertain the functional selectivity of the response and decipher its texture.

- **Logistics: cost, miniaturization and throughput.** Increasing the capacity to process a high number of samples in a cost and time effective manner will expand the applicability and utility.
- **Higher resolution and sensitivity of sensors** will allow the mass transport and crowding effect inherent to protein immobilization to be minimized. Likewise, it will mean a reduction in the usage of biological material.
- **Multiplexing.** One single compound preparation challenging different biological systems or reference surfaces in the same well means a more efficient and reliable procedure of ascertaining the specificity and selectivity of compound responses.
- **Robustness to unspecific and spurious signals,** for example, DMSO mismatches, temperature shifts, bulk effects, aggregating or insoluble compounds, unspecific binding to biological or sensor matrixes.
- **Unveiling the ultimate biological mechanism in the cells** that is producing the detectable signal.
- **Expand software and data management capabilities,** for example, analysis of raw data, correction of baselines, data export, robotics interfaces, clustering and recognition of kinetic profiles, and so on.

12.6 CONCLUSION

Plate-based label-free grating biosensors coupled to optical resonance detection constitute a versatile platform that can accommodate a broad range of applications: from formation of multicomponent biomolecular complexes to phenotypic alterations in native cells, from the detection of the interaction between small organic molecules and isolated proteins to the redistribution of mass within a cell upon activation of a particular receptor, from screening of compound libraries to hit validation or elucidation of the mode of action of lead compounds, from agonist trafficking to receptor panning. The drug discovery paradigm is shifting from magic bullets hitting single targets to the pharmacological exploitation of systems biology through the understanding of the biological complexity and deciphering drug pharmacology in a native texture. It is possible to envisage several places where to fit within drug discovery: fragment-based screening, novel hit identification strategies, hit validation, orthogonal readout, hit-to-lead, lead optimization support, and so on. Rather than replacing any of the existing technologies in use, it can enable, complement or simplify some of the methodological approaches currently available. Since it exploits a universal principle of detection (label-free, any target), it constitutes a valuable link between the direct label-free screening of any target for small compound binders and the understanding of the biological complexity in native cells. The amenability to classical HTS infrastructure in a cost effective manner opens the possibility of making complex assays accessible. Needless to say, not all that glitters is gold, and there exist technological challenges and uncertainties to address that might jeopardize the vast adoption of this incipient methodology by the community. In the forthcoming years it will be seen whether the hope was just hype or the promise is delivered.

REFERENCES

1. J.C. Venter, M.D. Adams, E.W. Myers, *et al.*, *Science* **291**, 1304 (2001).
2. J. Comley, *Drug Discovery World* **Winter 2004/5**, 63 (2004).
3. J. Comley, HTStec's Surveys: Binding and Cell-based Label-free Detection Trends (http://www.htstec.com/) (2008).
4. M.A. Cooper, *Drug Discovery Today* **11**, 1061 (2006).
5. B.T. Cunningham, P. Li, S. Schulz, *et al.*, *J. Biomol. Screen.* **9** (6), 481 (2004).
6. B.T. Cunningham and L. Laing., *Expert Reviews of Proteomics* **3** (3), 271 (2006).
7. S.L. McGovern, B.T. Helfand, B. Feng, and B.K. Shoichet, *J. Med. Chem.* **46**, 4265 (2003).
8. X. Xie, T. Bunch, and A.G. Frutos, LOPAC screen against trypsin using the Corning Epic system. *Poster at Society for Biomolecular Sciences (SBS) Conference* (2007).
9. L. Laing, P. Lowe, J. Gerstenmaier, *et al.*, SRU BIND microplate biosensor applied to screening and characterization of small molecule ligands to multiple proteins. *Poster at Society for Biomolecular Sciences (SBS) Conference* (2006).
10. L.L. Chan, M. Pineda, J.T. Heeres, *et al. ACS Chemical Biology* **3** (7), 437 (2008).
11. M.O. Shawn, X. Xinyin, and A.G. Frutos, *J. Biomol. Screen.* **12**, 117 (2007).
12. L. Minor, *American Drug Discovery* **2**, 14–18 (2007).
13. P.H. Lee, A. Gao, C. van Staden, *et al.*, *Assay Drug. Dev. Technol.* **6** (1), 83 (2008).
14. L. Minor, *Comb. Chem. High Throughput Screen.* **11**, 573 (2008).
15. Y. Fang, A.M. Ferrie, N.H. Fontaine, *et al.*, *Biophys. J.* **91**, 1925 (2006).
16. T. Kenakin, *Mol. Pharmacol.* **72**, 1393 (2007).

13

Use of Label-Free Detection Technologies in the Hit-to-Lead Process: Surface Optical Detection of Cellular Processes

F. Stuhmeier, J. Bradley, E. Fairman, E. Gbekor, P. Hayter, and S. Ramsey
Pfizer Global Research and Development, Sandwich, UK

Label-Free Technologies for Drug Discovery   Edited by Matthew Cooper and Lorenz M. Mayr
© 2011 John Wiley & Sons, Ltd

13.1 INTRODUCTION

The hit-to-lead optimization process is dominated by the use of highly purified enzymes and proteins and genetically engineered cell lines in homogeneous (no wash) plate-based assay formats. Most assays fall into two main categories: either binding or functional assays. Binding assays measure the binding of a compound to the biological target of interest, often through the displacement of a (labeled) high affinity ligand that is bound to the target. Functional assays measure the impact of the binding event on the functional activity of the target; they are often more complex than binding assays and depend on the use of antibodies, coupled enzyme reactions or ion sensing dyes to indirectly measure functional downstream effects of the initial binding event. The majority of binding and function-based assays depend on the use of fluorescent, luminescent or radioactive labels to generate a measurable signal.

Label-free assays for plate-based screening have several advantages over more established assay methods. The advantages for targets that are not embedded into a membrane, mainly enzymes, are well known, as methods like Surface Plasmon Resonance (SPR) have been in use for more than 15 years (1, 2). SPR measurements are unique as they enable a more or less direct measurement of the kinetics of the binding event; consequently, they are frequently used to determine the on- and the off-rates of enzyme inhibitors during the SAR (Structure–Activity Relationship) optimization process. SPR is also frequently used in the field of fragment screening against enzyme and protein targets, either as a primary screen or as a follow-up counter screen (3).

Label-free methods have also revolutionized the field of ion channel primary screening and SAR generation. For example, the availability of plate-based electrophysiology platforms enables direct functional characterization of hundreds of ion channel modulators per week. The resulting data do not only contain a wealth of detailed mechanistic information, they are also of superior quality when compared to other ion channel screening methods (4).

The use of label-free platforms based on optical or non-optical biosensors for the screening of cellular targets in recombinant and nonrecombinant cell lines is the latest development in the field of label-free screening. Several medium throughput capable platforms, based either on impedance or on surface optical technology, are now commercially available. A common feature of these platforms is that they measure what can best be described as an overall response of the cell to a stimulus, consisting of morphological changes, changes in the adhesion properties of the cell to the plate, and changes of the distribution of proteins in the cell and close to the cell membrane.

Label-free cell-based assays might have three potential advantages over conventional assays methodologies:

(i) Assay development, often considered a bottleneck in the early stage drug discovery process, might be easier and less time consuming, as the total number of assay relevant parameters is smaller for label-free cell-based assays than for conventional assays.

(ii) Label-free assays do not measure a specific event in the signal transduction cascade, but an overall cellular response to a stimulus. The data are information rich and can give insight into the specific nature of the signal transduction process. Therefore, it might be possible to use label-free assays to detect e.g. G-protein coupling multiplicity.

(iii) Label-free assays can be used with genetically unmodified cell lines and are therefore compatible with the use of primary cells in early-stage drug discovery.

Label-free assays for cellular targets, while currently not an integrated part of the modern drug discovery process, are actively being evaluated by most pharmaceutical companies. In this chapter, a brief overview of some of the label-free platforms that can be used for cellular assays is given firstly. Next, the outcome of a trial of the Corning Epic™ platform is summarized. Finally, the impact of label-free technologies on the screening of cellular targets is assessed.

13.2 OVERVIEW OF LABEL-FREE ASSAY PLATFORMS

The following is a brief review of bioimpedance and surface optical platforms, with the focus on medium throughput capable readers; medium throughput is defined operationally as sufficient throughput to allow the screening of at least 5000–15 000 data points per working day. This review only covers platforms that are also compatible with cell-based assays. Comprehensive overviews of the whole field of label-free screening (5–7) and of the use of plate-based electrophysiology in primary and secondary screening (8) are given elsewhere.

The electrical properties of cells have been investigated in great detail for more than 60 years (9), and several companies have developed and commercialized impedance-based instruments for a variety of biological applications. The basic principles of impedance measurements (10) are fairly similar for the different instruments. In the case of the CellKey[TM] system (MDS Analytical Technologies), electrodes are patterned at the bottom of a microplate, and cells are seeded as a monolayer on top of the electrodes. Then, an alternating voltage of a set frequency is applied to the cell and the resulting current is measured. This process is then repeated for a range of frequencies. At lower frequencies, the total current is dominated by current flow around and between the cells (extracellular current), while the total current at higher frequencies results mainly from the current flow across the cell membrane (transcellular current). The measurements are performed before the addition of a ligand to acquire a baseline, and then repeated after ligand addition. The analysis of the raw data can be complex (11), but the key point is that the impedance (Z), defined as the ratio of voltage to current ($Z = V/I$) changes due to the stimulation of the cell through the binding of the ligand to a receptor.

The 384 version of the CellKey[TM] system is currently the only impedance system that can be used for higher throughput SAR generation in 384 format. MDS Analytical Technologies claims that the system is capable of processing up to eight plates per hour on the high through-put mode (five minutes read time) or four plates per hour in the assay development mode (15 minutes read time). The temperature controlled system has an integrated compound addition unit, and there is no time delay between compound addition and start of the measurement process. The CellKey[TM] is positioned as a tool for pharmacological studies and pathway classification. Impedance measurements are not limited to classical SAR support. The ECIS[TM] systems from Applied BioPhysics – an early pioneer in the field of impedance measurements, with a very strong focus on academic applications – is positioned to support, among others, studies in toxicology (12), wound healing (13) and cell attachment (14), applications that are also supported by the xCELLigence[TM] system from Roche Applied Sciences and ACEA Biosciences.

The market for plate-based optical screening platforms is currently dominated by SRU Biosystems and Corning. The SRU Biosystems Bind reader is a small footprint stand-alone instrument based on photonic crystal sensor technology (15). The proprietary sensor, which is incorporated into the bottom of disposable 96-, 384- or 1536-well standard microplates, is illuminated from the bottom with white light. The sensor reflects energy within a narrow optical bandwidth, the wavelength being dependent on the index of refraction of the material in very close proximity (150 nm) to the surface of the sensor. The wavelength of the reflected light is altered by a small, but measurable amount by anything that binds to the surface, whether a cell, a small molecule or a protein. The effect is large enough to allow the quantification of cellular changes after the addition of an agonist ligand, and can also be used to measure the binding of compounds to proteins that are immobilized on the sensor. The SRU Biosystems Bind reader can be operated such that there is only a minimal time lag between the addition of a reagent to the plate and the start of the measurement, and the assay plate is freely accessible during the whole measurement process.

The Corning Epic™ reader is technically similar to the SRU Biosystems Bind™ reader, as the physics behind the measurement process is similar. There are, however, some differences: the reader unit in the Corning Epic system is temperature controlled at exactly 26 °C – the Bind™ reader is operated at ambient temperature – and also contains a stacker with a capacity of up to 20 plates. The Epic™ system can also be purchased with an integrated liquid handling system for the addition of compounds, making it amenable to medium throughput screens without the need of integrating it into a robotic screening platform. The Epic™ assay plate is not freely accessible during the data acquisition process, and there is a time lag of at least 45 seconds between addition of compounds to the plate and the start of the data acquisition process. This chapter is based on our results with the Epic™ system, some of our comments are influenced by our experience with the Bind™ reader.

13.3 SURFACE OPTICAL DETECTION OF CELLULAR PROCESSES

13.3.1 Experimental Details

Experiments were performed on the Corning Epic™ using Corning Epic™ 384 microplates in kinetic mode (acquisition of whole signal traces after compound addition for up to two hours). The instrument was temperature controlled at 26 °C and consisted of the reader and an integrated stacker carousel system; compounds were added externally using a CyBi™-Well 384 channel pipettor, as the Corning Epic™ system with the integrated liquid handling system was not available for the trial.

Briefly, freshly harvested or cryopreserved cells were plated in growth media in fibronectin coated 384 assay plates. Plates were stored overnight in a 37 °C incubator to allow adherence of the cells. The following morning, growth medium was exchanged with serum-free assay buffer, and cells were allowed to equilibrate in the instrument at 26 °C for about two hours. Next, a baseline measurement was performed, followed immediately by addition of compounds (antagonists). Plates were read for up to 60 minutes to detect any effect of the compounds on the cells, and to allow pre-incubation of the compounds with the receptor. Agonist was added after a second baseline measurement, and data were acquired for up to two hours (kinetic mode). The baseline is performed on each individual well, and the data (wavelength shift in pm) are referenced to the baseline measurement; it takes about two minutes to read a 384-well plate. The instrument can be operated in nonkinetic mode by reading a plate only once at a defined time after compound addition, thereby increasing the total throughput of the reader, but losing the information content in the traces. The cycle time of the Epic, defined as the time to load a plate, perform a baseline read, unload the plate, reload the plate after compound addition, perform the measurement and finally unloading the plate, is about five minutes, leading to a nominal throughput of about 40 000 wells in about eight hours operation.

The main factors influencing assay noise and window are the cell density, the serum concentration during the seeding period, and the equilibration time directly prior to the start of the data acquisition. Typical cell densities for 384-well plates are in the range of 10 000–15 000 cells per well at around 80% cell confluence, with typical equilibration times of at least 120 minutes before compound addition. Assay noise levels are also heavily influenced by the quality of the liquid handling set-up used to transfer the cells and the compounds into the assay plates, as the Corning Epic^{TM} measures a change in the index of refraction directly at the interface between the cells and the sensor. An assay window of approximately 150 pm wavelength shift is, in our experience, sufficient to set up a robust single point cell-based assay that meets standard quality requirements.

The assay quality is influenced by every factor that causes a change in the index of refraction of the assay solvent, or a change in the properties of the cells. Key factors to consider are (i) the concentration of DMSO, (ii) the composition of the buffer, and (iii) the temperature. (i) DMSO is known to have specific as well as nonspecific effects on cells. The effects are cell line dependent, and may impact cell viability, assay window, and the pharmacological response profile of the cell; cells can typically tolerate DMSO concentration of up to 0.50–0.75%. A mismatch between the DMSO concentration of the compound buffer and the concentration of the serum-free assay buffer can cause a sharp spike in the wavelength shift signal; the spike typically occurs directly after compound addition and is fairly short lived (up to 10 minutes), but might interfere with the interpretation of the change of the signal pattern after compound addition. Even a small mismatch of 0.1% can lead to a positive wavelength shift of up to 50 pm or more. (ii) It is recommended to use exactly the same buffer stock solutions for the solubilization of compounds and the preparation of the serum-free assays buffer, as small buffer mismatches can have an impact on the signal quality, typically leading to difficult to interpret changes and irreproducible results. (iii) Temperature fluctuations in the laboratory should be avoided; this is not so much an issue for the temperature controlled Corning Epic^{TM} system, but should be taken into account for the SRU Bind^{TM} system, which is not temperature controlled.

13.3.2 Results from Recombinant Cellular Assays

The purpose of the study was to evaluate the use of the Corning Epic^{TM} platform for SAR generation, identification of signal transduction pathways and primary screening, and to understand whether the technology is robust and mature enough to be operated by non-expert users in a screening environment. Several recombinant Gi-, Gs- and Gq-coupled GPCR cell lines were characterized with their endogenous agonist or related molecules; some of the cell lines were also characterized with a selection of antagonists. Resulting EC$_{50}$ values were compared with in-house data from functional assays. An extensive side-by-side comparison of the Epic with conventional assays was not performed, as this would have been outside the scope of this study.

The signal pattern for a Gs-coupled peptide hormone GPCR expressed in a CHO cell line is shown in Figure 13.1. This cell line also contained a cAMP-responsive β-lactamase reporter gene; the results from the β-lactamase assay were used for comparison. The observed pattern after GPCR stimulation with the endogenous agonist – an initial small decrease of the signal, followed by a continuous increase of the signal to up to 225 pm relative to the initial value at the time of the addition of the agonist – is in agreement with the pattern proposed by Fang et al. (16). The signal from unstimulated cells decreased by 45 pm relative to its initial value. The EC$_{50}$ values were determined for a range of chemically diverse agonists and compared to the EC$_{50}$ values previously determined with a β-lactamase reporter assay. The EC$_{50}$ values were time dependent,

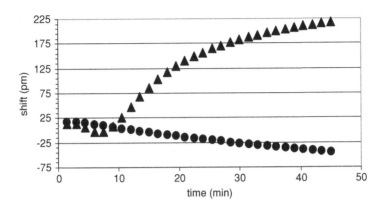

Figure 13.1 Time evolution of the wavelength shift for a Gs coupled peptide hormone GPCR. The stimulation of the receptor with a saturating concentration of the endogenous agonist causes a positive signal shift of approximately 220 pm 45 minutes after stimulation (triangles); the baseline (DMSO batched buffer without agonist) drifts by approximately 40 pm (circles). Values are the average of 40 wells each for the positive control (agonist wells) and the negative control (DMSO matched buffer wells) and were used to calculate the values in Figure 13.4.

making it imperative to study the time evolution of the signal during the assay development process (Figure 13.2). The correlation of the EC_{50} values from the Epic system, measured 45 minutes after compound addition, with the values determined in the β-lactamase assay is shown in Figure 13.3: 11 out of 25 compounds agreed within threefold and

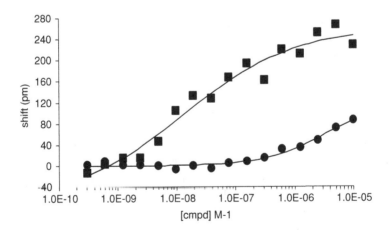

Figure 13.2 Representative agonist dose–response curves of the aforementioned Gs coupled peptide hormone GPCR, acquired 10 minutes (circles) and 45 minutes (squares) after compound addition to the cells. The EC_{50} value was time dependent and shifted from approximately 3 μM after 10 minutes to approximately 13 nM after 45 minutes.

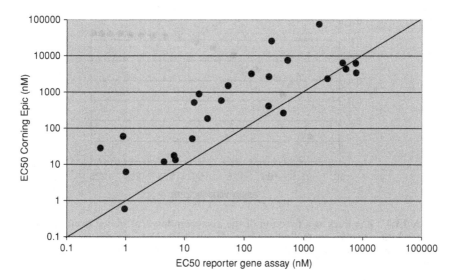

Figure 13.3 EC_{50} values from the Epic system (measured 45 minutes after compound addition) vs. EC_{50} values from a β-lactamase reporter assay (all values in nM). Overall correlation was acceptable: 11 out of 25 agreed within threefold and four out of 25 compounds within tenfold of previously determined values. The values for ten out of 25 compounds differed by more than tenfold.

four out of 25 compounds within tenfold of previously determined EC_{50} values. The values for ten out of 25 compounds differed by more than tenfold. The differences between the EC_{50} values were most likely related to the poor solubility of some of the compounds, or due to differences in the compound pre-incubation time in the different assays formats (four hours in the case of the β-lactamase assay). The assay was robust enough to enable single point screening, as an assay window of about 100–150-pm (Figure 13.4) is generally sufficient to set up a single point screen that passes standard quality requirements.

The signal pattern for Gq-coupled receptors, again a peptide hormone receptor in a β-lactamase CHO cell line, is shown in Figure 13.5. The pattern is qualitatively different from the Gs pattern: the signal increases significantly immediately after agonist addition, reaches a peak after less than ten minutes, and decreases slowly after. The EC_{50} for the standard agonist used to stimulate the receptor does not change over time (data not shown), in contrast to the results from the Gs coupled receptor. The pattern is identical to the observations by Fang *et al.* (16).

Functional assays for Gi coupled GPCRs are often less robust than Gs and Gq assays, as the intracellular cAMP concentration has to be elevated artificially with forskolin to generate an assay window. The Epic

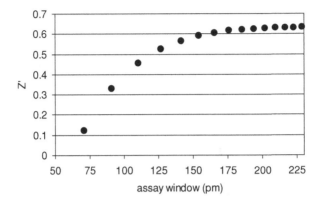

Figure 13.4 Z' values as a function of the assay window, calculated from the positive and the negative control values from Figure 13.1. Data are representative for all other GPCRs measured in this study: an assay window of about 100–150 pm is typically sufficient to set up a robust single point assay.

technology, on the other hand, allows the configuration of functional assays for Gi coupled GPCRs without the use of forskolin. The typical signal pattern for a Gi coupled GPCR is shown in Figure 13.6. The signal increases rapidly after agonist stimulation and continues to do so for an extended period; the pattern appears to be more complex and less continuous than the pattern for Gs and Gq coupled receptors,

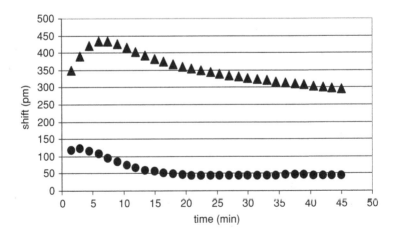

Figure 13.5 The signal pattern of a Gq coupled peptide hormone GPCR, acquired under similar conditions as the data in Figure 13.1. The signal peaked after about 10 minutes; the EC_{50} values were time independent (similar values whether they were measured after 10 minutes or 45 minutes).

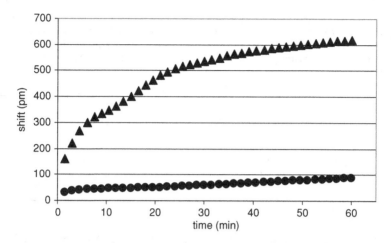

Figure 13.6 The signal pattern of a Gi coupled GPCR, acquired under similar conditions as the data in Figures 13.1 and 13.5; the EC_{50} values for various receptor selective agonist were again time independent.

and is again in good agreement with Fang *et al.* (16). Data quality was excellent, mainly due to the extremely large assay window of 500 pm; typical EC_{50} curves are shown in Figure 13.7. The EC_{50} values were time independent: we could not detect any shift in the values between five and 60 minutes after agonist addition. The EC_{50} values for a selection of

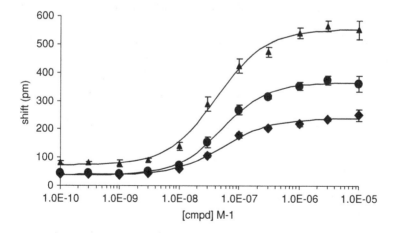

Figure 13.7 Representative agonist dose–response curves for the aforementioned Gi coupled receptor. Data were acquired five minutes (diamond), 15 minutes (circle) or 60 minutes (inverted triangles) after compound addition. The EC_{50} value of 50 nM was time independent.

Table 13.1 Comparison of EC_{50} values. The EC_{50} values from the Epic were in good agreement with the values from an AlphaScreen cAMP assay: six out of seven compounds were within twofold of previously established values, only one compound was significantly weaker in the Epic assay than in the AlphaScreen assay.

Compound	EC_{50} Epic (nM)	EC_{50} AlphaScreen (nM)
1	20	15
2	103	182
3	47	18
4	50	50
5	163	131
6	42	672
7	9	11

agonists were in agreement with the values from an AlphaScreen cAMP assay: six out of seven compounds were within twofold of previously established values, one compound, however, was significantly weaker in the Epic assay than in the AlphaScreen assays (Table 13.1). The assay protocols were quite similar, making it less likely that any differences were due to kinetic effects or poor aqueous solubility of the compounds.

We have not employed Epic™ in a large scale screening campaign, but experience with the system suggests that it would be compatible with medium or high throughput single point screening in nonkinetic mode. Two potentially complicating factors, however, have to be taken into account: (i) the time dependency of the signal and (ii) the requirement for a wash step. (i) The time dependency of the signal, and the need to acquire a well-specific baseline, make it necessary to schedule the compound addition and the data acquisition process: batch operation is possible only for small batch sizes, and only for targets with a favorable signal time dependency. (ii) The overall assay flow is not homogenous: it is possible to run in a homogenous mode (no exchange of growth media), but the data quality improves significantly by removing the growth media, and replacing it with serum free assay buffer for up to two hours before compound addition.

13.4 DISCUSSION

Label-free systems for cellular assays are not a part of the mainstream drug discovery process yet. We have decided to evaluate the different technologies in detail. In the following, we comment on the real and perceived advantages of optical label-free methods (Corning Epic™ and

SRU Biosystems Bind^{TM}) for the development and characterization of cell-based assays.

1. The assay development process for recombinant GPCR cell lines is, in our experience, simpler than the development of conventional assays. Key parameters to optimize for a given cell line are incubation and serum starvation times and the cell number. The data quality depends heavily on the quality of the liquid handling set-up that is used for the transfer of the cells and the compounds.

2. In total, 16 GPCR cell lines were evaluated on the Epic. The pharmacology was in general comparable to previously established values, the assay statistics were on average similar to FLIPR^{TM} type assays. Any significant differences in the pharmacological behavior of the compounds can be due to a variety of reasons, and would have to be investigated in much more detail. The quality for Gi coupled receptors was significantly higher than the quality of the corresponding conventional functional assays.

Our experience with (ligand-gated) ion channels is very limited; it is, however, unlikely that systems like the Epic^{TM} or the Bind^{TM} will be able to compete with the more specialized electrophysiology-based ion channel assay platforms for SAR generation, as these platforms provide a wealth of mechanistic high content information that is directly related to the molecular biophysics of the target of interest. We cannot comment of the use of platforms like the SRU Bind^{TM} or the Epic^{TM} for primary screening of ion channel targets.

3. Both the Corning Epic^{TM} and SRU Biosystems Bind^{TM} can be operated by non-expert users and are capable of achieving a throughput of about 40 000 data points per working day under optimal conditions. The total assay workflow is not homogeneous, making the systems less attractive from an HTS perspective for GPCR targets when compared to most homogeneous HTS compatible assay methods.

4. The Epic^{TM} can be used to identify different cellular signaling processes: the data patterns from recombinant cell lines overexpressing different GPCRs seem to be different for different G-protein coupling pathways, at least for the examples we have investigated. It is unlikely that these results can be generalized to all GPCRs and all cellular backgrounds: the cellular processes under investigation,

their kinetics and their cell line dependency are very complex, and the relationship between all these processes and the actual optical signal, which is heavily influenced by many factors and most likely related to overall morphological changes of the cell, changes in the cell adhesion properties, as well as changes in the mass redistribution in the bottom part of the cell (17), is not clearly established. Furthermore, there is clear indication, at least in the impedance literature, that impedance signal patterns can be difficult to interpret, therefore making it sometimes impossible to assign a specific pattern to a specific pathway (11). Not as many recombinant GPCRs were tested on the Bind^{TM} reader as on the Epic^{TM} reader; the Bind^{TM} reader was used mainly to investigate the use of surface optical technologies for primary cell assays. It was noticed, however, that the signal pattern for recombinant GPCR is somewhat different on the Bind^{TM} system when compared to the Epic^{TM}, most likely due to protocol differences or due to differences in the sensor surfaces. Both systems, the Epic^{TM} as well as the Bind^{TM}, are essentially phenotype assay systems and detect processes very much at the end of a signal transduction cascade, and can therefore be used to investigate pathways using pathway-specific probes and toxins.

5. The Bind^{TM} reader was used to perform an in-depth pharmacological characterization of a primary (smooth muscle) cell line (data not shown). The system performed very well, but the key in the use of primary cells in screening lies in the thorough characterization of the cells, using all tools available of modern molecular biology, and in the control of the growth conditions of the cells. The law of mass action does (of course) still apply for primary cells: a signal will not be seen if the expression level of the protein of interest is too low. Surface optical label-free systems are, nevertheless, potentially attractive tools for the development of assays for primary cells, if the instrument manufacturers provide designated low volume plates.

6. It is currently too early to say whether optical label-free systems will become mainstream for primary screening or SAR generation. These systems are attractive as additional tools for technically difficult target classes, and for the detailed mechanistic characterization of pharmacologically active substances in an orthogonal assay format. We can only speculate on the ability of label-free assays to detect compound classes of unknown mode of action, compounds that otherwise would have been missed in a conventional functional screen. To answer this question, it is necessary

to select several pharmacologically difficult targets, and to perform primary screens with tens or hundreds of thousands of compounds, followed by a detailed characterization of all the hits.

REFERENCES

1. R.L. Rich and D. M. Myszka, *Anal. Biochem.*, **361**, 1, (2006).
2. W. Huber, *J. Mol. Recognit.*, **18**, 273, (2005).
3. T. Neumann, H-D. Junker, K. Schmidt, and R. Sekul, *Curr. Top Med. Chem.*, **7**, 1630, (2007).
4. B.T. Priest, A.M. Swensen, and O.B. McManus, *Curr. Pharm. Des.*, **13**, 2325, (2007).
5. M. A. Cooper, *Nat. Rev. Drug Discov.*, **1**, 515, (2002).
6. M. A. Cooper, *Drug Disc. Today*, **11**, 1061, (2006).
7. M. A. Cooper, *Drug Disc. Today*, **11**, 1068, (2006).
8. J. Dunlop, M. Bowlby, R. Peri, *et al. Nat. Rev. Drug Discov.*, **7**, 358, (2008).
9. K. R. Foster and H. P. Schwan, *Crit. Rev. Biomed. Eng.*, **17**, 25, (1989).
10. R. McGuinness, *Curr. Opin. Pharmacol.*, **7**, 535, (2007).
11. G. J. Ciambrone, V. F. Liu, D. C. Lin, *et al. J. Biomol. Screen.*, **9**, 467, (2004).
12. C. Xiao and J. H. T. Luong, *Toxicol. Appl. Pharmacol.*, **206**, 102, (2005).
13. C. R. Keese, J. Wegener, S. R. Walker, and I. Giaever, *Proc. Natl. Acad. Sci. USA*, **101**, 1554, (2004).
14. C. Xiao, B. Lachance, G. Sunahara, and J. H. T. Luong, *Anal. Chem.*, **74**, 1333, (2002).
15. B. T. Cunningham and L. Lang, *Expert Rev. Proteomics*, **3**, 271, (2006).
16. Y. Fang, G. Li and A. M. Ferrie, *J. Pharmacol. Toxicol. Methods*, **55**, 314, (2007).
17. Y. Fang, A. M. Ferrie, N. H. Fontaine, *et al. Biophys. J.*, **91**, 1925, (2006).

14

Cellular Screening for 7TM Receptors Using Label-Free Detection

Jeffrey C. Jerman[1]*, Jason Brown[2], and
Magalie Rocheville[1]
[1]*Molecular Discovery Research*
[2]*Neurosciences Centre of Excellence in Drug Discovery,*
GlaxoSmithKline, Harlow, UK

Label-Free Technologies for Drug Discovery   Edited by Matthew Cooper and Lorenz M. Mayr
© 2011 John Wiley & Sons, Ltd

14.1 INTRODUCTION

Label-free detection is a powerful approach to the study of molecular interactions without the requirement for target modification. It offers potential advantages over conventional technologies by combining the direct probing of responses in real time with a high degree of sensitivity in native or un-tagged settings [1, 2]. The field is progressing rapidly, as evidenced by the increasing number of publications, system vendors, platforms, and underlying technologies launched to market every year. Label-free applications are numerous and can be grouped largely into cellular and biochemical (or noncellular) applications. In the case of whole cell assays, label-free responses are thought to be indicative of changes in cell morphology or behaviour in response to a stimulus. Such changes may occur via cytoskeletal re-arrangement, cell–cell interactions or otherwise [3–6]. The readout is noninvasive, cumulative, and signaling-route independent. Kinetic responses or 'fingerprints' elicited by a compound are unique and mechanistically informative. Default assay methodology is simple; core requirements include adequate cell adherence and the use of custom biosensor-coated plates. To date, the main types of cellular label-free readouts are optical and impedance-based. The former monitors dynamic cellular mass redistribution via changes in diffraction index from waveguide bottom coated-plates [7, 8]. The latter captures changes in trans and extracellular impedance currents via individual electrodes lining the bottom of plates [9–14]. Although the readouts differ, they appear equivalent in their biological resolution.

Cellular assays are at the core of screening activities for the numerous target classes pursued by drug discovery programmes. Several technologies have been employed to develop assays of high quality in multi-well plate formats. Typical reagent generation strategies have often favoured recombinant target expression and target tagging. Even so, there is a continuous desire to configure screening assays in ways to better resemble the physiological environment and a strong incentive for assays to deliver outputs with enhanced mechanistic texture. In turn, it is hoped that such assays will facilitate better decision making on compound progression at earlier points within screening cascades. The versatility of label-free detection is ideal in this respect and may help address these intents. The readout also presents a commonality of platform with multiple target classes and signalling end-points, which makes it appealing and generic. It holds potential to support a vast range of activities from small to high throughput screening, and this at endogenous level of target expression. Moreover, it displays a highly complex holistic signalling response akin to phenotypic tissue assays. Recent advances in the label-free area have been truly enabling for compound screening, in particular the emergence of 96- and 384-well plate formats and automated label-free platforms. This prompted us to consider its potential utility for drug discovery.

The aim of this chapter is to describe outputs from in-house label-free evaluations focused on cellular-based screening. Here, we investigated whether label-free is capable of delivering robust assays to assist both hit identification and follow-up compound profiling activities, and do so by comparison with outputs from existing/typical technologies. Experiments were performed on either optical (Corning Epic®, SRU Biosystems BIND®) or impedance-based (MDS Analytical Technologies CellKey™) platforms, selecting 7TM targets for which in-house reagents and tool compounds were readily available. 7TMs are intensively pursued targets in drug discovery efforts across the pharmaceutical industry and are linked to a plethora of disease indications accounting for over 40% of all clinically available drugs [15]. The emergence of label-free detection may provide a means of prosecuting 7TMs more effectively by exploiting physiologically relevant and predictive *in vitro* assays.

14.2 RESULTS AND DISCUSSION

14.2.1 Compound Profiling

The first objective of these studies was geared towards pharmacological profiling of small molecule S1P1 agonists to assess the correlation of outputs from label-free and classical technologies (Figure 14.1). S1P1 is a member of the EDG family of receptors reported to operate predominantly through the $G_{\alpha I}$-linked signalling route and routinely screened using membrane $GTP\gamma S^{35}$ filter binding. Label-free assays were developed on both the BIND® and CellKey™ platforms using an S1P1 recombinant cell line. Screening for a small number of agonist compounds in label-free mode revealed good apparent assay concordance compared with the classical GTPγS readout and R^2 values of 0.84 and 0.83 for impedance and optical systems, respectively. Absolute potency values from label-free

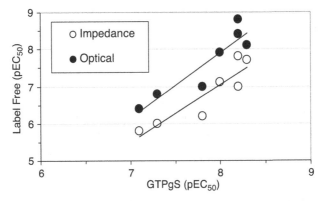

Figure 14.1 / Table 14.1 Potency values determined for a subset of agonist compounds tested against the S1P1-expressing adherent cell line. Apparent assay correlation was observed where comparing impedance-based (CellKey™), optical-based (BIND®) label-free detection with respect to the classical GTPγS[35] assay format.

	GTPγS (pEC$_{50}$)	Impedance (pEC$_{50}$)	Optical (pEC$_{50}$)
Native ligand	8.3	7.7	8.1
Compound 1	7.1	5.8	6.4
Compound 2	7.8	6.2	7.0
Compound 3	8.2	7.0	8.4
Compound 4	8.2	7.8	8.8
Compound 5	8.0	7.1	7.9
Compound 6	7.3	6.0	6.8

readouts were slightly off-set with a lower trend from impedance systems (~1 log shift) and generally closer agreement from the optical system. The capture of full temporal responses allowed further interrogation of underlying temporal/mechanistic profiles and analysis of the kinetic traces triggered by different small molecule compounds with respect to the natural agonist S1P. This led to some unexpected observations. Figures 14.2 and 14.3 depict examples of traces obtained BIND® (Figure 14.2) and CellKey™ (Figure 14.3) for compounds A and B alongside the S1P1 natural agonist. In keeping with that of S1P, compound A displayed negative responses at low concentrations and positive responses at higher concentrations. In sharp contrast, compound B gave positive deflections at all concentrations tested. Despite the observation that compound B elicited a distinct label-free or signalling profile to the natural agonist, comparative studies using the GTPγS assay format did not discriminate between any of these compound activities. A growing body

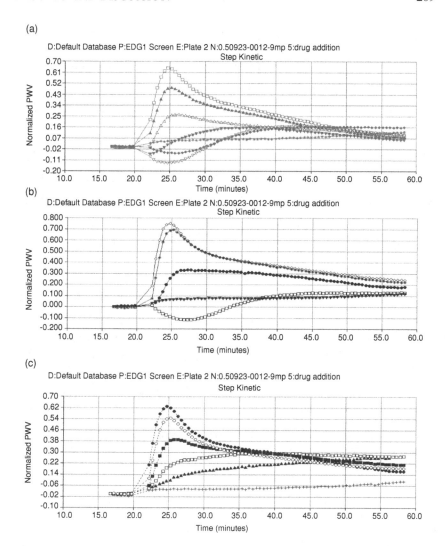

Figure 14.2 Representative kinetic profiles obtained for key agonist compounds tested against the S1P1-expressing adherent cell line with the BIND® system. Concentration–response curve (CRC) for natural S1P agonist (panel A); CRC for compound A (panel B); CRC for compound B (panel C).

of evidence suggest that numerous if not all 7TMs have a propensity for multiplicity of coupling. The concept of functional agonist selectivity also emerges, proposing stabilisation of unique 'agonist–receptor' active states [16]. For the S1P1 receptor, the observed label-free response for compound B may give clues towards its actions in recombinant and/or

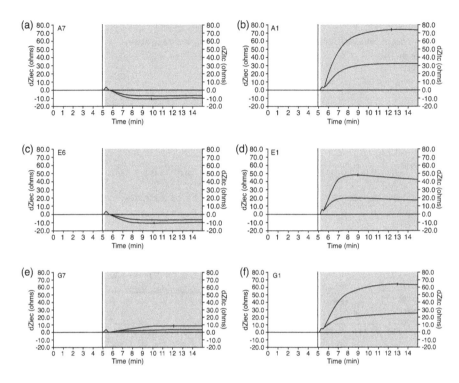

Figure 14.3 Representative label-free profiles obtained for key agonist compounds tested against the S1P1-expressing adherent cell line with the CellKey[TM] system. Dark responses over time represent Δ Ziec; lighter responses represent Δ Zitc. Natural S1P agonist at low (panel A) or high (panel B) concentration; compound A at low (panel C) or high (panel D) concentration; compound B at low (panel E) or high (panel F) concentration.

phenotypic native systems and that these may be distinct from that of the native ligand. However, the unique features of compound B may also be accounted for, at least in part, by the overexpression nature of the cellular system under study. More detailed experimentations are required to address these and related points. Collectively, these findings show that label-free can complement existing assay formats, providing unique insight into compound action and potential utility in compound ranking, chemical design and targeted signalling.

The second main objective of these studies was to compare assay formats for a receptor system known to be associated with multiple signalling routes. EP4 is a prostanoid receptor classified as a $G_{\alpha s}$ coupled receptor, which also displays $G_{\alpha q}$-mediated signalling amongst others. Compound profiling activities have been traditionally supported

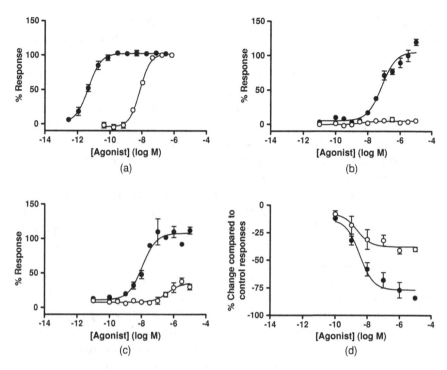

Figure 14.4 Compound profiling of the natural agonist PGE_2 (•) and compound X (○) against EP4-expressing cells using various technologies including, inhibition of forskolin-induced cAMP (panel A), intracellular calcium release via FLIPR (panel B), label-free using the BIND® system (panel C) and native tissue bath assay (panel D).

via cAMP detection methodologies using a recombinant cell line stably expressing EP4 and small molecule agonists have been identified during screening campaigns. A label-free EP4 assay was configured and known EP4 agonists profiled using the same recombinant cell line. Data were then compared to that from alternative assay formats including fluorescence imaging plate reader (FLIPR) (Ca^{2+} or $G_{\alpha q}$-linked signalling) and an established *in vitro* gut bath assay. Agonist concentration–response curve (CRC) characteristics from the label-free assay were largely unremarkable and, in terms of reproducibility, sigmoidal definition and slope were largely comparable to that of the other assay systems. However, unexpected results were obtained for some small molecule compounds, as exemplified by compound X (Figure 14.4). The natural ligand PGE_2 was active across all assay formats (cAMP, FLIPR, tissue bath). By contrast, compound X was found to be a full agonist in cAMP, partial agonist in the phenotypic native end-point and inactive in FLIPR. The finding that compound X was a partial agonist versus PGE2 in the label-free system and that such system was the only one matching tissue bath activity was particularly interesting. A frequent artefact of recombinant assays is to overestimate potency and efficacy compared to that of more relevant and intact systems as a consequence of expression and forced coupling. The correlation of both potency and efficacy observed with label-free and organ bath assays is evident despite the recombinant nature of the former. Although purely speculative, label-free assays may provide a more physiologically predictive output with respect to potency and efficacy even if employing recombinant reagents.

Regardless, the present study suggests that choice of assay format is critical for compound identification and optimisation. This study exemplifies the challenges in both assay design and selection in that compound X would not have been identified as worthy of progression if FLIPR alone had been employed. Conversely, FLIPR would not have seemed an unreasonable strategy in the absence of compound X based on the apparent activity of the native ligand. In the case of EP4, classes of small molecule agonists are emerging with or without 'additional' signalling ($G_{\alpha q}$/other) to the 'primary' $G_{\alpha s}$ output and more is required to probe the compound X mechanism(s) of action. The implication of such observations remains to be fully elucidated but it is inevitably desirable to configure screening assays in ways to predict activity at more physiological end-points, that is tissue assays. The advent of label-free as an all-inclusive holistic cumulative readout of cellular activity will complement results obtained from pathway-selective assay formats and go some way to making more informed decision regarding screen design.

In summary, assays can be readily developed for full curve analysis to probe target pharmacology. Cases of assay concordance and discordance are emerging, suggesting that the underpinning biology is complex and these data are a timely reminder of the fact that apparent pharmacology has both compound and system dependencies. Contributing factors may include receptor coupling, expression levels and stoichiometry, host background and cellular machinery. Holistic label-free readouts capture the cumulative, integrated response and can be compared to the classical limited-pathway reductionist approaches. Label-free readouts may offer better correlation with downstream tissue, whole organ or *in vivo* assay. Whether this provides an improved predictability of compound behaviours *in vivo* is presently unclear but it is hoped that label-free presents additional mechanistic texture to allow distinction between compound profiles and triage.

14.2.2 Hit Identification

U2OS cells are known to endogenously express the histamine H1 receptor, a prototypical $G_{\alpha q}$-linked 7TM receptor which causes an increase in calcium release from intracellular stores upon agonist stimulation [17]. Thus, histamine was used as positive response or high control for assay validation experiments. A label-free assay was first assembled on the Epic® system in single addition format and the validation phase rapidly completed. U2OS cells were recovered from cryo-preservation and directly seeded using a vial-to-assay plate thawing protocol. Cell density of 20 000 cells per well provided the highest signal with approximately 30-fold or greater response over basal and plate surface coating was found not be required. Full cell confluency was observed after 24 hours plating and uniform cell monolayer spread across wells. Assays were set-up in kinetic mode and assay temperature fixed to 26 °C throughout procedure to minimize nonspecific effects and drifts in label-free responses. Assay tolerance to DMSO showed acceptable limits up to 2% with histamine potency and signal window unaffected compared to control conditions.

Temporal resolution of the histamine responses in concentration–response curve mode was highly informative, allowing investigation of the merit of various data extraction methods prior to single-shot screening analysis. Label-free responses were found to be both concentration and compound dependent. At maximum effective concentration (EC_{100}), histamine profiles were characterized by a time-to-peak rate of approximately 15 minutes and a response which was largely sustained for the remaining reading duration. In contrast, time-to-peak was progressively delayed at lower concentrations by as much as a factor of two (30 minutes to peak at 1 μM). Acetylcholine, an unrelated compound known to cause Gq-linked signalling activation, was also tested in U2OS cells and distinct temporal response profiles were obtained despite putative signalling routes for these agonist being shared (data not shown). Comparison of analysis methods, using either maximum response over the entire read time versus a user defined single-point read of 15 minutes, also highlighted subtle differences in the derived curves and apparent potency estimates. Regardless, the apparent potency of histamine correlated well with that using conventional Ca^{2+} detection assay technology (FLIPR); label-free pEC_{50} 6.5 (end-read at 15 minutes), 6.8 (max peak response), 6.6 (AUC over 50 minutes) and 6.1 (AUC to peak), compared with pEC_{50} 5.9 from FLIPR.

Assay performance during single shot screening was investigated by testing a diverse set of 1408 low molecular weight compounds in agonist format (Figure 14.5). Full temporal acquisition was enabled to allow scrutiny of assay reproducibility, sensitivity of hit identification and the temporal profile of selected hits. Figure 14.5 depicts kinetic responses obtained from the testing of diverse compound chemotypes and actives were characterized by a mixture of profiles ranging between positive, negative and neutral wave shifts. The onset, sustainability and magnitude of response varied greatly, with time-to-peak values in the vast majority of cases differing from that of histamine. By themselves, these unique profiles may potentially denote different signalling events via a single target of interest and/or may point towards multiple routes elicited by distinct targets endogenously present in U2OS cells. Only one compound appeared to display a signature resembling that of histamine with a positive wave shift maximum response peaking at 14 minutes (Figure 14.5). Subsequent follow-up experiments on this compound, using alternative technologies such as Ca^{2+} detection (FLIPR) and cAMP accumulation, confirmed that this response was unlikely to be mediated by H1 receptor activation (data not shown).

The data set was analysed using two single time point extraction methods (Figure 14.6, Table 14.2). For the early time point of 15 minutes, signal-to-noise ratios remained excellent and consistent between days, across days and on multiple plate runs. Average peak shift values were 0.32+3.93 pm and 70.06+6.22 pm for low and high controls, respectively, defining an average Z' value of 0.68 (Figure 14.6, panel A). Sample responses displayed a normally distributed population around the low controls. Apparent hit rate was very low at less than 1% using a 10% activity cut-off with and no obvious incidence of false positives (Table 14.2). Correlation rate was high with 75% of actives repeating across days. These results indicate a highly robust and clean assay with fit-for-purpose performance for single shot screening. A second round of comparative data analysis was performed using a later endpoint of 50 minutes to assess whether common or alternative hits would be identified (Figure 14.6, panel B). Assay 'variability' was higher and average Z' values of 0.23, typically below the acceptable cut-off of 0.4. Sample variance around the low controls was also greater and activity cut-offs consequently high. Of particular note was a general lack of correlation between actives from this analysis and that of the earlier time point of 15 minutes. The analysis method employed and time point(s) selected appeared to have significant bearing on the likelihood of selecting particular actives.

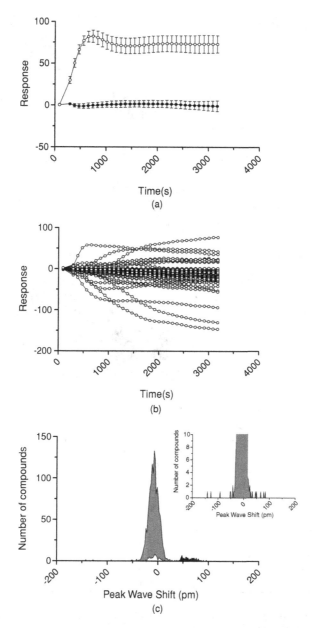

Figure 14.5 Representative traces of the temporal profiles obtained from single shot testing of diverse chemotypes in U2OS cells. Output of a single plate from the screening carried out to assess assay performance and reproducibility using the optical Epic® system. Panel A shows mean high (○) and mean low (●) control responses, n = 16 ±SD; panel B shows sample response profiles; panel C and insert show the frequency and distribution of peak responses from all cpds over the duration of the read; sample (grey), low controls (white) and high controls (black).

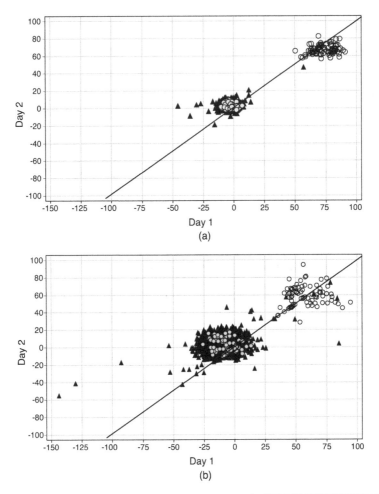

Replicate	Rob mean	Rob SD	Rob Cut-off (%)	N hits	HR
Day 1 at 15 min end-point	0.27	3.60	11.08	11	0.78
Day 2 at 15 min end-point	−0.16	3.24	9.56	10	0.71
Day 1 at 50 min end-point	−2.4	11.87	33.19	17	1.21
Day 2 at 50 min end-point	−1.93	10.11	17	13	0.92

Figure 14.6 / Table 14.2 Correlation of label-free responses obtained from single shot testing against U2OS cells. Data were generated on two separate test occasions using the optical Epic® system. The diagonal line indicates unity. Data were extracted and analysed from both single-point read of 15 minutes post-compound addition (panel A) and a later single-point read of 50 minutes (panel B). Low controls (●), high controls (○); normalized sample responses (▲).

In summary, the findings suggest that endogenously expressed 7TM can be exploited to develop label-free assays. Acquisition of full response profiles can be highly valuable to the process of hit identification, leading to a greater data interrogation. The comparison of common and different temporal profiles may point towards shared or alternative mechanisms of action, apparent potency and efficacy estimates; apparent hit rate can also be affected by the choice of data extraction method. The strategy of obtaining full profiles is not without cost in throughput as well as complexity in analysis. However, additional texture in hit identification and follow-up study may be exploitable and elucidate alternative/additional signalling routes as well as highlighting 'off-target' activities. Targeted drug design may be enabled to develop compounds and therapeutics that act similarly, or distinctly, from particular agonist types, for example, native agonists. These results highlight the challenging prospect associated with the cherry-picking of relevant label-free actives for follow-up studies and homologous or heterologous label-free signatures may underpin distinct modes of action and complex integrated biology.

14.3 CONCLUSIONS AND PERSPECTIVE

Label-free detection, whether impedance or optical-based, emerges as a novel yet powerful tool in the drug discovery process. Its applicability spans multiple screening activities, notably hit identification and follow-up compound profiling. High quality, sensitive and robust cellular assays can be readily developed in single shot and full curve modes using recombinant and/or endogenously expressing receptor systems. Whilst initiated, the area of label-free screening remains young and more evidence is required before conclusions can be confidently drawn on the alignment of label-free and classical 'pathway-selective' assays. Obtaining full temporal profiles provides a wealth of detailed information but typically comes at some cost in throughput and complexity in analysis. The running of a high throughput screen campaign may not need to be supported by full kinetic-read mode, rather reduced-point readouts may suffice for established systems, or even end-point analysis where the temporal responses have been validated. However, it is also clearly possible for hits to be missed or misclassified without some understanding of the high content read. Data analysis is challenging but scrutiny is crucial to enable proper data interpretation and maximize on the impact of label-free approaches. Data are underpinned by a complex biology, particularly for 7TM targets believed to have multiple signalling routes, both G-protein dependent and independent. Intriguingly the label-free arena is emerging alongside a renewed consensus and interest in the pleiotropic nature of 7TMs.

Can label-free data be exploited to further drug discovery? The reading of holistic signalling as opposed to targeted signalling may be one step in the direction of improving physiological relevance but certainly the noninvasive nature of label-free detection lends itself to the study of phenotypic native receptor systems such as primary cultured cells. The value of label free in compound progression remains to be fully addressed and promises to be the focus of years to come. Predictability of the detection of *in vivo* readouts is not yet fully understood. Advances in label-free technology have enabled systems capable of being employed as generic platforms for the pharmacological study of compounds through primary to mechanistically intact and predicable assays. The exact nature of this predictability remains to be addressed but great promise is held in the ability of label-free systems to progress the 'best' compounds and to reduce compound attrition, and ultimately that of drugs in late stage clinical trials.

14.4 MATERIALS AND METHODS

14.4.1 Materials

Histamine-hydrochloride, sphingosine-1-phosphate (S1P) and prostaglandin E2 (PGE$_2$) were supplied by Sigma-Aldrich. Low molecular weight compounds were all obtained from in house supplies, including a subset of tool compounds and a 1408 structurally diverse compound set used for assay robustness testing. The human osteosarcoma (U2OS) cell line was purchased from American Type Culture Collection (ATCC) and scaled-up batches prepared for cryo-preservation in which to support a vial-to-plate recovery protocol prior to assay. DMEM/F12 media supplemented with 10% fetal bovine serum (FBS) was purchased from InVitrogen and used for cell plating. A cell line stably expressing S1P1 receptor as well as human embryonic kidney-293 (HEK-293) cells stably expressing EP4 receptor were generated in house. Both were previously validated and are used for screening in GTPγS^{35} filter binding and HTRF-cAMP assay formats, respectively. DMEM/F12 media supplemented with 10% FBS, 500 mg/ml neomycin (InVitrogen) and 3 µM indomethacin (Sigma-Aldrich) was prepared for the EP4-cell line. Both 96- and/or 384-well formats of label-free plates were provided directly by Corning, MDS Analytical Technologies and SRU Biosystems.

14.4.2 Methods

14.4.2.1 Epic® Label-Free Assay Protocol

U2OS cells were thawed from frozen and seeded onto custom 384-well biosensor-coated plates at 20 000 cells per well, then incubated overnight at 37 °C and 5% carbon dioxide. At the time of assay, cells were gently washed using a Biomex-FX and supplemented with HBSS/HEPES assay buffer (pH 7.4) pre-equilibrated at 26 °C containing 2% DMSO. From then on, temperature was kept constant at 26 °C for the duration of the experiment. Plates were transferred to a cell incubator for two hours prior to being loaded onto the Epic System and baseline read measurement taken for 4.5 minutes (baseline read). Cell plates were unloaded and compounds pre-diluted to 2% DMSO with assay buffer were added 'off-line' using a CybiWell. Cell plates were finally re-loaded for 'online' kinetic readings at 90 second intervals for 50 minutes (stimulation reads). A dynamic mass redistribution (DMR) signal was derived from the average of three scans per well per time point. The EpicViewer software was used for data visualisation and extraction, supporting different analysis modes, including maximal or minimal response, signal change, area under the curve, and this over the entire read time or according to user defined start/stop end points. Final assay concentration for the robustness compound set was 5 μM and a DMSO-containing plate was included within each run to assess false positive detection rates. Histamine was used as high control at 40 μM final assay concentration and compared to buffer as low control. Assay tolerance to DMSO was investigated by monitoring the effect of increasing content from 0 to 5% throughout assay procedure on the histamine potency and signal to noise ratio.

14.4.2.2 CellKey™ Label-Free Assay Protocol

Freshly grown cells overexpressing either S1P1 or EP4 receptors were seeded into custom 96-well microplates containing interdigitated electrodes at 50 000 cells per well and incubated overnight at 37 °C (5% CO_2). At the time of assay, cell plates and compound plates were loaded onto the CellKey system, which integrates temperature control, fluid exchange (head pipetor) and impedance reading capabilities. The temperature condition of 37 °C was applied throughout the assay procedure. Cells were gently washed twice and supplemented with HBSS/HEPES assay buffer (pH 7.4) containing 0.1% BSA and allowed to equilibrate for 30 minutes. Impedance was measured continuously throughout a baseline period of five minutes followed by compound addition and post-addition steps lasting 30 minutes. Compounds pre-diluted in assay buffer were added online at a dilution ratio of 1:10 to minimize buffer disturbance. Final concentrations of DMSO ranged from 0 to 0.01% for some compounds which were paired with appropriate vehicle controls. Changes in both transcellular (ΔZitc) and extracellular (ΔZiec) impedance values were monitored. Data were extracted from the instrument software using onboard propriety methodology and exported as required using the max–min of ΔZiec signal response over the period measured.

14.4.2.3 BIND® Label-Free Assay Protocol

Freshly grown cells overexpressing S1P1 were seeded into custom 96-well biosensor-coated plates at 50 000 cells per well and incubated overnight at 37 °C (5% CO_2). From assay start, experimental steps were carried out at room temperature using bench-top automation. Cells were gently washed twice using a Biomex-FX and supplemented with HBSS/HEPES assay buffer (pH 7.4) containing 0.1% BSA, then allowed to equilibrate for 30–60 minutes on the bench. Plates were loaded onto the BIND instrument and set for continuous reading at 50 second intervals. Baseline responses were first acquired for 5–10 minutes followed by manual addition of pre-diluted compounds online to the cell plate at a dilution ratio of 1:6 to minimize buffer disturbance. Final concentration of DMSO ranged from 0 to 0.01% for some compounds and paired with appropriate controls. Data were extracted and exported by the onboard software tool wizard; typically maximum minus minimum signal response over the measured period.

14.4.2.4 Non Label-Free Assay Protocols

Changes in intracellular cAMP levels were measured using a HTRF-LANCE assay format (Perkin-Elmer) according to generic guidelines from vendors. Changes in intracellular calcium levels were monitored using the fluorescence imaging plate reader (FLIPR) assay format as previously described [18]. Membrane GTPγS^{35} filter binding (Amersham) was set up from generic conditions as previously reported [19].

14.4.3 Data Analysis and Statistics

Concentration response curves were fitted using a four parameter logistic fit using the Prism 4.0 software (GraphPad, San Diego, CA). Standard deviation (SD) was calculated from triplicate data points unless otherwise stated. Correlation coefficient (R^2) values were derived from linear regression and analysis of single shot testing performed using Excel expressing responses as a percentage low and high assay controls. Robust percentage cut-off was calculated from $3\times$ the SDs of the low controls following outlier exclusion. Hit rate was calculated as percentage of the number of actives over the total number of compound tested. Correlation rates were compared between replicates across the two days of testing. Robust Z' were calculated as the difference between the low and high controls as a function of their SDs after statistical outlier exclusion. [20].

ACKNOWLEDGEMENTS

The authors would like to thank the people involved in making these evaluations possible: Sue Brown from GSK and Peter Lowe, Tim Kinnings and Lance Laing from SRU Biosystems for the BIND® system evaluation; Katherine Cato and Martin Wood from GSK and John Proctor and Kevin McCormack from MDS Analytical Technologies for the CellKey™ system evaluation; Angela Dunne, Isabel Coma, Dion Daniels, Phil Green, Christos Moraitis, Julio Martin and Alan Wise from GSK and Volker Eckelt, Alice Gao, Silvie Bailly, Lucinda Gedge and Ute Vespermann from Corning for the Epic® system evaluation. Special thanks to the Corning team at Fontainebleau, France, for its diligence as well as sharing of its laboratory facilities.

REFERENCES

1. M. A. Cooper, *Drug Discov Today* **11**, 1068 (2006).
2. M. A. Cooper, *Drug Discovery World* **7**, 68 (2006).

3. S. Siehler, *Biotechnology J* **3**, 471 (2008).
4. B. Xi, N. Yu, X. Wang *et al. Biotechnology J.* **3**, 484 (2008).
5. Y. Fang, A. G. Frutos and R. Verklereen, *Comb Chem High Throughput Screen.* **11**, 357 (2008).
6. L. Minor, *Comb Chem High Throughput Screen.* **11**, 574 (2008).
7. Y. Fang, *Assay Drug Dev Technol.* **4**, 583 (2006).
8. P. Lee, A. Gao, C. Van Standen *et al. Assay Drug Dev Technol.* **6**, 83 (2008).
9. G. J. Ciambrone, V. F. Liu, D. C. Lin *et al. J Biomol Screen.* **9**, 467 (2004).
10. J. M. Atienza, N. Yu, S. L. Kirstein *et al. Assay Drug Dev Technol.* **4**, 597 (2006).
11. E. Verdonk, K. Johnson, R. McGuinness *et al. Assay Drug Dev Technol.* **4**, 609 (2006).
12. N. Yu, J. M. Atienza, J. Bernard *et al. Anal. Chem.* **78**, 35 (2006).
13. R. McGuiness, *Current Opin Pharmacol.* **7**, 535 (2007).
14. M. F. Peters, K. S. Knappenberger, D. Wilkins *et al. J Biomol Screen.* **12**, 312 (2007).
15. J. Drews, *Science* **287**, 1960 (2000).
16. T. Kenakin, *Trends Pharmacol Sci* **28**, 407 (2007).
17. R. Ames, P. Nuthulaganti, J. Fornwald *et al. Receptor Channels* **10**, 117 (2004).
18. M.D. Wood, J.C. Jerman and D. Smart, *Recent Research Developments in Neurochemistry*, **3**, 135–142 (2000).
19. J. M. Watson, S. Brough, M. C. Coldwell and T. Gager, *Br J Pharmacol* **125**, 1413 (1998).
20. J. H. Zhang, T. D. Y. Chung and K. R. Oldenburg, *J Biomo. Screen* **4**, 67 (1999).

15

Novartis Evaluation of the ForteBio Octet RED: A Versatile Instrument for Direct Binding Experiments

Eric Martin[1], John Wang[1], Isabel Zaror[1], Jiamin Yu[1], Kelly Yan[1], Mike Doyle[1], Paul Feucht[1], Kevin Shoemaker[1], Bob Warne[1], Mike Chin[1], Blisseth Sy[1], Lukas Leder[2], Marco Meyerhofer[2], Charles Wartchow[3], and Danfeng Yao[3]

[1]*Novartis Institutes for Biomedical Research, Emeryville, CA, USA*
[2]*Novartis Institutes for Biomedical Research, Basel, Switzerland*
[3]*FortéBio, Inc., Menlo Park, CA, USA*

Label-Free Technologies for Drug Discovery   Edited by Matthew Cooper and Lorenz M. Mayr
© 2011 John Wiley & Sons, Ltd

15.1 INTRODUCTION

In the drug discovery process, label-free biophysical analysis of small molecule binding to a validated therapeutic target is emerging as an important research tool. Primary biochemical screening with small molecule libraries often generates numerous hits, including false positive results. As a result, the binding of these compounds to a target must be validated in a secondary assay to differentiate true hits from compounds that do not bind to the target, that bind to the target protein nonspecifically, or with nonstoichiometric binding.(1–3). An additional application is the screening of small molecule fragments (with molecular weight as low as ~ 150 Daltons), which potentially increases the number of hits generated in the discovery process (4).

The Octet RED is an eight-channel instrument designed for the determination of kinetic constants (K_D, k_{on}, k_{off}) and saturable binding capacity for small molecules with molecular weights greater than ~ 150 Daltons in a 96-well plate format. Advantages of this format include ease of use, fast assay development, less sensitivity to DMSO concentration, and the ability to assay soluble analytes even in the presence of insoluble components.

The FortéBio Octet instrument platform detects the binding of molecules to the tips of disposable fiber-optic biosensors with biolayer interferometry (BLI). This technique generates an interference pattern by monitoring visible light reflected from two surfaces within each fiber-optic biosensor. When a binding event occurs at the tip of a biosensor in solution, the "optical thickness" of this layer changes, and the interference pattern shifts to a higher wavelength. as shown in Figure 15.1. These

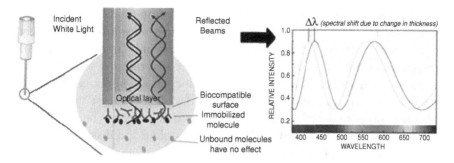

Figure 15.1 In BioLayer Interferometry, white light shines through a 0.5mm fiber-optic pin. Reflections return from the optical layer and the solvent interface. A layer of protein attached to the tip of an optic fiber creates an interference pattern at the detector, dependent on the "optical thickness" of the layer. Ligand binding changes the "optical thickness" and shifts the interference spectrum.

changes are monitored in real time. The instrument uses a linear array of eight sensors that simultaneously read a column of a 96-well plate.

In a typical experiment, up to 96 high density Super Streptavidin (SSA) coupled biosensors are pre-equilibrated in a sensor tray containing assay buffer. Eight pins at a time are dipped into the columns of a 96-well plate oscillating at 1000 rpm. Temperature control is achieved by heating the bottom of the plate to a desired temperature (usually a few degrees above the ambient temperature). This plate contains biotinylated protein target, a biotin derivative (for blocking unoccupied binding sites on SSA), assay buffer, and compounds. An example plate layout is shown in Figure 15.2. After protein loading in column one, responses are measured for

	1	2	3	4	5	6	7	8	9	10	11	12
A	Target	Biotin	Buf.	Dis 1	Dis 7	Dis 13	1 low	1 hi	7 low	7 hi	13 low	13 hi
B	Target	Biotin	Buf.	Dis 2	Dis 8	Dis 14	2 low	2 hi	8 low	8 hi	14 low	14 hi
C	Target	Biotin	Buf.	Ref. Buf.	Ref. Buf.	Ref. Buf.	Ref. Buf.	Ref. Buf.	Ref. Buf.	Ref. Buf.	Ref. Buf.	Ref. Buf.
D	Target	Biotin	Buf.	Dis 3	Dis 9	Dis 15	3 low	3 hi	9 low	9 hi	15 low	15 hi
E	Target	Biotin	Buf.	Dis 4	Dis 10	Dis 16	4 low	4 hi	10 low	10 hi	16 low	16 hi
F	Target	Biotin	Buf.	Ref. Buf.	Ref. Buf.	Ref. Buf.	Ref. Buf.	Ref. Buf.	Ref. Buf.	Ref. Buf.	Ref. Buf.	Ref. Buf.
G	Target	Biotin	Buf.	Dis 5	Dis 11	Dis 17	5 low	5 hi	11 low	11 hi	17 low	17 hi
H	Target	Biotin	Buf.	Dis 6	Dis 12	Dis 18	6 low	6 hi	12 low	12 hi	18 low	18 hi

Figure 15.2 An example sample plate layout to optimize assay conditions. Two sets of eight streptavidin sensors are used (not shown): the first will be loaded online with target protein (Trgt) in column one. The second will skip the target column to be used as bare streptavidin reference sensors. Biotin is used to block unoccupied streptavidin sites. A buffer well (Buf) is used for equilibration of the sensors. 18 compounds (1–18) are assayed at two concentrations (high and low concentrations). Each compound has its own dissociation well. Rows C and F are blanks used for reference subtraction.

baseline, association, and dissociation of the compound by dipping the sensor into wells containing assay buffer, compound solution, and assay buffer, respectively. At least one row contains only assay buffer, and responses in this row are used for reference corrections. A second set of reference sensors blocked with biotin or biocytin are also analysed, and the data are used to remove systematic artifacts. To increase the number of compounds analysed in a single run, protein loading can be performed manually at the bench, and wells used for baseline and dissociation can be used more than once.

15.2 METHODS

15.2.1 Production of Proteins

15.2.1.1 Proteins "E" and "P"

The cDNA from proteins "E" and "P" were cloned into pET-based expression vectors. Protein "E" was a fusion protein with N-terminal Avi- and His$_6$-tags. Protein "P" was a fusion protein with N-terminal His$_6$-tag and a C-terminal Avi-tag. Expression of the proteins was performed in $E.$ $coli$ cells under standard conditions. The proteins were purified by metal ion affinity chromatography (IMAC) and size exclusion chromatography (SEC). Pure protein "E" was then biotinylated site-specifically with recombinant biotin ligase (BirA) and biotin at its N-terminal Avi-tag (sequence of 15 aa recognized by BirA). The molecular weight of biotinylated protein "E" is about 31 kDa. The N-terminal fusion tag of protein "P" was cleaved, and it was biotinylated site-specifically at its C-terminal Avi-tag with recombinant BirA ligase and biotin. The molecular weight of biotinylated protein "P" is about 37 kDa.

15.2.1.2 Proteins "D" and "K"

His-tagged Proteins "D" (35 kDa) and "K" (33 kDa) were overexpressed and purified using IMAC, ion exchange, followed by SEC. Homogenous (>95%) Proteins "D" and "K" were further chemically biotinylated with Sulfo-NHS-LC-Biotin (Pierce) following manufacture's protocol.

15.2.2 Protein Loading and Small Molecule Binding Analysis

For initial assay development, loading of biotinylated protein on streptavidin sensors and subsequent small molecule binding were performed on the instrument in a single run. Once conditions were established for protein loading, protein loading was performed in batch at the bench, before the assay, to maximize the use of sample wells in the assay plate. In this case, multiple sensors were incubated in a 96-well plate, or in every other well of a 384-well plate to minimize protein usage. The pre-loaded (with target protein) sensors were then transferred to the instrument and the assay started without the protein-loading columns. Protein concentrations of 25–100 μg/ml were typically required to ensure maximal loading of protein in 10–20 minutes.

In a typical experiment where proteins were loaded from the instrument, sixteen Super Streptavidin (SSA) Biosensors (product no: FortéBio 18-0011) were rehydrated by placing them in a sensor plate containing assay buffer. The first column of eight sensors was loaded with protein and the second set was a blank control. Biotinylated protein, biotin (or biocytin), assay buffer, and 35 compounds were placed in a 96-well plate, as shown in Figure 15.3. The sensors and sample plate were placed on the instrument. Both sets of eight sensors were run sequentially across the sample plate in a single experiment. A typical instrument protocol included loading biotinylated protein onto the first set of sensors to saturation (column 1, 10–20 min), blocking with a biotin derivative (column 2, 10 μg/ml, 2 min), sensor equilibration (column 3, 10–20 min), followed

Sensor Map			Sample Plate Map											
	1	2		1	2	3	4	5	6	7	8	9	10	11	12
A	SSAv	SSAv	A	Biotin-Protein	Biocytin	AB	AB	AB	AB	AB	C	C	C	C	C
B	SSAv	SSAv	B	Biotin-Protein	Biocytin	AB	AB	AB	AB	AB	C	C	C	C	C
C	SSAv	SSAv	C	Biotin-Protein	Biocytin	AB	AB	AB	AB	AB	C	C	C	C	C
D	SSAv	SSAv	D	Biotin-Protein	Biocytin	AB	AB	AB	AB	AB	C	C	C	C	C
E	SSAv	SSAv	E	Biotin-Protein	Biocytin	AB	AB	AB	AB	AB	C	C	C	C	C
F	SSAv	SSAv	F	Biotin-Protein	Biocytin	AB	AB	AB	AB	AB	C	C	C	C	C
G	SSAv	SSAv	G	Biotin-Protein	Biocytin	AB	AB	AB	AB	AB	C	C	C	C	C
H	SSAv	SSAv	H	Biotin-Protein	Biocytin	AB	AB	AB	AB	AB	AB	AB	AB	AB	AB

Figure 15.3 Typical sensor and sample plate maps for protein loading and small molecule analysis on the Octet RED instrument. (Abbreviations: AB, assay buffer; SSAv, Super Streptavidin biosensors; C, compound.)

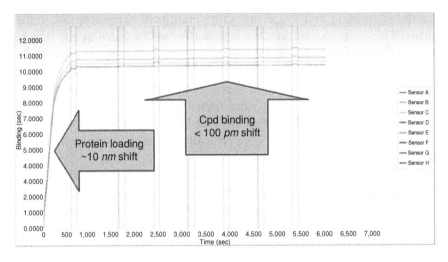

Figure 15.4   Eight parallel sensor graphs for the active sensors: (1) load protein, (2) block unused streptavidin sites with biocytin, (3) equilibrate, (4) bind compound, (5) dissociate compound, repeat (4) and (5) with additional compounds. Sensors in rows C and F represent buffer blanks for reference subtraction. They show no absorption/desorption, but do show some small baseline shifts due to well artifacts.

by compound analysis. One cycle of baseline, association, and dissociation occurs in columns three, eight and three respectively, the next cycle occurs in columns four, nine and four, and so forth. In this example, one buffer column is used twice without interference from carry-over of solution or the presence of compound from the previous run. Figure 15.4 shows the raw data for eight sensors, including protein loading and several cycles of compound binding. The second biocytin blank sensor set is similar, except that the protein loading step is skipped.

15.2.3 Referencing

Reference corrections were required to remove potential optical artifacts and drift from the raw data prior to data analysis. In the experiment described above, two data sets were generated, one for the sensors with the target protein and one with control sensors merely blocked with the biotin derivative. Reference corrections were performed by first subtracting the data set for the control sensors from the sensors with protein target, to correct for systematic artifacts including optical variances due to plate reflections, and for artifacts due to the presence of the analyte, including nonspecific binding to the sensor. Then, the row containing only buffer was subtracted to correct for drift, possibly due to gradual loss of protein over time. Thus, a reference-corrected data set is obtained by subtracting sensor data sets as follows: $(A1 - A2) - (C1 - C2)$, where A1 is a sensor containing protein that binds compounds in row A, A2 is the biocytin-blocked streptavidin control sensor that is subsequently run in the same wells as sensor A1 to measure system artifacts in row A, C1 is the sensor containing protein target that is run in parallel to sensor A1 in a control row of buffer, and C2 is the biotin-blocked streptavidin control sensor that is run in parallel to sensor A2, which measures system artifacts in row C of the sample plate. This process is known as "double reference subtraction". Figure 15.5 shows the results of each step in the correction. After these corrections are performed, the data set is ready for analysis.

15.2.4 Data Analysis

Data analysis tools provided by FortéBio include visualization of the reference correction process, the ability to generate responses in the association phase and dissociation phase, the ability to perform steady state analysis of responses for a concentration series to obtain the affinity constant K_D, the ability to fit individual curves to obtain observed rate constants (k_{obs}), the association rate constant (k_{on}) and the dissociation rate constants (k_{off}). Kinetics constants are also obtained through "global analysis", which derives a single set of parameters including R_{max}, k_{on}, k_{off}, and K_D from a set of association and dissociation curves from a concentration series (5).

15.2.5 Binding Studies

15.2.5.1 Proteins "E" and "P"

Biotinylated protein "E" (31 kDa, 100 μg/ml) was attached to Super Streptavidin Biosensors in 50 mM Tris buffer, pH 7.4, containing 150 mM NaCl and 10% glycerol for 10 minutes with 1000 rpm shaking. Typical responses on the Octet RED instrument were 10 nanometers. A preliminary screen of 12 compounds including a positive and negative control compound was performed at 1 and 10 μM in 50 mM HEPES pH 7.5 containing 5 0mM KCl, 3 mM DTT and 1% DMSO to obtain a preliminary affinity constant. Kinetic parameters were then obtained from five-point dilution series (2X–3X). Responses ranged from

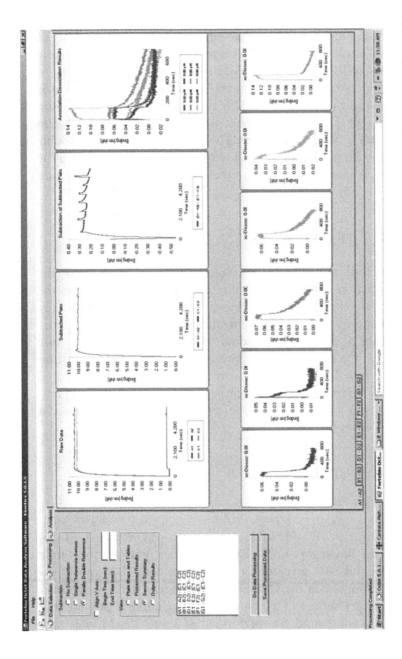

Figure 15.5 The first panel shows the raw data both for sensor graphs with large signals from protein loading, and the much smaller signals for the control sensors (bare streptavidin) without protein loading. Row A contained binding compounds and row C contained only buffer. A1 – A2 subtracts row A's bare streptavidin pin from the pin with loaded protein to correct for plate artifacts and nonspecific binding to the sensor substrate. (A1 – A2) – (C1 – C2) subtracts the reference buffer row C to correct for gradual protein loss, evaporation, and other artifacts.

~0.05–0.3 nm. Protein "P" binding assays were conducted similarly, but with 25 mM HEPES pH 7.5, 50 mM NaCl, 1 mM EDTA, 5 mM DTT, 1% DMSO.

15.2.5.2 Proteins "D" and "K"

To determine kinetic and equilibrium K_D for small molecule binding to Protein D, compounds were diluted into six concentrations and dispensed in columns 7–12 for measuring association, whereas buffers were dispensed in columns 1–6 for measuring dissociation. Biotinylated Prot "D" was diluted to 100 μg/ml and loaded onto SSA sensors off-line before starting the assay. All assays were conducted in 50 mM HEPES buffer pH 7.5, 10 mM MgCl$_2$, 150 mM NaCl, 2 mM DTT and 5% DMSO. K_D values were then calculated by kinetic analysis (k_{on}, k_{off}, and K_D) or by equilibrium binding analysis.

Protein "K" binding was conducted similarly except that biotinylated Protein "K" was diluted to 50 μg/ml before loading onto SSA sensors off-line. The assays were conducted with 50 mM Tris-HCl buffer pH 7.5 containing 15 mM MgCl$_2$ and 0.1% Tween 20. DMSO concentration was 5% in most of the assays.

15.3 RESULTS AND DISCUSSION

15.3.1 Protein "E"

Protein "E" was the first target tested in the evaluation and was the only blind test. Twelve "fragment size" ligands had been previously tested by Novartis in Basel on a Biacore T100. The disguised protein and compounds were sent to FortéBio with coded names. FortéBio was told the protein molecular weight, and told one positive control and one negative control to help develop the assay conditions. The molecular weights of these "fragment sized" compounds varied from 162 to 330. The Octet Red affinities varied from about 10 μM to 0.5 μM. Figure 15.6 compares Octet RED and Biacore sensorgrams for the smallest compound, "E2", with molecular weight = 162 Da. This shows ample signal-to-noise and good agreement among both instruments for a small fragment, but note that E2 is quite potent for its size.

The Octet RED confirmed that two compounds were nonbinders. Results for k_{on}, k_{off}, and kinetic K_D for the remaining 10 compounds

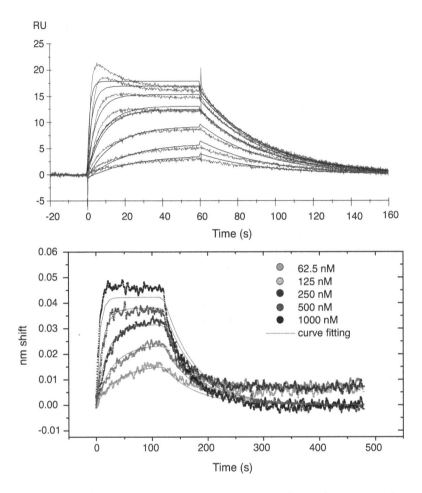

Figure 15.6   Sensor graphs for the Biacore T100 (upper plot) and Octet RED (lower plot) for compound "E2", MW = 162, the smallest fragment binding to protein "E."

are given in Table 15.1. All FortéBio values from the Octet RED agreed within 4× of the Biacore values determined at Novartis, with somewhat better agreement in k_{off} than k_{on}. This was considered a good result, so Novartis accepted an instrument for internal testing at Novartis in Emeryville, and all further tests were performed there.

15.3.2 Protein "D"

K_D was measured for 14 drug-sized compounds against Protein "D" over three different dates. Four compounds were measured on two dates and,

Table 15.1 Blind comparison of FortéBio kinetics with Biacore for Protein "E."

Ligand	MW	Octet RED[a]			Biacore[b]		
		k_{on} (1/M*s)	k_{off} (1/s)	K_D (μM)	k_{on} (1/M*s)	k_{off} (1/s)	K_D (μM)
E1	258.3	9920	0.0055	0.56	27000	0.011	0.40
E2	162.2	146000	0.020	0.14	65500	0.030	0.46
E3	267.7	25000	0.031	1.24	28900	0.096	3.31
E4	282.3	3000	0.015	4	8870	0.051	5.7
E5	296.4	5880	0.003	0.64	9670	0.0024	0.25
E6	330.8	1050	0.007	7.9	688	0.0038	5.57
E8	295.4	4720	0.0069	1.46	7290	0.0093	1.28
E9	269.3	7050	0.083	11.78	26500	0.123	4.63
E10	269.3	16500	0.0042	0.26	13000	0.0054	0.42
E11	221.3	37000	0.062	1.68	45300	0.085	1.88
E12	324.4	NB	NB	NB	NB	NB	NB
E13	300.4	NB	NB	NB	NB	NB	NB

[a]Performed at ForteBio. [b]Performed at Novartis in Basel.

of these, three replicated well. The fourth, "556", gave an unexpectedly low value on the second day. Table 15.2 compares these results with EC$_{50}$ values from an enzymatic screen. Molecular weights varied from 359 to 546 and affinity varied over 0.01–2 μM. Two of the compounds, which were each tested on two dates, were also tested by Biacore and isothermal titration calorimetry (ITC). For these two compounds, all five

Table 15.2 Results for Protein "D" comparing enzymatic IC$_{50}$, FortéBio K_D, Biacore K_D, and ITC K_D.

ID	MW	Enzyme IC50 (μM)	FortéBio 20-Feb-08	Octet RED 21-Feb-08	K_D [μM] 28-Feb-08	Biacore K_D (μM)	ITC K_D (μM)
511	399	0.014	0.029	0.027		0.04	0.018
91	359	0.12	0.18	0.15		0.13	0.12
966	546	0.015	0.056	0.017			
374	500	0.025		0.099			
450	497	0.057		0.17			
74	461	0.16	0.62				
944	424	0.2	0.62				
556	489	2.1	0.91	0.04			
160	374	0.04			0.22		
294	511	0.014			0.035		
152	496	0.11			0.47		
136	470	0.22			0.56		
453	410	0.17			0.22		
306	513	0.08			0.12		

experiments are in near perfect agreement. IC_{50} and FortéBio K_D for 13 of the 14 compounds agreed within a factor of five. IC_{50} and FortéBio K_D did not agree for "160". It was only measured once, and the discrepancy was not pursued. Overall, FortéBio K_D measurements for Protein "D" were considered to agree well with the other experiments.

15.3.3 Protein "K"

Protein "K" is a kinase which was available in both an active phosphory-lated form and an inactive dephosphorylated form. Two possible kinase binding modes are possible, classified as type I and type II, with the former preferring the phosphorylated protein conformation and the latter preferring the dephosphorylated conformation. Ordinary enzymatic assays using catalytically active protein can be less sensitive to type II binders, because the compound must bind the phosphorylated enzyme and force it into an inactive-like conformation, or select the smaller population of that conformation. A "dephos" enzymatic assay is available, in which the compounds are first incubated with the dephosphorylated enzyme, which is then activated and an IC_{50} quickly measured. This approach is potentially misleading, however, because the enzymatic test must always ultimately be performed on catalytically activate enzyme. Biophysical methods can directly measure binding to an inactive enzyme. Six "drug-sized" compounds (MW = 494–558) were tested against both protein forms. They had been previously tested in both "phos" and "dephos" enzymatic assays. The results are shown in Table 15.3. The enzymatic and biophysical assays agree in all cases.

Encouraged by these results, the Octet RED was applied as a secondary screen for two fragments that had been previously identified by

Table 15.3 Octet RED K_D is consistent with enzymatic IC_{50} for phosphorylated and dephosphorylated protein "K."

	Enzymatic IC_{50} (µM)			Octet RED K_D (µM)		
MW	Phos	Dephos	Type	Phos	Dephos	Type
494	0.004	0.04	I	0.001	0.14	I
459	0.003	0.02	I	<0.005	0.05	I
517	0.1	0.02	II	0.14	0.06	I/II
489	0.17	0.03	II	0.21	0.03	II
558	0.58	0.12	II	4.3	0.60	II
519	1.19	0.18	II	5.6	0.09	II

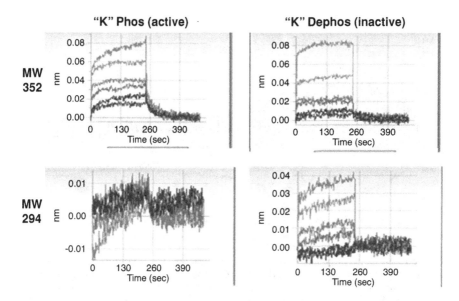

Figure 15.7 The 352 Dalton fragment binds equally to the phosphorylated and dephosphorylated forms, suggesting that it binds in a region which is similar in both conformations, most likely near the "hinge". The 294 Dalton fragment preferred the dephosphorylated protein, suggesting type II binding. The concentration range is 6–200 μM. (Note the different scales.)

NMR to bind protein "K". Figure 15.7 shows that the 352 Dalton fragment bound equally to the phosphorylated and dephosphorylated forms, suggesting that it binds in a region which is similar in both conformations, most likely near the "hinge". The 294 Dalton fragment preferred the dephosphorylated protein, suggesting type II binding.

15.3.4 Medium Throughput Screening

Medium throughput screening was also examined with proteins "K" and "D". In these experiments, 54 compounds were on a single plate, each at a single concentration of 100 μM. The protein was loaded off-line and every three compounds must share a single buffer well for desorption. Control experiments confirmed that carryover was less than 0.04% per dip into the buffer, so cross-contamination was not a problem (data not shown). Figure 15.8 shows the superimposed curves for sample experiments, including some typical artifacts. The "upside-down" curve is an artifact due to reference subtraction for a compound with higher

131

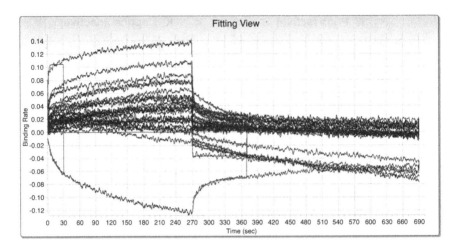

Figure 15.8 Superimposed sensor graphs for plates of 54 compounds measured at a single concentration for medium throughput screening. Most samples show the expected binding curve shapes, but some never reached saturation, indicating nonspecific binding. One curve is negative, an artifact from reference subtraction of a compound that bound strongly to the biocytin blank.

affinity for the streptavidin blank sensor than for protein "K" itself. Several sensor graphs do not reach a steady state plateau, but continue to climb. This indicated nonspecific binding to the protein at these high concentrations, and makes the graphs difficult to analyse. For this reason, the method is most suitable for soluble, non-aggregating compounds. Based on our results, we recommend screening at two concentrations, 50 and 200 μM, visually examining all curves, and following up promising "hits" with full titrations.

15.3.5 Protein "P"

The examples above show successful protein targets for which the Octet RED generally agreed with other biophysical and biochemical experiments, and, indeed, the results from the Octet RED might be preferred to the established methods. Other proteins were also studied during the course of this three-month evaluation, but these were the systems which gave good results quickly, with no construct optimization and very little assay optimization. Not all protein systems behaved so well. Some studies were complicated by nonspecific binding – especially at higher concentrations, where the protein continued to absorb ligand beyond

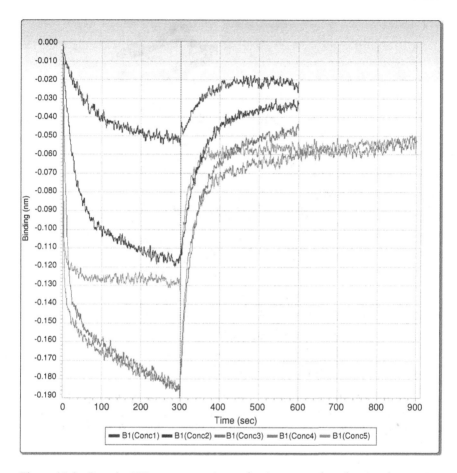

Figure 15.9 Protein "P" gave a consistent dose/response, but the signals were inverted for all compounds tested. Unlike the inverted peak in Figure 15.8, this was not an artifact of reference subtraction, but was clearly seen in the uncorrected target sensor graph. Protein "P" gave normal signals on Biacore T100. According to the simple physical model of biointerferometry, this would indicate a decrease in "optical thickness."

1:1 stoichiometry. A more interesting problematic case was protein "P". Protein "P" gave perfectly normal behavior on the Biacore T100, but gave inverted sensor graphs on the Octet RED. Figure 15.9 shows how protein "P" appeared to give a consistent dose/response, but the curves were increasingly negative with higher concentration. This is unlike the inverted curve in Figure 15.8, which was due to subtracting a positive signal from the strong binding to the biocytin blank, which was larger than the positive signal from binding to the protein target. The

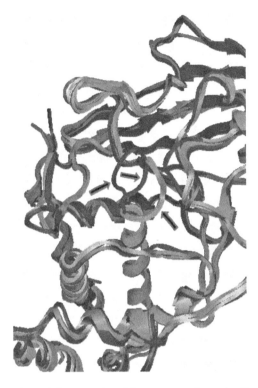

Figure 15.10 Overlay of five protein "P" structures from the Protein Data Bank. Apo structures are the lighter ribbons and ligand-bound co-structures are the darker ribbons. The collapse of two loops upon protein binding might account for a decrease in "optical thickness."

protein "P" signals are actually negative on the target sensor, before any corrections.

What can this mean? The simple physical model presented in Figure 15.1 would dictate that the "optical thickness" is decreasing rather than increasing upon ligand binding. One possible scenario would be that a buffer component larger than the sample ligand is weakly bound to the protein receptor site, and is displaced by ligand binding. However, systematically eliminating each buffer ingredient could not identify any such constituent. Another possibility is that the protein undergoes a conformational change upon binding that decreases its optical thickness. Interestingly, there are several crystal structures of protein "P" published in the RCSC Protein Data Bank. Figure 15.10 shows an overlay of the active sites of these proteins. The lighter ribbons are of apo structures, and the darker ribbons are from ligand-bound co-structures. There does indeed appear to be a systematic collapse of two loops upon protein binding. Whether this can account for the negative signals is pure speculation. It does raise questions of what "optical thickness" really means at a molecular level, especially given the dynamic nature of proteins.

15.4 CONCLUSION

The FortéBio Octet RED was found to be a flexible instrument useful for many types of experiments. We have used it for secondary direct binding assays, such as the phosphorylated and dephosphorylated assays for protein "K", and to follow up primary cellular assays and complex primary coupled assays that involve several proteins. It gave binding constants and kinetics consistent with other enzymatic and biophysical methods. Use as a primary, medium throughput assay for fragment-based screening was possible, albeit with some caveats. Well behaved fragments could be tested, but saturation of the binding curves was often not achieved, particularly for less soluble fragments at high (>100 μM) concentrations. This complicated analysis of the sensor graphs, but suitable results were achieved by screening at two concentrations, and following up all potential hits with full titrations. The instrument was also used for protein quantitation with an anti-his antibody, and for protein measurements in cell lysates (data not shown). These macromolecular measurements do not require the enhanced sensitivity of the Octet RED and Super Streptavidin sensors, but it is convenient that both small molecules and cell lysates can be studied on a single instrument.

During the course of the evaluation, three other proteins were tried that did not work as well as those presented here (data not shown). Proteins "R" and "F" gave inconsistent results, working for half the small molecules tested, but failing to reach saturation for the remainder. Protein "M" was very sticky, binding super-stoichiometrically both to itself and to all ligands. Due to time constraints, very little effort was made to optimize the assay conditions or protein constructs, so it is unknown whether these outcomes might be improved.

In all cases, both successful and unsuccessful, the biggest limitation appeared to be sensor graphs that did not reach saturation, presumably due to nonspecific binding. Soluble, non-aggregating compounds appeared to work best. More experience with assay optimization might improve this, or more sophisticated curve-shape analysis might deconvolute multiple binding events. Assessment of these difficulties requires a more comprehensive study where compounds and targets are compared directly. An additional limitation is that temperature control requires the instrument to be operated several degrees above ambient temperature. At this temperature, evaporation limits the length of a single run to about 2–3 hours.

The instrument is very convenient to operate. The eight-channel, 96-well format provides good throughput. The disposable pins permit testing potentially dirty or reactive samples, and it is comforting to periodically get a fresh protein surface. The relatively high DMSO tolerance is sufficient for samples stored in variable concentrations of DMSO solution. In cases where the Octet works well, we consider it the method of choice. In problematic cases, we are lucky enough to have access to alternative methods. Overall, the evaluation was considered a success; the Octet RED is considered a valuable addition to our arsenal of biophysical methods, and the instrument was purchased.

REFERENCES

1. Z. Wu, D. Liu, and Y. Sui, *J Biomol Screen* **13** (2), 159–167 (2008).
2. J. Zhang, X. Wu, and M. Sills, *J Biomol Screen* **10** (7), 695–704 (2005).
3. A. Gianetti, B. Koch, and M. Browner, *J Med Chem* **51** (3), 574–580 (2008).
4. M. Hämäläinen, A Zhukov, M. Ivarsson, *et al. J Biomol Screen*, **13** (3), 202–209 (2008).
5. T. Morton and D. Myszka, *Energetics of Biological Macromolecules*, Methods in Enzymology series (eds G. Ackers and M. Johnson), Vol. **295**, 268–294 (1998)

16

The Pyramid™ Approach to Fragment-Based Biophysical Screening

Glyn Williams
Astex Therapeutics Ltd, Cambridge, UK

16.1 INTRODUCTION

The screening of protein targets using simple, low molecular weight organic compounds ('fragments') at high concentrations began more than ten years ago as an exploratory exercise within a number of academic

Label-Free Technologies for Drug Discovery   Edited by Matthew Cooper and Lorenz M. Mayr
© 2011 John Wiley & Sons, Ltd

and pharmaceutical research groups [1]. Some researchers wished to explore the chemical preferences of protein active sites which interact with simple molecules, in order to make more informed choices when selecting groups to modify existing leads, while others wished to develop and improve scoring functions which were intended to quantitate these interactions. Few groups believed that the low molecular weight molecules themselves could become the basis for potent and selective drug candidates.

Amongst the pharmaceutical groups that first published data on the use of fragment hits as starting points for drug design, those at Abbott and Vertex stand out. Abbott Laboratories identified hits from changes in NMR chemical shifts, using an NMR method (^{15}N-^{1}H HSQC), which selectively detects signals from the amide groups of a ^{15}N-labelled target protein [2]. Molecules that bound to the target protein, FKBP, perturbed a limited number of amide signals that could be assigned to residues in and around the binding site. The ability to locate fragment binding sites, even approximately, along with knowledge derived from known binders assisted in the rational chemical design of elaborated and linked fragments, which ultimately led to more potent inhibitors. However, the method was limited to small (<30 kDa) proteins which could be expressed at high levels for isotope-labelling.

Vertex also used an NMR-based method to detect hits, but one which relied on detecting changes in the NMR relaxation properties of the fragments themselves when bound to a protein target [3]. This approach removed any restrictions on the protein size and relaxed some of the requirements for high-level protein expression. However, it also sacrificed information on the binding site(s) of the fragments. Vertex's response to this was to select fragments from a pool of privileged fragments called 'scaffolds', which were designed to represent the core structures of known drugs and drug-like leads and which contained chemical handles which could be synthetically modified. Once scaffolds which bound to the target had been identified, they could be rapidly elaborated into combinatorial libraries that explored, albeit blindly, the possible interactions in the binding site.

16.2 ASTEX AND THE PYRAMID™ APPROACH

Astex Therapeutics was formed (as Astex Technology) in 1999 with the sole purpose of pursuing an X-ray structure-guided approach to drug discovery, starting from fragments. While a range of biophysical methods would be used, it was clearly recognised from the outset that structural information would be key to understanding the interactions that were made with the target protein and, more importantly, key to ensuring that hits could be rapidly and efficiently elaborated into diverse chemical series.

Historically, X-ray diffraction has been the method of choice for providing accurate structural data for protein–ligand complexes. By developing automated methods for data collection and structure solution, Astex has 'industrialised' the process of obtaining complex structures and in doing so demonstrated that it provides a robust and sensitive method for fragment-based screening [4, 5].

One of the concerns expressed by others was that fragments which bind with millimolar affinities may not demonstrate the ordered binding modes that are required for detection using a diffraction method. However, despite their low affinities, fragment hits generally have ligand efficiencies (defined loosely as the amount of binding free energy per atom) that are as high as, or higher than, the most potent inhibitors. Thus, at the atomic level, the interactions they make with their protein target are strong and may well be close to optimal. The reason for their low affinity is simply that these interactions are few in number and must overcome the loss of a large amount of rotational and translational entropy when the fragment binds to the protein. When the fragment is elaborated and makes more interactions with the protein, the entropic penalty remains approximately constant while the binding enthalpy increases. However, the initial interactions remain key and usually contribute disproportionately to the overall free energy of binding. In effect, fragment screening seeks out the strongest interactions that can be made between the protein and the chemical groups represented in the library, since only these will overcome the large entropic cost in binding (ΔG_{rigid}). This cost has been estimated as 15–$20 \, kJ.mol^{-1}$ [6]. The approximate energetic analysis described in Figure 16.1 should make this clear.

The numerical values given in Figure 16.1 were taken from the detection and development of fragment hits against the atypical kinase, PKB. A number of chemical lead series were generated from the fragment hits: one such series has been described [7].

The concept of ligand efficiency or binding free energy per (non-hydrogen) atom has proved to be extremely useful [8]. It provides a size independent parameter that can be used to ensure that the optimisation of the initial hit proceeds in such a way that the final product will conform to Lipinski's rule for the molecular weight of orally-active

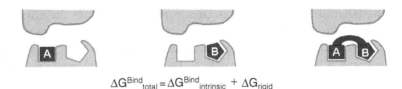

$$\Delta G^{Bind}_{total} = \Delta G^{Bind}_{intrinsic} + \Delta G_{rigid}$$

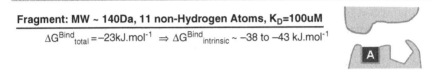

Fragment: MW ~ 140Da, 11 non-Hydrogen Atoms, K_D=100uM

$\Delta G^{Bind}_{total} = -23kJ.mol^{-1} \Rightarrow \Delta G^{Bind}_{intrinsic} \sim -38$ to -43 kJ.mol^{-1}

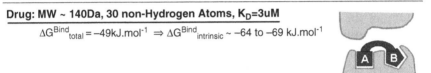

Drug: MW ~ 140Da, 30 non-Hydrogen Atoms, K_D=3uM

$\Delta G^{Bind}_{total} = -49kJ.mol^{-1} \Rightarrow \Delta G^{Bind}_{intrinsic} \sim -64$ to -69 kJ.mol^{-1}

- **Despite a 33000 fold increase in potency and threefold increase in MW, the intial fragment still supplies ~60% of the intrinsic binding energy of the drug**

Figure 16.1 Experimental estimates for ΔG_{rigid} can be obtained by comparing the affinities of linked molecules and their fragments. Best current estimate is 15–20 kJ.mol^{-1}, that is three orders of magnitude in K_D. Reproduced by Permission of Astex Therapeutics.

drugs [9]. It is defined here as:

$$LE = \frac{-\Delta G_{bind} \, (kcal/mol)}{number \, of \, non\text{-}hydrogen \, atoms}$$

Some important, ligand-efficient examples of fragment binding are shown in Figure 16.2.

One important contribution of the combination of fragment screening and X-ray structure determination is to reveal interactions that are surprisingly ligand efficient. For example, the amino-pyrazine shown above bound to CDK2 (PDB = 1WCC) was predicted to be a classical 'kinase hinge' binder and was expected to form two hydrogen bonds to the kinase activation loop via its adjacent ring nitrogen and amino groups. In fact, the presence of the sterically demanding and electron withdrawing chloro atom has favoured an alternative binding mode in which three hydrogen bonds are formed by the second ring nitrogen and two adjacent aromatic protons. These interactions are not weak – a ligand efficiency

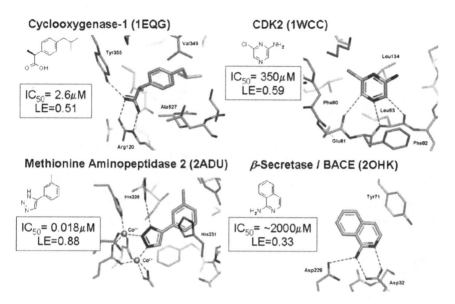

Figure 16.2 What do ligand-efficient interactions look like? Reproduced by Permission of Astex Therapeutics.

of 0.59 represents twice the free energy of binding per non-hydrogen atom that is required to remain within 'Lipinski space'. However, the incorporation of CH–––O hydrogen bonds into a drug design strategy might have been overlooked without these data. The apparent strength of the interaction may also be a reminder that binding is opposed by the free energy required to desolvate the interacting groups and that a reduction in this term can partially compensate for the formation of a weaker hydrogen bond to the protein.

The Astex Pyramid screening approach is to use a number of orthogonal biophysical methods to identify fragments which bind with low (millimolar) affinity to the protein target. These methods will include a crystallographic screen in which suitable crystals of the target are soaked in solutions containing fragments, followed by identification of any hits using difference Fourier maps. In a typical Pyramid screen, an NMR method will also be employed in which binding is detected from changes in the NMR properties of the fragment. Often the NMR method will include a competition step in which the fragment displaces or is displaced by ligands that bind at well defined sites. In this way additional hits can be grouped and prioritised for X-ray structural studies. The Pyramid process is shown schematically in Figure 16.3.

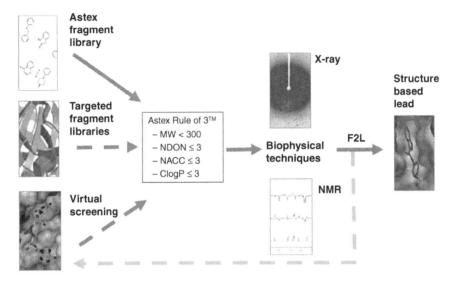

Figure 16.3 The Astex Pyramid^{TM} Approach. Reproduced by Permission of Astex Therapeutics.

16.3 DESIGN OF FRAGMENT LIBRARIES

The content of fragment screening libraries is a subject of intense interest and commercial importance. In a general sense it is clear that, by virtue of their smaller size and lower complexity, fragments are more able to explore the range of possible interactions in a protein binding site than larger, more complex molecules, albeit at a cost in binding affinity [10]. However, in order practically to exploit this theoretical advantage, the fragment library must contain the widest possible range of functional groups combined in molecules that allow geometric and physical variations (e.g. charge, dipole, hydrophobicity). In some cases, the molecules may also need to be tailored to a particular detection technique or philosophy of chemical elaboration.

The current Astex fragment library is the product of several years experience and many rounds of structure-based screening. The general rules for selecting suitable fragments have been elaborated as the 'Astex Rule of Three' (molecular weight <300 Da, number of hydrogen bond donors <3, number of hydrogen bond acceptors <3, clogP <3) [11]. However, additional factors, such as aqueous and non-aqueous solubility, stability, novelty, chemical tractability and 'drug-likeness', will also play a part in the selection process. Using our methods, fragment screening has reliably yielded multiple hits which could be elaborated into several, distinct chemical series. As the fragment library has evolved, the diversity of the hits has been improved and this has enabled more efficient optimisation by transferring SAR information back and forth between different chemical series.

During the screening and optimisation process, all information is combined into an Oracle database that includes biophysical, structural and bioassay data and allows it to be accessed by all members of the company. Sophisticated tools have been developed to allow non-experts to view and interpret to X-ray structural data (including electron densities) and to contribute to the chemical design process by performing docking experiments. This is exemplified by the use of Astex Viewer™, a molecular viewer optimised for protein complexes, which has been made freely available [12].

16.4 BIOPHYSICAL METHODS IN PYRAMID™

Using our methods, the improved sampling of chemical space that is possible when using a diverse fragment library is translated into hit rates between 5 and 15% for a range of druggable targets, including kinases, proteases and ATP-ases. Thus, the number of hits is rarely a concern [13]. The hits generally have good ligand efficiencies (LE >0.3) and affinities for the target between 10 mM and 100 µM. However, efficient drug design requires that these hits are not only reliably detected but also characterised by their affinities and the interactions that they make with the target. Astex has addressed this by integrating multiple biophysical methods into the Pyramid screening cascade, as outlined below:

- The end product is an **X-ray structure** of the fragment hit complexed to a relevant protein construct.
- Ideally, hits will be characterized by their **affinities/ligand efficiencies** (14, 15).
- Two, or even three, assay methods are applied **in parallel**, selected from X-ray, NMR, ITC and bioassay.
- **Hit rates** are established during 'Pre-Pyramid' experiments and appropriate cocktail sizes are chosen (X-ray, NMR).
- **Affinities** are estimated (ITC/NMR/Bioassay); hits may need elaboration or selection of follow-ups before coming on-scale in a bioassay.

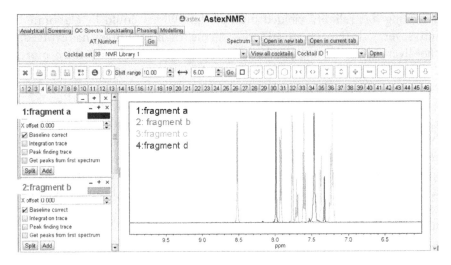

Figure 16.4 NMR Cocktailing. Reproduced by Permission of Astex Therapeutics.

The early estimation of hit rates from a trial screen is important, since it allows optimum cocktail sizes to be chosen for the subsequent full screen. When screening by X-ray, fragments can be mixed together in a way that maximizes the diversity of molecular shapes within each cocktail, thus simplifying the identification of any hits from that cocktail. In an NMR experiment where the proton spectrum of the fragments is observed, cocktails of compounds are designed in such a way that the overlap between their proton spectra is minimized. The result for a cocktail of four fragments is shown in Figure 16.4.

Data from a typical NMR screening experiment are shown below in Figure 16.5. This experiment used a Water-LOGSY pulse sequence [16] in which binding of azaindole to a kinase target was detected by a change in the sign of the magnetization transfer between the solvent (water) and the ligand in the presence of the kinase (lower and middle traces). This effect could be reversed by the addition of a tight-binding inhibitor (upper trace).

16.5 APPLICATION OF PYRAMID™ TO HSP90

A number of companies, including groups at Active Sight, Astex and Vernalis, have applied their methods to screen for inhibitors of the chaperone, HSP90. As these data begin to be published, this target is likely

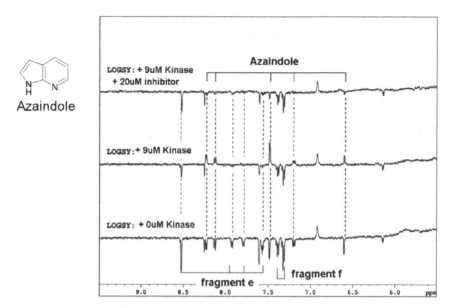

Figure 16.5 Water-LOGSY pulse sequence in cocktails. Reproduced by Permission of Astex Therapeutics.

to provide a useful means of benchmarking the various approaches and chemical libraries used in the screening.

At Astex, a crystal system was established in which the N-terminal, ATP-ase domain was shown to be soakable, using a variety of targeted fragments generated by combining in-house experience and proprietary modelling. X-ray screening of the entire fragment library revealed novel hits, some of which generated substantial conformational changes in the ATP domain. In parallel, an NMR screen gave a good hit rate (7.5%) in which hits could be ranked according to their displacement of the weakly bound product, ADP.

Follow-up of selected hits using crystallography generated more than 30 fragment structures from which more than 10 distinct chemical series were identified. Several of these series were progressed into a chemistry programme, which ultimately led to the identification of a clinical candidate within two years. An important component of the programme was the use of isothermal titration calorimetry to generate affinity data for the developing series. Data for one of these series are shown in Figure 16.6.

While not central to the development of the series, it is interesting to note the changes in enthalpy and entropy during the process of optimisation. Variations in ΔH and $T\Delta S$ are typically two to threefold greater

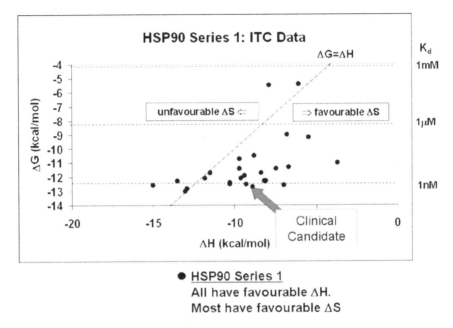

Figure 16.6   ITC Data: HSP90, Series 1. Reproduced by Permission of Astex Therapeutics.

than their combined effect on ΔG, demonstrating the well known phenomenon of enthalpy–entropy compensation. The molecule selected as the clinical candidate has both favourable enthalpy and entropy of binding. Equipotent molecules in the same chemical series can display very different enthalpies and entropies. In this case, structure-guided design has led to optimised leads with a range of thermodynamic signatures which may be valuable in further development [17].

16.6 SUMMARY AND CONCLUSIONS

The combination of X-ray crystallography and NMR spectroscopy provides a good platform for fragment-based drug discovery [18]. The use of multiple biophysical methods to detect fragment hits increases the probability of their detection and affords opportunities to identify fragments which display unusual mechanisms of action and to eliminate false positives. The inclusion of X-ray structural data, obtained during screening or as part of the hit validation process has revealed unexpected, ligand efficient interactions and enabled rapid and successful progression of fragment hits into clinical candidates with good potency and tailored selectivity.

The additional information obtained from using multiple techniques is rarely redundant. Integration of the methods allows the best set of techniques for screening to be selected at an early stage. It also allows reliable estimates of hit rates, likely ligand efficiencies and 'druggability' of the chosen target or site. Where there are discrepancies between the detection methods, these are usually related to the effects of differences between the affinities or physicochemical properties of individual compounds. Some of the possible reasons for different outcomes in X-ray and NMR screening experiments are:

- Ligand-detected NMR hits are not always observed in an X-ray soaking experiment.
  - Mainly due to solubility/potency ratio or ionic strength;
  - Ligand concentration: NMR experiment will detect hits at fragment concentrations $\leq K_D$. Good occupancy in X-ray requires concentrations > 5 times K_D;
  - NMR hits may show competition but could also be allosteric;
  - binding to protein may have multiple modes (static disorder).
- X-ray hits are not always observed in NMR screens.
  - If fragment solubility is not an issue, X-ray soaks at very high concentration reveal weak hits ($K_D > 5$–$10\,mM$);
  - NMR experiments at high fragment concentration would require high protein concentrations; also
  - some fragments have poor NMR properties.
- Confirmational and entropic differences (+pH, salt etc.) between Xtal and solution can alter K_D

Additional biophysical methods such as calorimetry and thermal unfolding have been incorporated into the Pyramid approach, to provide information on the overall strength of binding (ligand efficiency) or the consequences of small changes in the fragment (group efficiency). The knowledge gained from seven years of fragment screening, including more than 25 Pyramid screens covering a diverse set of target proteins can be summarised as follows:

- Fragments
  - Seldom move
  - Can induce conformational movement
  - Difficult to predict binding mode
  - Generate multiple hits per target (typically 5–20)

- Hits
  - ○ Multiple hits per target making a limited number of interactions
  - ○ Individual interactions are readily explored
  - ○ Usually transformed into several lead series
  - ○ Series progression depends on multiple factors
  - ○ Can usually transfer SAR between series

ACKNOWLEDGEMENTS

The author wishes to acknowledge the contributions of the entire Astex team of Crystallographers, Structural Biologists, Biologists, Computational Chemists, Chemists and Biophysicists. Central to the overview presented here has been the vision of the Astex founders, Harren Jhoti, Tom Blundell and Chris Abell, the computational tools developed by Ian Tickle, Mike Hartshorn and Paul Mortenson, the fragment library design carried out by Chris Murray and Miles Congreve and the careful experimental work performed by the biophysics group of Hayley Angove, Joe Coyle, Finn Holding and Rob van Montfort.

REFERENCES

1. Verlinde, C.L.M.J., Kim, H., Bernstein, B.E. *et al.* in *Structure-based drug design* (ed. P. Veerapandian), Marcel Dekker, Inc., New York, pp 365–394 (1997).
2. Shuker, S.B., Hajduk, P. J., Meadows, R.P., and Fesik, S.W., *Science*, **274**, 1531–1534 (1996).
3. Fejzo, J., Lepre, C.A., Peng, J.W. *et al. Chemistry and Biology*, **6**, 755–769 (1999).
4. Blundell, T. L., Jhoti, H. and Abell, C., *Nature Reviews Drug Discovery*, **1**, 45–54 (2002).
5. Mooij, W.T.M., Hartshorn, M.J., Tickle, I.J. *et al. ChemMedChem*, **1**, 827–838 (2006).
6. Murray, C.W. and Verdonk, M.L. in *Methods and Principles in Medicinal Chemistry* Vol. 34 (Fragment-Based Approaches in Drug Discovery, eds Jahnke, W. and Erlanson, D.A.), Wiley-VCH Verlag GmbH, 55–66 (2006).
7. Caldwell, J.J., Davies, T.G., Donald, A. *et al. J. Med. Chem.*, **51**, 2147–2157 (2008).
8. Abad-Zapatero, C. and Metz, J.I., *Drug Discovery Today*, **10**, 464–469 (2005).
9. Lipinski, C.A., Lombardo, F., Dominy, B.W. and Feeney, P.J., *Adv. Drug Delivery Rev.*, **23**, 3–25 (1997).
10. Carr, R. and Hann, M., *Modern Drug Discovery*, **5**, 45–48 (2002).
11. Congreve, M., Carr, R., Murray, C. and Jhoti, H., *Drug Discovery Today*, **8**, 876–877 (2003).
12. http://www.openastexviewer.net/web/

13. Hajduk, P., Huth, J.R., and Fesik, S.W., *J. Med.Chem.*, **48**, 2518–2525 (2005).
14. Hopkins, A.L., Groom, C.R. and Alex, A., *Drug Discovery Today*, **9**, 430–431 (2004).
15. Kuntz, I.D., Chen, K., Sharp, K.A. and Kollman, P.A., *Proc. Nat. Acad. Sci. USA*, **96**, 9997–10002 (1999).
16. Dalvit, C., Fogliatto, G., Stewart, A. *et al. J. Biomolecular NMR*, **21**, 349–359 (2001).
17. Freire, E., *Drug Discovery Today*, **13**, 869–874 (2008).
18. Jhoti, H., Cleasby, A., Verdonk, M. and Williams, G., *Curr. Opin. Chem. Biol.*, **11**, 1–9 (2007).

17

Characterisation of Antibodies Against the Active Conformation of $G_{\alpha i1}$ Using the SRU-BIND® Label-Free Detection System

Melanie Leveridge, Chun-Wa Chung and Trevor Wattam
GlaxoSmithKline, Stevenage, UK

Label-Free Technologies for Drug Discovery   Edited by Matthew Cooper and Lorenz M. Mayr
© 2011 John Wiley & Sons, Ltd

17.1 INTRODUCTION

G-protein coupled receptors (GPCRs) account for approximately 30% of all launched drug targets and are historically the most successful therapeutic target family (1). These receptors signal through guanine nucleotide-binding proteins (G-proteins). G-proteins themselves are heterodimeric proteins consisting of three subunits (α, β and γ) (2). In the inactive state, the G-protein α subunit is bound to guanosine 5'-diphosphate (GDP); however, receptor activation by ligand promotes the release of GDP and its replacement by guanosine 5'-triphosphate (GTP) (3) (Figure 17.1). This results in a conformational change that enables both the α and β/γ subunits of the G-protein to modulate effector enzymes, which in turn synthesise secondary messengers and activate other downstream processes (4). Finally, GTPase enzymes hydrolyse the terminal phosphate of GTP, essentially terminating the process and returning the system to an inactive state (3).

Assays which quantify GTP exchange at the level of the G-protein permit a direct measurement of GPCR activation. However, current assays require the use of radioactivity, for example the widely used $[^{35}S]$ guanosine 5'-[γ-thio]triphosphate ($[^{35}S]$GTPγS) binding assay (5). In this assay $[^{35}S]$GTPγS replaces endogenous GTP. Guanosine 5'-[γ-thio]triphosphate (GTPγS) is a poorly hydrolysable analogue of GTP (6), and $[^{35}S]$GTPγS labelled Gα subunits therefore accumulate in proportion to the level of receptor activation and can be measured. Due to the need for radioactivity in this and other assays of G-protein activation, there is a desire to identify alternative methods. Work has, therefore, been ongoing to identify antibodies capable of binding only the active conformation of native G-proteins (7). Such antibodies would enable radiolabel-free plate-based assays and high content imaging assays of GPCR activity in both recombinant cells

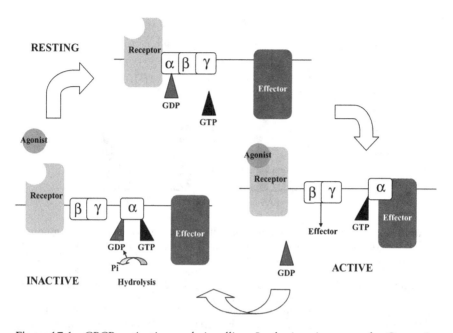

Figure 17.1 GPCR activation and signalling. In the inactive state, the G-protein α subunit is bound to guanosine 5′-diphosphate (GDP). However, receptor activation by ligand promotes the release of GDP and its replacement by guanosine 5′-triphosphate (GTP). This results in a conformational change that enables both the α and β/γ subunits of the G-protein to modulate effector enzymes, which in turn synthesise secondary messengers and activate other downstream processes. Finally, GTPase enzymes hydrolyse the terminal phosphate of GTP, essentially terminating the process and returning the system to an inactive state.

and primary tissues. They may also enable truly 'label-free' assays of GPCR activation.

To date, three monoclonal antibodies have been identified which display marked selectivity towards either a constitutively active mutant or GTPγS-bound form of $G\alpha_{i1}$, $G\alpha_{i2}$, $G\alpha_{i3}$ and $G\alpha_o$ (7) (Figure 17.2). These antibodies have been characterised by immunocytochemistry and sodium dodecyl sulfate polyacrylamide gel electrophoresis (SDS-PAGE) (7) and have also been shown to detect agonist activation of both transfected and endogenous G-proteins (data not published).

The aim of the work described here was to determine the affinity of these three antibodies for the active and inactive conformations of $G\alpha_{i1}$, with a view to establishing a GPCR activation assay in a label-free format. Experiments were performed using the SRU Biosystems Biomolecular Interaction Detection (SRU BIND®) label-free detection system, which uses a guided-mode resonant filter (GMRF) biosensor incorporated into standard microplate formats (8). This biosensor reflects only a single

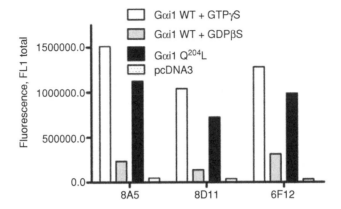

Figure 17.2 Antibody producing plasma cells were harvested from mice immunised with GTP-loaded $G\alpha_{i1}$ and used to generate hybridomas. 763 hybridoma supernatants were mixed with fluorescently labelled secondary antibody and HEK293 cells transfected under each of the following four conditions: (1) HEK293T cells transfected with wild-type (WT) $G\alpha_{i1}$ cDNA and incubated with $100\,\mu$M GTPγS to maintain the $G\alpha_{i1}$ in the active (GTP-bound) conformation (white bars). (2) HEK293T cells transfected with wild-type $G\alpha_{i1}$ cDNA and incubated with $100\,\mu$M GDPβS to maintain the $G\alpha_{i1}$ in the inactive (GDP-bound) conformation (grey bars). (3) HEK293T cells transfected with constitutively active $G\alpha_{i1}$ Q^{204}L cDNA (black bars). (4) HEK293T cells transfected with empty pcDNA3 (dotted bars). The mixtures were then added to a 384-well plate and screened using the ABI 8200 cellular detection system (Applied Biosystems, Foster City, CA, USA), which is based on fluorescence microvolume assay technology (FMAT). Of the 763 hybridoma clones screened, three showed selectivity toward conditions in which $G\alpha_{i1}$ was expressed and in the active (GTP-bound) conformation. These were 8A5, 8D11, and 6F12. (Taken from [7].)

wavelength at a time, referred to as the peak wavelength value (PWV). When a binding event occurs on the surface of the biosensor, there is an increase in the PWV and hence real time binding can be measured by a change in PWV over time. This system has been shown to enable very rapid and accurate characterisation of protein–protein binding interactions (8), and was therefore a suitable platform for studies of G-protein binding to the anti-$G\alpha_i$ monoclonal antibodies.

17.2 MATERIALS AND METHODS

17.2.1 Materials

For experiments performed on the SRU BIND® label-free detection system, immobilisations were performed in a 96-well SA1 streptavidin-coated BIND® microplate (SRU Biosystems, Woburn, MA, USA). Plates were read on an SRU BIND® plate reader (SRU Biosystems). Biotin conjugated, affinity purified anti-mouse immunoglobulin G (IgG) F(c) was purchased from Rockland (Gilbertsville, PA, USA). Monoclonal test antibodies 8A5, 8D11, 6F12 and a mouse IgG1 isotype control antibody were supplied by GlaxoSmithKline Bio-Reagents Department (Stevenage, UK) (7). Throughout the experiments all antibodies were diluted in phosphate buffered saline (PBS) (Invitrogen, CA, USA). Myristoylated recombinant rat $G\alpha_{i1}$ subunit was purchased from Merck KGaA (Darmstadt, Germany) and diluted in an assay buffer consisting of 100 mM NaCl, 20 mM HEPES and 3 mM $MgCl_2$, pH 7.5 (all chemicals from Sigma-Aldrich, St. Louis, MO, USA). The rat $G\alpha_{i1}$ was then incubated with either 2 mM guanosine 5'-[γ-thio] triphosphate (GTPγS) or 2 mM guanosine 5'-[β-thio] diphosphate (GDPβS), both from Sigma-Aldrich. All serial dilutions were performed in a 96-well polypropylene microplate, V-well (Greiner Bio-one, Stonehouse, UK).

For experiments performed on the BIAcore™ 3000, immobilisations were performed on a CM5 sensor chip, (Biacore, Uppsala, Sweden). An amine coupling kit (1-ethyl-3-(3-dimethylaminopropyl), carbodiimide hydrochloride (EDC), N-hydroxysuccinimide (NHS), 1.0M ethanolamine-HCl pH 8.5), (Biacore) was used to immobilise an anti-mouse IgG (Fc) specific reagent (anti-mIgG) (Biacore), diluted to 30 μg/ml in 5 mM sodium acetate buffer pH 4.5. Monoclonal test antibodies 8A5, 8D11, 6F12, as well as rat $G\alpha_{i1}$ were immobilised in HBS-EP run buffer (10 mM HEPES pH 7.4, 150 mM NaCl, 3 mM EDTA, 0.005% v/v Surfactant P20) (Biacore). The sensor chip was regenerated using 100mM Phosphoric acid regeneration buffer.

17.2.2 Methods

17.2.2.1 Immobilisation of Biotin Conjugated Purified Rabbit Anti-mouse IgG F(c)

A 96-well SA1 streptavidin-coated BIND® microplate was washed once thoroughly with distilled water. The plate was dried by inverting and gently tapping on a paper towel. 100 μl PBS was added to each well of the plate and emptied onto a paper towel. This process was repeated twice. A third addition of 100 μl per well of PBS was added and the plate read continuously on the SRU BIND® plate reader for 30 minutes to equilibrate (or until the response had reached a plateau). After 30 minutes the PBS was removed using a multichannel pipette and replaced with 50 µl per well of biotin conjugated rabbit anti-mouse IgG F(c) at a concentration of 40 µg/ml in PBS. The plate was read continuously on the SRU BIND® plate reader until equilibrium was reached, usually 90 minutes. The antibody was removed from the plate and the plate washed by adding and removing 100 µl per well of PBS three times.

17.2.2.2 Titration of Conformation Specific Anti-Gα_i Antibody Clones 8A5, 8D11 and 6F12 onto Immobilised Rabbit Anti-mouse IgG F(c)

A one in two, eight point serial dilution in PBS of each of the test antibodies 8A5, 8D11 and 6F12, as well as the mouse IgG1 isotype control, was performed down one column of a 96-well polypropylene plate. A starting concentration of 100 µg/ml was used. 50 µl of this dilution series for each of the four antibodies was transferred into two columns of the BIND® microplate, onto which the biotinylated rabbit anti-mouse IgG F(c) was already immobilised (Section 17.2.2.1). The plate was left to read continuously for one hour on the BIND® plate reader. After one hour the unbound antibodies were removed from the plate and the plate washed by adding and removing 100 µl per well of PBS three times. Data were exported to Excel via the experimental management software system (EMS) export wizard and plotted in GraFit version 5.0.8 (Erithacus Software Ltd) to enable calculation of K_D values.

17.2.2.3 Titration of Recombinant Rat Gα_{i1} Subunit onto Immobilised Test Antibodies

A working stock of 500 nM recombinant rat Gα_{i1} was made up in assay buffer. This stock was split and pre-incubated for one hour with either 2 mM GTPγS or 2 mM GDPβS to lock the Gα_{i1} into either the active (GTP-bound) or inactive (GDP-bound) conformation. After one hour, a one in two serial dilution of the pre-incubated 500 nM stock was performed down one column of a 96-well polypropylene plate in either assay buffer with 2 mM GTPγS added, or assay buffer with 2 mM GDPβS added, according to the pre-incubation. A 96-well BIND® microplate was set up with 40 µg/ml of biotinylated rabbit anti-mouse IgG F(c) immobilised on the surface of eight columns of the plate (Section 17.2.2.1) and with 25 µg/ml of each of the mouse IgG monoclonal test antibodies 8D11, 8A5, 6F12 and mouse IgG1 isotype control immobilised

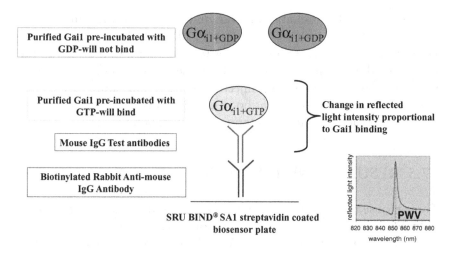

Figure 17.3 Schematic of an SRU BIND® assay to determine affinity and specificity of three monoclonal antibodies 8A5, 8D11 and 6F12 for active and inactive conformations of rat $G\alpha_{i1}$. A biotinylated rabbit anti-mouse IgG F(c) antibody, plus each of the three test antibodies 8A5, 8D11 and 6F12, were first immobilised to the surface of an SA1 streptavidin-coated BIND® 96-well microplate. A titration of rat $G\alpha_{i1}$ which had been pre-incubated in either 2 mM GTPγS or 2 mM GDPβS was added and binding detected using the SRU BIND® plate reader.

onto two columns each of this rabbit anti-mouse IgG F(c) surface. A concentration of 25 µg/ml was chosen based on the data from the antibody titration (Section 17.2.2.2) and immobilisation was performed as per Section 17.2.2.2. 50 µl per well of either the 2 mM GTPγS buffer or 2 mM GDPβS buffer (one column of each buffer type per antibody) was added to the BIND® plate and left to equilibrate. After one hour, the buffer was removed and replaced with 50 µl of each of the two $G\alpha_{i1}$ dilution series in four columns of the plate, such that each test antibody was combined with one GTPγS dilution and one GDPβS dilution. An assay schematic is shown in Figure 17.3. The plate was read continuously on the BIND® plate reader for two hours and data were exported using the EMS export wizard.

17.2.2.4 Binding of Antibodies 8A5, 8D11 and 6F12 to Purified Rat $G\alpha_{i1}$ Subunit on the BIAcore™ 3000

An anti-mouse IgG capture surface was prepared on a CM5 sensor chip using standard amine coupling conditions. Each antibody sample was then diluted to 10 μg/ml in run buffer, and injected over the anti-mouse IgG capture surface for two minutes to allow sufficient antibody to be captured. This was followed by a two minute injection of the rat $G\alpha_{i1}$ diluted in run buffer to 4 μg/ml. The sensor chip surface was then regenerated with a three minute injection of 0.1M phosphoric acid before repeating the cycle for each antibody sample. Report points were taken pre and post each injection to determine the level of binding for injection.

17.3 RESULTS AND DISCUSSION

Three mouse monoclonal antibodies have been identified that recognise only the active, GTP-bound conformation of $G\alpha_{i1}$, $G\alpha_{i2}$, $G\alpha_{i3}$ and $G\alpha_o$ (7). These antibodies may enable nonradioactive plate-based assays for high throughput screening (HTS), compound profiling, and also label-free assays of GPCR activation. The aim of the work described here was to further characterise these antibodies by determining their affinity for the active and inactive conformations of $G\alpha_{i1}$, with a view to establishing a GPCR activation assay in a label free format. To enable this, an assay was set up using the SRU BIND® label-free detection system (8).

40 μg/ml of a biotin conjugated purified rabbit anti-mouse IgG F(c) in PBS was immobilised onto an SA1 streptavidin-coated 96-well BIND® microplate. 90 minutes incubation was sufficient to reach equilibrium, and at this time a mean normalised peak wavelength value of 2.13 nm $^+/_-$ 0.15 nm was achieved. The CV across the plate was 7.21% (data not shown).

A titration of each of the anti-$G\alpha_i$ monoclonal antibodies (8A5, 8D11 and 6F12) was performed to determine the optimum concentration for immobilisation of these antibodies onto the rabbit anti-mouse IgG F(c) coated surface. A mouse IgG1 isotope control antibody was also included. This antibody does not recognise nor bind to $G\alpha_i$ regardless of its conformational state, hence acts as a negative control. A clear concentration dependent change in peak wavelength value was observed upon addition of all four antibodies to the plate (Figure 17.4), and all bound to the rabbit anti-mouse IgG F(c) coated surface with an affinity in the region of 50 nM (Figure 17.4), which is similar to values quoted by SRU Biosystems for a mouse IgG monoclonal antibody binding to a rabbit anti-mouse IgG F(c) coated surface (personal communication from SRU Biosystems). The similarity in K_D values between each of the anti-$G\alpha_i$ antibodies and the mouse IgG1 isotope control is consistent with the fact that they are all mouse immunoglobulin G (IgG) antibodies, and

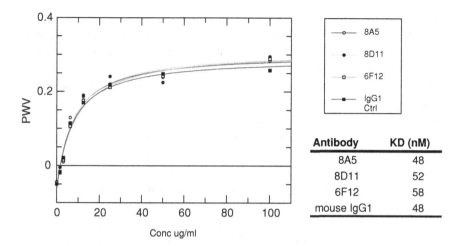

Figure 17.4 Titration of monoclonal antibodies 8A5, 8D11, 6F12 and mouse IgG1 onto a rabbit anti-mouse IgG F(c) coated SA1 BIND® microplate. Having immobilised the antibodies, the plate was read continuously for one hour on the BIND® plate reader. A concentration dependent change in peak wavelength value was observed upon addition of each of the four test antibodies. Data were exported using the EMS export wizard and plotted using Grafit. The K_D of each of the four test antibodies binding to the rabbit anti-mouse surface was found to be approximately 50 nM.

therefore all have molecular weights of ~150 kDa. The shift in PWV generated on the SRU BIND® is in this case proportional to the molecular weight of the test antibody relative to that of the rabbit anti-mouse IgG F(c) to which it is binding (BIND® Technical Note 301). An antibody concentration of 25ug/ml was chosen for further work, as this concentration allows maximum signal generation without saturation of the biosensor surface. Saturation of the surface can lead to steric interactions between immobilised molecules and subsequent inhibition of binding (9).

Having determined the optimal concentration for test antibody immobilisation, the affinity of each of these antibodies for GTP and GDP bound $G\alpha_{i1}$ was determined. Each of the test antibodies 8A5, 8D11 and 6F12, together with the negative control mouse IgG1 isotype control, were immobilised onto two columns each of a 96-well SA1 BIND® microplate which had been pre-coated with rabbit anti-mouse IgG F(c). To one of these columns a serial dilution of GTPγS-loaded $G\alpha_{i1}$ was added, and to the other column a serial dilution of GDPβS-loaded $G\alpha_{i1}$ was added. GTPγS is a poorly hydrolysable analogue of GTP which maintains the G-protein subunit in the active conformation by preventing hydrolysis of GTP by GTPase enzymes (6). GDPβS is a poorly hydrolysable analogue of GDP and, therefore, maintains the G-protein in an inactive conformation in the same way. The three antibodies used in this experiment have been shown to recognise only the active, GTP-bound conformation of Gα$_i$ (7). One would therefore expect to see high affinity binding of the GTPγS-loaded Gα$_{i1}$ to the test antibodies, but low affinity or no binding of the GDPβS-loaded Gα$_{i1}$. The G-protein was not expected to bind to the mouse IgG1 isotype negative control under any conditions.

Over a two hour period following addition of rat Gα$_{i1}$, an increase in peak wavelength value was observed in columns of the plate containing GTPγS-loaded Gα$_{i1}$. However, the magnitude of response was between 0.08 and 0.10 nm at the highest concentration of Gα$_{i1}$ for all four antibodies tested, including the mouse IgG1 isotype negative control. In addition, a similar level of response was observed in columns containing GDPβS-loaded Gα$_{i1}$ (Figure 17.5). These data suggest that

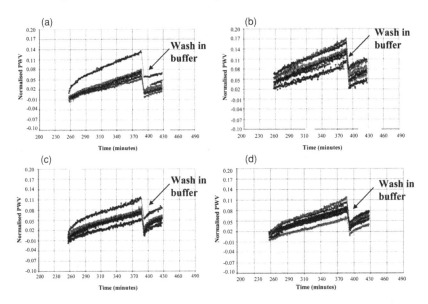

Figure 17.5   Serial dilutions of rat Gα$_{i1}$ binding to monoclonal antibody 8A5 and a mouse IgG1 control antibody are shown as follows: (a) rat Gα$_{i1}$ pre-incubated and diluted in 2 mM GTPγS buffer binding to conformation dependent antibody 8A5; (b) rat Gα$_{i1}$ pre-incubated and diluted in 2 mM GTPγS buffer binding to a mouse IgG1 negative control antibody; (c) rat Gα$_{i1}$ pre-incubated and diluted in 2 mM GDPβS buffer binding to conformation dependent antibody 8A5; (d) rat Gα$_{i1}$ pre-incubated and diluted in 2 mM GDPβS buffer binding to a mouse IgG1 negative control antibody. The same results were observed for the other conformation dependent antibodies 8D11 and 6F12 (data not shown).

any binding observed was nonspecific. The shape of the BIND® trace in each case also indicates nonspecific binding, as the peak wavelength value continues to increase even after two hours. If a true binding event had occurred, the peak wavelength value should increase upon addition of $G\alpha_{i1}$ at a rate dependent on the K_a of $G\alpha_{i1}$ and eventually reach equilibrium. One would expect the maximum change in PWV before equilibrium is reached to be ~0.07 nm upon addition of $G\alpha_{i1}$, based on its molecular weight (40 kDa) relative to that of the test antibodies (150 kDa), assuming a stoichiometry of 1:1. In fact, the response continues to rise beyond 0.10 nm after two hours. In addition, the majority of binding is lost upon washing. Both of these occurrences are further indicative of a non-specific binding event.

This apparent high level of nonspecific binding was unexpected, as the plate was re-equilibrated for one hour with either 2 mM GTPγS or 2 mM GDPβS buffer prior to addition of the $G\alpha_{i1}$ dilution series, to minimise bulk shifts in the refractive index. It is possible that the GTPγS/GDPβS were at such high concentrations in the buffer (2 mM) that, in fact, a total re-equilibration did not occur in the hour allocated. There are also other factors which may cause nonspecific binding, such as changes in pH, temperature and salt concentrations (10), so further optimisation of the method may be possible.

It is also possible that true binding events did occur upon addition of the $G\alpha_{i1}$, but were masked by the nonspecific binding events in the plate. To determine whether this was indeed the case, an experiment was also performed on the BIAcore™ 3000 Surface Plasmon Resonance (SPR) Spectrometer, which measures the change in refractive index when soluble antigen binds to an antibody immobilised on a modified gold film (11). Each of the anti-$G\alpha_i$ monoclonal antibodies 8A5, 8D11 and 6F12 were immobilised in turn onto a BIAcore™ chip. GTPγS-loaded $G\alpha_{i1}$ was then flowed over this chip. No binding was observed on the BIAcore™ 3000 for any of the three test antibodies (Figure 17.6), suggesting that the lack of true binding observed with the BIND® assay was genuine. This also confirms that any changes in peak wavelength value that were observed on the SRU BIND® were indeed the result of nonspecific binding.

17.4 CONCLUSIONS

This work has successfully demonstrated the use of SA1 streptavidin-coated BIND® microplates for the immobilisation of a biotinylated rabbit

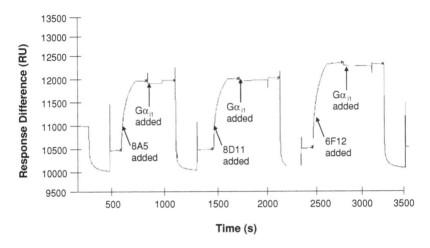

Figure 17.6 BIAcore^{TM} trace showing binding of GTPγS-bound Gα$_{i1}$ to immobilised antibodies 8A5, 8D11 and 6F12. An initial increase in response is observed upon addition of antibody, which equilibrates rapidly. However, upon addition of the Gα$_{i1,}$ no increase in response is observed for any of the three antibodies tested, indicating that the antibodies are not binding to the antigen.

anti-mouse IgG F(c) and subsequent immobilisation of the four mouse IgG monoclonal test antibodies. It was possible to show clear concentration dependent changes in peak wavelength value upon addition of four mouse IgG antibodies (8A5, 8D11, 6F12 and mouse IgG1 isotype control), with K_D values in the region of 50 nM when binding to a rabbit anti-mouse IgG F(c) coated surface. These values are consistent with data generated by the manufacturer (personal communication from SRU Biosystems).

However, it was not possible to demonstrate binding of rat Gα$_{i1}$ to the immobilised antibodies in either its active or inactive conformation. Antibodies 8D11, 8A5 and 6F12 have previously been shown to bind specifically to the active, GTP-bound conformation of Gα$_{i,}$ (7). Although the presence of nonspecific binding events in the BIND$^{®}$ assay may have masked the specific binding of this antigen to the antibodies of interest, the lack of binding observed on the BIAcore^{TM} 3000 suggests that specific binding did not occur and that the antibodies have either extremely low or no affinity for the GTPγS-loaded Gα$_{i1}$ under the conditions tested.

There are a number of possible reasons for the lack of binding, including the possibility that insufficient GTPγS was added to convert the Gα$_{i1}$ to its active conformation. This is, however, unlikely because a concentration of 2 mM GTPγS was included in the buffer; this is well above physiological levels of GTP ($\sim$150 μM) (12). The most likely explanation for the lack of binding is that the assay conditions employed altered the tertiary structure of the $G\alpha_{i1}$ in some way. SDS-PAGE experiments have shown that the antibodies are unable to detect denatured G-protein, indicating that they are sensitive to its tertiary structure (7). All previous experiments with these antibodies have been conducted with G-protein in a cellular environment, including the fluorometric microvolume assay technology (FMAT) screen used to select the three hybridoma clones of interest (8A5, 8D11 and 6F12) (Figure 17.2). It is therefore possible that the antibodies were selected for binding to a cellular conformation that cannot be mimicked in a biochemical situation. Experiments using cell membrane preparations were performed in an attempt to mimic a more 'cellular' environment (data not shown); however, these proved difficult due to the crude nature of the samples. Future experiments could exploit the constitutively active mutant $G\alpha_{i1}$ $Q^{204}L$, which has previously been shown to bind to the test antibodies in a cellular assay with an affinity equal to or greater than GTPγS-loaded $G\alpha_{i1}$ (7). This mutant could be used to develop a cell-based label-free assay of antibody binding.

In addition to continued efforts to develop and optimise a truly label-free assay of G-protein activation using the three anti-$G\alpha_i$ antibodies 8A5, 8D11 and 6F12, work is continuing to identify additional applications of these reagents for the study of G-protein binding, such as a nonradioactive GTPγS plate-based assay or TR-FRET system.

ACKNOWLEDGEMENTS

The authors would like to thank Ian Kinghorn (GlaxoSmithKline Bioreagents department, Stevenage) for provision of the anti-$G\alpha_{i1}$ and mouse IgG1 isotype control antibodies, and Peter Lowe (SRU Biosystems) for help with the SRU BIND® protocols. We would also like to acknowledge Robert Lane and Graeme Milligan at the University of Glasgow for the initial work to identify the conformation specific antibodies. Finally, we would like to thank Stephen Rees (GlaxoSmithKline Screening and Compound Profiling Department) for his assistance compiling this chapter.

REFERENCES

1. E. Jacoby, R. Bouhelal, M. Gerspacher and K. Seuwen, *Chem. Med. Chem.* 1, 761 (2006).

2. A. G. Gilman, *Biosci. Rep.* **15**, 65 (1995).

3. G. Milligan and E. Kostenis, *Br. J. Pharmacol.* **147**, S46 (2006).

4. M. Frank, L. Thumer, M. J. Lohse and M. Bunemann, *J. Biol. Chem.* **280**, 24584 (2005).

5. C. Harrison and J. R. Traynor, *Life. Sci.* **74**, 489 (2003).

6. A. G. Gilman, *Annu. Rev. Biochem.* **56**, 615 (1987).

7. R. J. Lane, D. Henderson, B. Powney *et al. FASEB J.* **22**, 1924 (2008).

8. B. T. Cunningham, P. Li, S. Schulz *et al. J. Biomol. Screen.* **9**, 481 (2004).

9. P. Schuck, *Annu. Rev. Biophys. Biomol. Struct.* **26**, 541 (1997).

10. L. L. Chan, B. T. Cunningham, P. Y. Li and D. Puff, *Sens. Actuators B.* **120**, 392 (2007).

11. M. Malmqvist and R. Karlsson, *Curr. Opin. Chem. Biol.* **1**, 378 (1997).

12. J. Jeon, S. Cho, C. Kim *et al. Biochem. Biophys. Res. Commun.* **294**, 818 (2002).

18

SPR-Based Direct Binding Assays in Drug Discovery

Walter Huber

F.Hoffmann-La RocheAG, Pharma Research Basel, Basel, Switzerland

Label-Free Technologies for Drug Discovery   Edited by Matthew Cooper and Lorenz M. Mayr
© 2011 John Wiley & Sons, Ltd

18.1 INTRODUCTION

The identification of high quality hit and lead compounds is of outmost importance in the discovery of new drug molecules. High quality data on the interaction of target biomolecules with potential hits or leads are essential in selecting the best chemical classes for chemical optimization. During the last decade direct, label-free binding assays have come more and more into the focus of the researchers in the pharmaceutical industry. They represent an orthogonal assay format with widespread application along the whole drug discovery pathway (1). Main applications are primary and secondary screening as well as hit and lead confirmation. The present work discusses the advantages of applying surface plasmon resonance (SPR)-based assays in:

 i. Fragment screening
 ii. Lead selection

18.2 SCREENING USING SPR-BASED DIRECT BINDING ASSAY

The pharmaceutical industry is constantly exploring new and innovative methods to discover small molecule drug candidates. One of such methods, fragment-based screening, has become a promising alternative in pharmaceutical research (2). It involves the selection, screening and optimization of fragments of a compound lead. Fragment libraries for screening contain molecules of low complexity and low molecular weight (90–300 Da), but high chemical diversity. Since only low affinity and potency can be expected for such small molecules special screening methods are required. Surface plasmon resonance (SPR) has become an important tool for screening fragments (3, 4, 5), in addition to other technologies such as NMR (6) and X-ray (7).

18.2.1 What is Required for Fragment Screening

18.2.1.1 Assay Quality

The quality of an SPR-based direct binding assay is described as for HTS assay by measures that characterize the robustness and the reproducibility of the assay. For determining the reproducibility of a screen, a set of compounds is tested in replicate. It is important that all experimental steps of a given screen, such as sample preparation, injection mode, washing procedures, and data evaluation, are included in the determination of such measures. The statistical data of the correlation (for instance slope and standard error) are indicative for the reproducibility of the data.

The Z' factor introduced by Zang is a well accepted measure for the robustness of HTS screens. It is calculated according to Equation 18.1:

$$Z' = 1 - \frac{3\sigma_s + 3\sigma_b}{R_s - R_b} \qquad (18.1)$$

In this equation, the indices s and b denote the variation (σ) or the average response (R) of the positive (s) and a negative (b) control. R_s is determined at saturation concentration of the positive response. With certain limitations, the Z' factor can be used as well for expressing the robustness of an SPR-based fragment screen. Since it compares the variation of the signals with the signal window and since the latter is dependent of the molecular weight of the compound, Z' factors are only relevant measures for robustness if they are determined for controls that have a molecular weight comparable to the average molecular weight of the compounds to be tested. It has been discussed that molecular weight dependent Z' factors can be used to determine the minimum molecular weight and the percentage of compounds of a given library for which statistically relevant (3) data could be expected for that screen. The definition of the Z' factor by Equation 18.1 points at the parameters that have to be optimized to increase the Z' factor of an assay (3).

18.2.1.2 The Screening Cascade

The screening cascade in an SPR-based fragment screen is not fundamentally different from screening cascades in high throughput screening. It contains a series of assays that enable the application of different filter criteria for the selection of true positive binders. An overview on the most commonly used filters is given in Table 18.1.

Single concentration affinity filter: The measured responses at the given concentration should be located in a window that is defined by the average responses and the respective standard deviation of negative and positive controls. Often, the lower limit of a positive response is taken as three times the standard deviation of a negative control. The upper limit of such a window is less well defined. Many of the compounds show over-stoichiometric binding when being screened at high concentration. Gianetti *et al.* point out that non-optimal behavior with respect to

Table 18.1 Overview on selection filters and the respective assay types in screening assays.

Filter	Filter criteria	Type of assay performed
Affinity filter	Response at screening concentration >3× standard deviation of negative control	Single concentration binding assay with wild-type protein
Promiscuity filter	Curve shape during association and/or dissociation, super-stoichiometry, etc.	Single concentration binding assay with wild-type protein
Specificity filter	Response ratio of responses measured on target and on suitable reference protein (active site mutation, blocking)	Single concentration assay with parallel immobilization of wild-type and reference protein
	Displacement of test compound by reference compound	Competition assay with control analyte molecule
Dose response filter	Ratio of responses at different concentrations	Screening at two different concentrations
	Shape of dose response (saturation, slope, etc.)	Dose response assay with concentration series

stoichiometry does not, *per se*, disqualify compounds as good binders (8). They differentiate between "super-stoichiometric" binders (>5 times the saturation response of positive control) and nonstoichiometric binders. It can be argued that there is a fair chance to find good binders within the nonstoichiometric class, but none within the super-stoichiometric one and they discuss reasons why nonstoichiometry can occur for such compounds.

Promiscuity filter: The term promiscuous binders has recently been applied to a class of compounds that often show up in high throughput screens as false positive hits due to their ability to inhibit a broad spectrum of different protein classes. The investigation of promiscuous binding indicates that in solution they often form soluble or colloidal aggregates that often envelop the protein. Gianetti *et al.* (8) recently demonstrated that such promiscuous binding can easily be identified in SPR experiments, and that the time resolution of the assay reveals a number of mechanisms by which such promiscuous binders can inhibit the protein function. The classification scheme presented in this work can be used during the evaluation of single concentration data to rapidly characterize and eliminate such compounds.

Specificity filters: In SPR technology any adsorption of material to the sensing surface will lead to a signal response. The observed signals often result from an overlap of specific binding to desired binding sites on the target biomolecule and nonspecific binding to any place on the surface of the biomolecule or even anywhere on the surface of the sensor. Special care is required to design an experimental set-up that can distinguish clearly between specific and nonspecific binding. Most of the approaches are based on preparing reference channels by immobilizing proteins that are structurally related to the target, but which show no specific binding to control analytes. Another possibility is to perform competition experiments with compounds that bind to the binding site of the target (3, 4, 9, 10).

Ideal proteins to be used as references are those that can be obtained by site directed mutagenesis, that is, by impairing or modifying the targeted site of a given protein via the exchange of one or several essential amino acids. Such a modification influences the binding behavior of compounds to the targeted site without modifying nonspecific binding. Another possibility for preparing an ideal reference channel is to block the target site of the protein with a covalent inhibitor. For instance, inhibitors that form selectively covalent bonds with the activated serine in serine proteases are well known in the literature. Recently, an approach was described that used an inactive form of the active protein (a zymogen) as reference protein (3).

An alternative approach to confirm specific binding is to perform competitive binding assays with a reference compound that binds specifically to the target site (3, 9, 10). In this case, the binding experiments have to be performed with pure test analyte solution, with the reference compound solution, and with mixtures of both. Generally, the compound concentrations in mixtures are the same as those in the solutions that contain analyte and reference alone. In case of noncompetitive binding (different binding sites), the sensor signal that results from the mixtures is simply the sum of the sensor signals that were measured in contact with the solutions that contain the two compounds alone. In case of competitive binding, the resulting signal of the mixture is intermediate between the two signals measured for the solutions containing one of the compounds alone. If the competitor is added at saturation concentration the signal of the mixture corresponds to the signal observed for the competitor solution. The signal that can be expected for the mixture can be estimated by calculating the fractional occupancies of the binding site by competitor and test analyte (3). They can be derived by applying the law of mass action under the assumption that the concentration of the compounds in solution is not changed upon binding (this assumption is only applicable when working with a flow system).

Dose response filters: Dose response filters have high stringency but often also involve the highest workload. They are based on data recorded for dilution series of compounds (8–10 concentrations per compound).

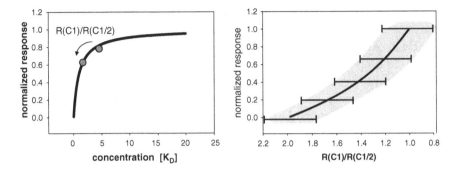

Figure 18.1   The ratio of the responses measured at two different concentrations as an early filter criterion for the selection of positive hits. The concentration behavior of an ideal binder follows a Langmuir isotherm (left). The concentration is given in units of K_D and the responses are normalized responses ($R/R_{saturation}$). The ratio of the responses (R1/R2) measured for the two concentrations ($2 \times C2 = C1$) is continuously changed from 2 ($C \ll C_{saturation}$) to 1 ($C = C_{saturation}$) along this isotherm (black line in the right graph). Compounds with ideal dose response behavior should be located on this line or given a certain experimental error in a closed area around this line (gray area in right graph).

Exclusion criteria are the fit of the experimental data points to theoretical curves with respect to curve slope and saturation behavior. Sigmoidal dose response (response versus logarithm of concentration) or hyperbolic (response versus concentration) functions are both used as theoretical fit functions.

Due to the throughput limitations of most of the presently available SPR systems, complete dose response curves can only be recorded for a restricted number of compounds. In the case of a target for which specificity filters cannot be applied, a first screen could deliver several hundreds of positives; hit rates in primary screens of 10–20% are frequently observed in primary fragment screens. In such cases a rough dose response filter can be applied to data from only two concentrations per compound. It can be shown (Figure 18.1) that the ratio of two responses (R1/R2) measured for a compound at two different concentrations (C1 and C2) varies with the degree of saturation that is reached at one of the concentrations. Based on this theoretical background, the behavior of a compound can therefore be roughly tested by simply measuring the response at two different concentrations and comparing the resulting response ratio with the theoretically expected one (Figure 18.1).

The number of filters might vary from target to target because it strongly depends of the possibilities that are offered by the target to develop the assays needed for the application of the filter. Often binding sites for ligands are not well defined, or positive control ligands to perform competition assay are missing. In this case, no reference proteins can be prepared via blocking or mutagenesis and no competition assay can be performed. In such cases, selection of positive hits relies only on the use of filters such as affinity promiscuity and dose response.

Often, many of the filter criteria can be covered by a single assay. With the flexibility offered by the modern SPR instruments, many reference proteins can be immobilized in parallel with the target protein, making data for selectivity, promiscuity and affinity criteria available in one single assay. The temporal sequence of different assays in a screening cascade is guided by efficiency consideration, that is, assays with lower time demand per tested compound are generally located at the top of the cascade whereas more time consuming assays are at the bottom when filtering has already reduced the number of test compounds. In general, the more complex an assay the more stringent the filter criteria related to it, that is, the filtering becomes more and more stringent along the screening cascade.

18.2.2 Bace-1 Fragment Screen (11)

Bace-1 has been identified by several independent approaches as the first enzyme of an enzymatic cascade that produces β-amyloid from β-amyloid precursor protein, and which plays a role in the development of Alzheimer's disease. Bace-1 is considered as a prime target for the development of Alzheimer's disease therapeutics (12). Bace-1 is classified as a challenging target in drug discovery due to its structural features of a eukaryotic aspartic protease and its high conformational flexibility around the active site. The fact that Bace-1 inhibitors have to traverse the blood–brain barrier adds another level of complexity for drug discovery. To identify new lead molecules of low molecular weight a fragment strategy was applied.

18.2.2.1 The Assay Set-Up

SPR measurements were performed on a Biacore S51 instrument. For the primary screen full length Bace-1 was immobilized (~12 000 RU) by standard amine coupling chemistry on a CM5 sensor. A mutant protein (D39A) was used as a reference protein in the reference channel. Binding experiments were performed using acetate buffer (50 mM, pH 4.6,

150 mM NaCl, 3 mM EDTA, 0.005% P20 and 4% DMSO) as running buffer. Compounds were dissolved in DMSO at a concentration of 100 mM and subsequently diluted in acetate buffer to adjust the final DMSO content (4%) and the respective compound concentration (200 μM). Hits from the primary screen were further investigated for specific binding to the active site by competition experiments using a high affinity ($K_D = 40$ nM) inhibitor of Bace-1 derived from the substrate (pGlu-Val-Asn-statin-Val-Ala-Glu-Phen-am) as competitor compound.

18.2.2.2 Results from the Assay

Figure 18.2 shows a sensogram monitored for the above described set-up with wild-type and mutant protein immobilized in parallel when contacted with a known high affinity (60 nM) small molecule inhibitor. The figure clearly shows that the set-up is highly suitable to identify compounds that bind specifically to the active site of Bace-1.

Figure 18.3 shows a graphical presentation of the screening results obtained from 96 compounds dissolved in a 96-well plate. It is clear from this representation that such a specificity filter is necessary to cut down the number of compounds that are submitted to competition and dose response assays and to crystallization trials. Applying only the affinity (response $>3\times$ standard deviation) and promiscuity filter would lead on this plate to a hit ratio of about 60%. Applying the specificity filter that considers the ratio of the responses of wild-type and mutant protein reduces this number to 2.1%. In the present screen only 300 fragments

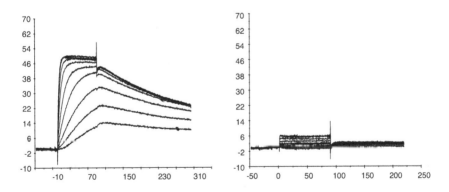

Figure 18.2 Sensogram monitored for the binding of an active compound to wild-type (left side) and an active site mutated (D93A) protein. The set-up is used to indicate active site binding of compounds.

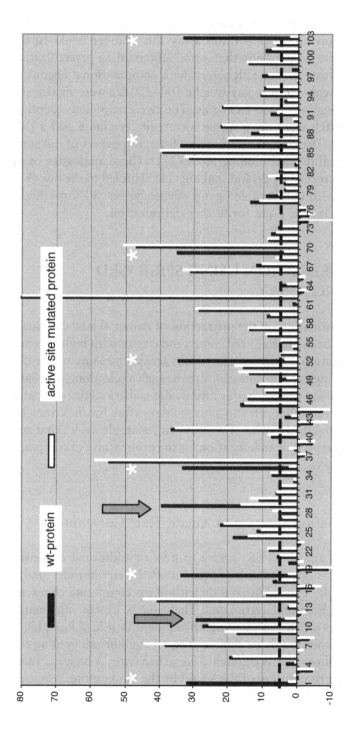

Figure 18.3 Binding responses observed for 96 fragments. Black and white bars indicate the response for the wild-type and the mutated (D93A) protein, respectively. The control compounds injected are marked with a white asterisk. The 3 × standard deviation line is indicated with a black dashed line. Compounds fulfilling the selection criteria (affinity and specific active site binding) are marked with gray arrows.

were screened. 19 compounds passed the affinity, promiscuity and specificity filters. Applying a competition assay this number could further be reduced to five compounds that were submitted to crystallization. From a combination of this SPR screen with computational chemistry, 48 compounds with a molecular weight 100–150 Da were finally submitted for soaking into Bace-1 crystals. The two compounds identified from this approach were the tyrosine metabolite tyramine and a thiopheneacetonitril. The compounds bind in different pockets of the active site and have well defined binding-modes (11). Close analogues of the tyramine were screened by crystal soaking (11). This led to the discovery of compounds with comparable ligand efficiency, but 30 times higher affinity, a good starting point for further optimization.

18.3 LEAD SELECTION USING SPR-BASED BINDING ASSAY

The detailed information on the interaction of potential lead candidates forms the basis for the selection of compound classes with high potential for lead optimization. Beside the data from activity measurements, data from direct binding experiments can support such a selection. SPR-based direct binding assays deliver, beside affinity data, also kinetic parameters (on-rate and off-rate) that offer an additional measure for the characterization of potential lead classes. The following example shows that such kinetic data can represent an indication for the promiscuity of compound classes.

18.3.1 Information Content of Kinetic Rate Constants

The kinetic rate constants (k_{on} and k_{off}) add an additional dimension to the one dimensional ranking of compounds by equilibrium binding constants (13, 14). This additional dimension for compound characterization has long been underestimated. The value of kinetic information becomes obvious when representing all the data in a k_{on}/ k_{off} plot (9, 10, 15). Compounds that have similar or equal equilibrium binding constants (K_D) can show totally different kinetic behavior. A high k_{on} rate is indicative of fast recognition of the ligand by the binding site, whereas a low k_{on} rate can indicate conformational changes that have to occur for an optimal fit of a ligand. High and low k_{off} rates, on the other hand, indicate low and high kinetic stability of the once formed complex. This kind of information is of help to the chemist in the selection and optimization of suitable hits and leads. This type of kinetic-based compound differentiation was used to support lead compound class selection for lead optimization in the Dipeptidylpeptidase-IV (DPP-IV) project.

18.3.2 Lead Selection for DPP-IV

DPP-IV is an accepted target for the treatment of diabetes type II (16). Drug discovery programs are looking for inhibitors that bind to the active site of the enzyme. Kinetic analysis was used to differentiate lead classes with respect to selectivity, reversibility and kinetics of binding.

18.3.2.1 The Assay Set-Up

SPR measurements were performed on a S51 Biacore instrument using a CM5 sensor. DPP-IV was immobilized on the two spots of one flow-through channel. The protein on one measuring spot was treated with an inhibitor that binds covalently and selectively to the serine in the active site of this serine protease (17). This set-up enabled the characterization of compounds with respect to active site selectivity of binding. The concentration series monitored for the kinetic characterization were recorded for five different concentrations of the compound (Figure 18.4)

18.3.2.2 Results from the Assay

The compounds characterized with the set-up described above belonged to three different structural classes: cyanopyrrolidines, benzoquinolizines and pyrrolidinones (Figure 18.5). About 200 compounds were characterized by kinetic rate constants. All of them showed inhibitory effect in an enzymatic assay. The results of the SPR characterization are graphically depicted in Figure 18.5. The figure shows that compounds with similar or equal K_D (points that are located on the same diagonal line) can have totally different time/response curves and, therefore, totally different kinetic rate constants. Rate constants of such compounds can be different by several orders of magnitude. It is interesting to note that the three classes investigated cluster in different areas of the k_{on}/k_{off} plot. There are two classes, the cyanopyrrolidines and the benzoquinolizines,

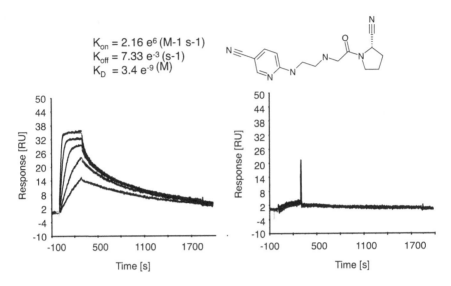

Figure 18.4 Responses monitored for a compound at five different concentrations (125, 62.5, 31.25, 15.625, 7.8 nM) for the active protein (left) and the DPP-IV with the covalently blocked active site (right). The set-up can be used to test for active site specific binding.

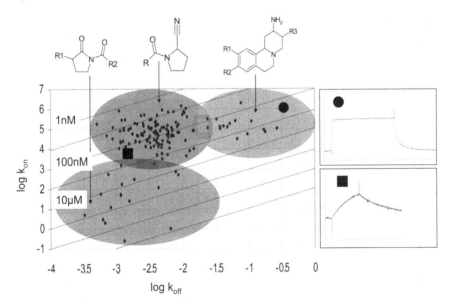

Figure 18.5 k_{on}/k_{off} plot for compounds binding to DPP-IV. The insert shows the binding curves at equal concentration $(C = K_D)$ for two compounds with similar K_D (twofold difference) but totally different k_{on} (100-fold difference) and k_{off} rate (100-fold difference).

with similar on-rates. They differ mainly in k_{off}. The cyanopyrrolidines that cluster in the upper left corner have slow off-rates, resulting in compounds with K_D values in the nanomolar range. This is probably the class from which potential drug molecules could emerge if all other prerequisites for developing a successful medicine are fulfilled. The ben-zoquinolizines in the upper right corner differ from the cyanopyrrolidine class by their fast off-rates. This class can be optimized mainly through structural modifications that slow down the dissociation process, be-cause it appears from the comparison with the cyanopyrrolidines that an increase in K_D is mainly obtained by a decrease in k_{off}. The third class, the pyrrolidinones, contains compounds with similar K_D values as the benzoquinolizines. There are compounds in the two classes that differ in K_D by less then a factor of two but have a 100-fold difference in k_{on} and/or k_{off}. At a first glance, this different behavior could be due to conformational changes that are necessary for binding and inhibitory effect. In this case, however, it could clearly be demonstrated by analyti-cal ultracentrifugation that the unusual kinetic behavior originates from the solution behavior of the compounds. Compounds that exhibit such behavior have been classified recently in the literature as "promiscuous binders" or "frequent hitters" (8).

18.4 CONCLUSION

The two examples presented demonstrate that SPR-based binding assays have become a useful tool for hit and lead finding, as well as hit and lead validation. One of the main advantages of the technology is the high information content of a binding event monitored in real time. In screening approaches, applications such as fragment screening the shape of the time dependent response curve can be used as an additional filter criterion for elimination of promiscuous compounds. In lead selection the quantitative analysis leads to kinetic rate constants that are used as additional information for the differentiation of potential leads. One of the main disadvantages is the fact that the target biomolecules have to be immobilized. The development of an assay set-up can sometimes fail due to instability of the proteins on the surface. In addition, careful characterization of the binding behavior of the immobilized protein and comparison with binding behavior in free solution is a must before start-ing any screening or validation activities. Due to the limited throughput of the technology, applications in screening are presently restricted to a few thousands of compounds.

ACKNOWLEDGEMENTS

The author thanks Josiane Kohler (F.Hoffmann-La RocheAG) for performing the SPR measurements, Jörg Benz, Armin Ruf, Michael Hennig, and Andreas Kugelstatter (F.Hoffmann-La RocheAG) for performing the protein crystallographic work and D.Schlatter, Ralph Thoma, and Fiona Grüninger (F.Hoffmann-La RocheAG) for preparing the proteins.

REFERENCES

1. Cooper, M.A. (Ed.) *Label-Free Biosensors: Techniques and Applications*, edn 1, Cambridge University Press, New York, 2009, 1.
2. J. S. Albert, N. Blomberg, A. L. Breeze, *et al.*, *Curr. Top. Med. Chem. (Sharjah, UAE)*, 7, 1600 (2007).
3. S. Perspicace, D. Banner, J. Benz, *et al.*, *J. Biomol. Screenin*, 14, 337 (2009).
4. M. D. Hämäläinen, A. Zhukov, M. Ivarsson, *et al.*, *J. Biomol. Screenin*, 13, 202 (2008).
5. H. Nordstroem, T. Gossas, M. D. Hämäläinen, *et al.*, *J. Med. Chem.*, 51, 3449 (2008).
6. S. B. Shuker, P. J. Hajduk, R. P. Meadows, and S. W. Fesik, *Science*, 274, 1531 (1996).
7. M. J. Hartshorn, C. W. Murray, A. Cleasby, *et al.*, *J. Med. Chem.*, 48, 403 (2005).
8. A. M. Giannetti, B. D. Koch, and M. F. Browner, *J. Med. Chem.*, 51, 574 (2008).
9. W. Huber and F. Mueller, *Curr. Pharm. Des.*, 12, 3999 (2006).
10. W. Huber, *J. Mol. Recognit.*, 18, 273 (2005).
11. A. Kuglstatter, M. Stahl, J.-U. Peters, *et al.*, *Bioorg. Med. Chem.*, 18, 1304 (2008).
12. I. D. Hills and J. P. Vacca, *Curr. Opin. Drug Discovery Dev.*, 10, 383 (2007).
13. K. Andersson and M. D. Hämäläinen, *J. Chemom.*, 20, 370 (2007).
14. K. Andersson, R. Karlsson, S. Loefaas *et al.*, *Expert Opin. Drug Discovery*, 1, 439 (2006).
15. P.-O. Markgren, W. Schaal, M. D. Hämäläinen, *et al.*, *J. Med. Chem.*, 45, 5430 (2002).
16. R. Thoma, B. Löffler, M. Stihle, *et al.*, *Structure*, 11, 947 (2003).
17. K. Augustyns, G. Bal, G. Thonus, *et al.*, *Curr. Med. Chem.*, 6, 311 (1999).

19

Kinetic Binding Mechanisms: Their Contribution to an Optimal Therapeutic Index

David C. Swinney
iRND3, Institute for Rare and Neglected Diseases Drug Discovery, Belmont, CA, USA

Label-Free Technologies for Drug Discovery Edited by Matthew Cooper and Lorenz M. Mayr
© 2011 John Wiley & Sons, Ltd

19.1 INTRODUCTION

Why is a drug's binding mechanism important to individuals that practice drug discovery and development? The short answer is because an optimal binding mechanism can help determine the therapeutic index and the utility of a medicine. In the current environment of increasing drug attrition rates and efforts to decrease attrition rates, it is surprising that so little effort is spent optimizing the mode of action of a compound. This chapter describes how binding mechanisms, binding kinetics and conformation can contribute to a medicine's therapeutic index and provide opportunities to differentiate medicines.

Much of pharmacological and physiological action requires an interaction between two molecules that leads to a desired response. This point is well recognized as a basis for pharmacological action. Paul Ehrich noted in 1913 that a substance will not work unless it is bound, "corpora non agunt nisi fixata" (1). However, it is important to realize that binding alone is not always sufficient for a substance to communicate the desired message to physiology (2–7). The bimolecular interaction of binding must also lead to effective communication of a message that is robust and safe. Two similarly structured molecules can bind to an enzyme with similar affinity; however, only one will bind in an orientation suitable for the catalytic reaction. Two similarly structured molecules can bind to a receptor with similar affinity; however, one will initiate the response (agonist), whereas the other will block the response (antagonist). Obviously the simple act of binding is required but not sufficient for the desired response.

19.2 WHY ARE BINDING MECHANISMS AND KINETICS IMPORTANT TO DRUG ACTION?

Kinetic binding mechanisms will influence a drug's therapeutic index by shaping dose–response relationships for efficacy and safety (Figure 19.1) (3–5). Kinetic binding mechanisms will determine the biochemical efficiency by which binding is coupled to physiology (3). For example, the concentration of drug required for the efficacy of a rapidly reversible competitive inhibitor will be shifted to higher concentrations in the presence of endogenous effector. The response will require higher concentrations of drug, as a result of the inefficient communication of binding to the physiological response. The higher drug concentrations may also increase the potential for side effects and, thereby, decrease the therapeutic index.

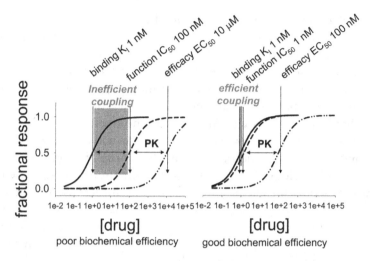

Figure 19.1 Contributions of binding affinity (fractional occupancy), binding mechanism (coupling efficiency) and pharmacokinetics to dose–response relationships. The dose–response relationships quantitatively describe the contribution of binding affinity (solid line), binding mechanism and biochemical coupling efficiency (dashed line) and pharmacokinetics (dash-dot-dot-dash line) to a therapeutic response. The dose–response curves are shifted to higher drug concentrations depending on mitigating factors, such as how effectively binding is coupled to the response (dashed line) and the pharmacokinetics (dash-dot-dot-dash line). These curves demonstrate that a drug with good biochemical coupling efficiency (right panel) will elicit a response at lower concentrations than a drug with poor biochemical coupling efficiency (left panel) when the pharmacokinetics (PK) are similar. The curves simulate one-site binding, in which the binding curves (solid lines) show the response when K_I equals 1 nM, the dashed lines show the response when the biochemical coupling efficiency is 1 (right) and 0.01 (left) and the dash-dot-dot-dash lines show the change in responses when only 1% of the drug is free and available for binding to the target (presumably 99% is bound to serum proteins). (Reproduced with permission from Wolters Kluwer Pharma Solutions (4), copyright 2008.)

The impact of inefficient communication was exemplified in a recent publication by Yun *et al.* concerning the EGF receptor (8). The diminished ATP affinity of oncogenic EGF receptor mutants was used to open a "therapeutic window", that is, it rendered them easier to inhibit relative to the wild-type EGF receptor and other kinases. Resistance mutations in the ATP binding site were subsequently observed to restore the affinity of the kinase for ATP to wild-type levels, enabling ATP to compete more effectively with the inhibitor.

Some kinetic binding mechanisms are intrinsically efficient at coupling binding to function (3). These mechanisms include noncompetitive inhibition and irreversible inhibition. The greater efficiency is apparent in overlapping dose response curves for binding and functional assays

(Figure 19.1). The studies by Yun *et al.* also provided an explanation as to why EGF receptor covalent irreversible inhibitors are insensitive to the resistance mutations (8). Given the lack of competition with ATP, the dose–response curves for the irreversible inhibitors are not shifted to higher concentrations (Figure 19.1). The most significant impact for selection of an optimal kinetic binding mechanism is the presence/potential for mechanism-based toxicity, also termed on-target toxicity (3). A drug with no potential for mechanism-based toxicity will maximize its therapeutic index via kinetic mechanisms in which drug binding is efficiently coupled to physiology. Mechanisms that maintain or decrease the concentrations required to achieve the physiological response will be more efficient. Kinetic mechanisms that are irreversible, insurmountable, noncompetitive, full agonistic or slow dissociating will be safer because lower drug concentrations are required for efficacy. Lower drug concentrations minimize off-target toxicity and result in an increased therapeutic index. In general, drugs used against nonhuman targets, as is the case for most anti-infective agents, will not have mechanism-based toxicity and these kinetic mechanisms are superior in this context. These mechanisms are generally contraindicated for targets in which there is mechanism-based toxicity (Figure 19.2).

For most human targets there is potential for mechanism-based toxicity. Therefore, the challenge is to identify kinetic mechanisms that minimize this potential while retaining the desired response. Competition with an endogenous effector (surmountable with rapid kinetics), uncompetitive inhibition, partial agonism, functional selectivity, and allosteric partial antagonism all involve a kinetic binding mechanism in which the physiological environment can help to shape the dose–response curves in such a manner as to minimize mechanism-based toxicity while retaining sufficient drug efficacy (Figure 19.2) (3–5).

19.3 HOW CAN KINETICS CONTRIBUTE TO AN OPTIMAL MECHANISM?

To help address this question binding kinetics are categorized into four classes depending upon how they communicate binding to pharmacological responses: reversible equilibrium, in which the response will be directly related to the equilibrium binding constant; covalent irreversible inhibition; reversible non-equilibrium; and slow reversible association kinetics associated with conformational change. All of these must be

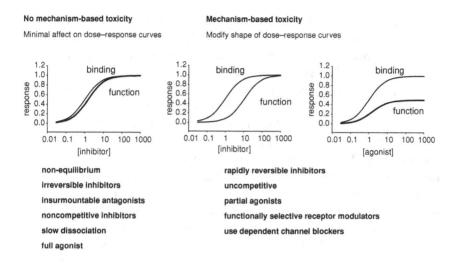

Figure 19.2 A primary driver of the impact of binding mechanism on the therapeutic index is the potential for mechanism-based toxicity. The curves show the relationship of concentration to binding versus function. When there is no mechanism-based toxicity, the binding should be efficiently coupled to function and the dose–response curves will optimally be overlapping (left). When there is potential for mechanism-based toxicity the functional curves may be shifted to the higher concentrations to limit mechanism-based toxicity (center). This is what would be expected with rapidly reversible competitive inhibitors at equilibrium. A decrease in maximal response as seen with partial agonists is another mechanism to minimize mechanism-based toxicity (right). (Reproduced with permission from Wolters Kluwer Pharma Solutions (4), copyright 2008.)

considered in the context of communication of a pharmacological message that maximizes efficacy while minimizing toxicity.

19.3.1 Reversible Equilibrium

Equilibrium is reached when the magnitude of the dissociation rate constant is sufficiently fast as compared to competing rates that the concentrations of the reactants and products have no net change over time. The outcomes from reversible equilibrium binding are under thermodynamic control. Reversible equilibrium binding is commonly seen for substrate competitive inhibitors as described above for ATP competition with the EGF receptor (8). The competition will result in a rightward shift in dose–response curves (higher concentrations of drug are required to achieve efficacy); this shift may decrease the therapeutic index if the increase in drug concentrations required for efficacy increases toxicity.

The rightward shift in dose–response curves may not always be a bad thing. If there is a potential for mechanism-based toxicity then a rightward dose–response curve shift may limit the toxicities and enable the drug to be therapeutically useful provided sufficient efficacy can be achieved. Specific examples highlighting the ability of competitive reversible equilibrium kinetics to minimize mechanistic toxicity have been described for the D_2 dopamine receptor antagonist by Kapur and Seeman (9) and the N-methyl-D-aspartate (NMDA) receptor antagonist memantine by Lipton (10). Long residency times of drug candidates with these targets resulted in undesirable side effects. The side effects were reduced with the use of rapidly reversible equilibrium inhibitors. It was postulated that rapid reversibility allows the drug to compete effectively with the high levels of endogenous effector produced by activation of the system. Lipton has highlighted this as a drug discovery strategy, using the NMDA receptor as an example, based on the principle that drug action should be activated by the pathological state that the drugs are intended to inhibit (11).

Reversible equilibrium binding is rarely sufficient to communicate a safe, robust response. The examples above with NMDA and dopamine receptors show how binding must be coupled to the activation of the system to achieve a therapeutically safe response. An analysis of US Food & Drug Administration (FDA) approved medicines between 2001 and 2004 revealed that many different biochemical mechanisms are used to couple binding to physiology in order to communicate efficacious and safe pharmacological responses (Table 19.1) (2).

19.3.2 Covalent Irreversible Inhibition

A number of drugs are irreversible inhibitors (Table 19.2). Irreversible inhibition is desirable in the absence of mechanism-based toxicities because they limit the rightward shift in dose response curves caused by high concentrations of endogenous activators (Figure 19.1 and 19.2). The general liability of irreversible inhibitors is the potential lack of specificity. Drugs targeting monoamine oxidize (MAO) (12), acetylcholinesterase (13) and H^+K^+ ATPase (14) are among the irreversible inhibitors finding therapeutic use (Table 19.2). Irreversible H^+K^+ ATPase inhibitors such as omeprazole are prodrugs, thus specificity is achieved by metabolic activation at the site of action. The mechanism-based toxicity associated with irreversible inhibition of MAO and cholinesterase has limited the use of irreversible inhibitors for these targets. Aspirin is

Table 19.1 Mechanisms of Drugs Approved by the US FDA between 2001 and 2004.

Mechanism	NMEs
Involves a drug stabilized conformational change	*Agonist* almotriptan, apomorphine, eletriptan, formoterol, frovatriptan, travoprost *Partial agonists* tegaserod, aripiprazole *Active antagonist* eplerenone, fulvestrant, pegvisomant *Conformational inhibition* fondaparinux, gemifloxacin, imatinib, pimecrolimus, epinastine, enfuvirtide *Allosteric or noncompetitive* rifaximin, cinacalcet *Uncompetitive-like*-tadalafil, vardenafil, memantine
Irreversible and reversible non-equilibrium	*Chain termination* adefovir, emtricitabine, telithromycin, tenofovir *Irreversible* azacitidine, cefditoren, dutasteride, ertapenem, nitisinone *Slow dissociation* bortezomib, rosuvastatin, valdecoxib, aprepitant, desloratadine, olmesartan, tiotropium, duloxetine, palonosetron, oxaliplatin
Reversible equilibrium binding	atazanavir, erlotinib, ibandronate, gefitinib, miglustat, seraconazole, voriconazole, abarelix, alfuzosin, bozentan, solifenacin, atomoxetine

an irreversible inhibitor of cyclooxygenases, whereas nonsteroidal anti-inflammatory drugs (NSAIDs) such as ibuprofen and naproxen are reversible inhibitors. It is aspirin's irreversible mechanism of inhibition that enables its use as an anti-platelet drug (15).

19.3.3 Reversible Non-Equilibrium

The potency advantages of covalent irreversibility are limited by the potential lack of specificity. Slow dissociation kinetics in a non-equilibrium system produce kinetic irreversibility, pseudo irreversibility or insurmountability (different terms for the same pharmacodynamic behavior)

290 KINETIC BINDING MECHANISMS

Table 19.2   Drugs with slow or irreversible dissociation rates.

Drug	Target	Dissociation ($t_{1/2}$)
Candesartan	Angiotensin II receptor 1	11.5 h
Tiotropium	Muscarinic m3 receptor	34.7 h
Desloratadine	Histamine H1 receptor	>6 h
Maraviroc	CCR5	10.5 h
Lapatinib	EGF receptor	300 min
Buprenorphine	μ-opioid receptor	166 min
Olmesartan	Angiotensin II receptor 1	72 min
Amlodipine	L-type calcium channel	77 min
Aprepitant	Neurokinin 1 receptor	154 min
Oseltamivir	Viral neuraminidase	33–60 min
Darunavir	HIV-1 protease	>240 h
Aspirin	Cyclooxygenase	Irreversible
Omeprazole	H^+K^+ ATPase	Irreversible
Lansoprazole	H^+K^+ ATPase	Irreversible
Clavulanate	β-lactamase	Irreversible
Sulbactam	β-lactamase	Irreversible
Tazobactam	β-lactamase	Irreversible
Selegiline	Monoamine oxidase	Irreversible
Tranylcypromine	Monoamine oxidase	Irreversible
Celecoxib	Cyclooxygenase 2	Irreversible
Finasteride	Steroid 5α-reductase	Mechanism-based
Formestane	Aromatase	Mechanism based
Procarbazine	Guanine alkyltransferase	Irreversible
Orlistat	Pancreatic lipase	Irreversible
Vigabatrin	GABA transaminase	Irreversible

Data from: Tummino and Copeland 2008 Table 2 (7), Swinney 2008 Table II (4) and Swinney 2004 Table 1 (3).

that can provide the potency advantage of a covalent irreversible inhibitor without the selectivity liability. This type of irreversibility is not associated with the formation of irreversible covalent bonds. A recent analysis by Van Liefde and Vauquelin identified a correlation between insurmountable behavior and slow dissociation rates for the angiotensin II receptor 1 blockers known as sartans (15). The insurmountable behavior of the sartans (valsartan, olmesartan and candesartan) is correlated with increased clinical efficacy measured by an increased maximal effect on diastolic blood pressure as compared with the surmountable antagonist losartan (16) and better survival rates on the time to all causes of death in 6876 patients aged 65 years and older (17, 18).

Reversible non-equilibrium kinetics differentiate the L-type calcium channel blocker nifedipine, a dihydropyridine, from verapamil (19). Dihydropyridine binding is voltage dependent, whereas verapamil binding is facilitated by the repetitive depolarization of the channel, a phenomenon described as use or frequency dependence. Verapamil's frequency dependent block is the basis for the use of verapamil in supraventricular tachyarrhythmias, whereas dihydropyridines are used primarily to treat hypertension. Channel blockage by verapamil is enhanced by increased frequency of stimulation. This facilitates accumulation of verapamil-bound channels due to verapamil's slower rate of dissociation as compared to the frequency of channel stimulation. Verapamil does not have time to dissociate in the time it takes for the channel to open and close during the repetitive fast stimulations. The importance of use dependent block is also seen with cardiac sodium channel blockers. The use dependent behavior causes increased drug binding and, consequently, increased sodium channel blockade at faster stimulation rates. The kinetics of drug association and dissociation from the sodium channel differ for the sodium channel drugs flecainide, lidocaine and procainamide (20). The unblocking rate is a key determinant of the steady state block of the sodium channels. When heart rate increases, the time available for unblocking decreases, and steady state sodium channel block increases.

19.3.3.1 Case Study: Cyclooxygenase Inhibitors

Inhibitors of cyclooxygenase 1 and 2 (COX1 and COX2) provide examples of molecules that bind to the same binding site but have different utilities depending on their kinetic mechanisms. Mechanisms of inhibition include reversible equilibrium (exemplified by ibuprofen against COX1 and COX2, and celecoxib for COX1), irreversible (exemplified by aspirin against COX1 and COX2, and celecoxib against COX2), and reversible non-equilibrium (exemplified by the slow binding inhibitor indomethacin against COX1 and COX2).

As noted above, aspirin has anti-platelet activity whereas the other COX inhibitors do not (15). All COX inhibitors bind to the arachidonic acid binding site, but only aspirin covalently inactivates the enzyme by acetylation of Ser530 (21). The irreversible action of aspirin in platelets leads to long lasting anti-thrombotic effects because platelets do not have the capacity to make new enzyme.

Up to 40% of patients treated with selective or nonselective COX inhibitors experience dyspeptic symptoms, abdominal pain, and heartburn, sometimes with severe impairment of their quality of life (22). The relative risk of gastrointestinal (GI) toxicity for aspirin, indomethacin, ibuprofen, and celecoxib was reported as aspirin ≈ indomethacin > ibuprofen > celecoxib. A meta-analysis of the GI safety risk by Henry and coworkers showed that ibuprofen was safer than indomethacin and aspirin; however, this advantage disappeared at higher doses of ibuprofen (23). Endoscopic studies by Lanza also showed greater GI toxicity for aspirin and indomethacin than ibuprofen; these results also showed a dose dependent increase in toxicity with ibuprofen (24, 25). Endoscopic studies showed celecoxib to be almost free of GI side effects (26).

The GI side effects are thought to result from inhibition of prostaglandin formation by COX1, whereas the antipyretic, analgesic and anti-inflammatory actions are principally related to COX2 (27, 28). This hypothesis was the driving rationale for the development of the COX2 selective inhibitors. Accordingly, safer NSAIDs should have a decreased inhibitory affect on COX1 at the clinically approved doses. The affect on COX1 can be evaluated by determining the fractional occupancy of the enzyme at clinical doses. For a system at equilibrium the magnitude of the inhibition should parallel the fraction occupancy. The fraction occupancy at C_{max} drug concentrations (corrected for free fraction) associated with the clinical doses for indomethacin, ibuprofen and celecoxib, all translated to high fractional occupancy of COX1, with no rank correlation between occupancy and GI toxicity (Table 19.3). Ibuprofen and celecoxib had the highest occupancy, but the lowest GI toxicity. It should be noted that the COX2 inhibitors are rapidly reversible inhibitors of COX1, the selectivity of COX2 over COX1 arises from the pseudo irreversible inhibition of COX2 (29). These data suggest that the GI toxicity is not strictly correlated with occupancy of the COX1 active site.

Table 19.3 Calculated occupancies for NSAIDs binding to COX1 in humans.

Drug	Free C_{max}	K_I	Occupancy (%)
Ibuprofen	1.6 μM	0.24 μM	98
Indomethacin	0.056 μM	0.032 μM	64
Aspirin			87
Celecoxib	54 μM	11 μM	83

The fractional occupancy was calculated from the relationship [drug]/(K_I + [drug]). Free C_{max} values were determined from total plasma concentration reported in clinical trials corrected for protein binding. Ibuprofen C_{max} was determined following a 600 mg dose assuming 1.5% free fraction; indomethacin from a 50 mg dose with 1% free fraction; aspirin dependent acetylated enzyme activity after 320 mg dose was used as a measure of irreversibility; celecoxib from a 200 mg dose assuming 2.6% free fraction. See reference (30) for further details.
(Reproduced with permission from Bentham Science Publishers Ltd (30), copyright 2006.)

The transient availability of arachidonic acid for the synthesis of prostaglandins by the COX enzymes creates a non-equilibrium kinetic window and provides the rationale for a kinetic hypothesis for differentiation of drug induced GI toxicity (30). The substrate, arachidonic acid, is released in a bolus from membrane phospholipids following activation of upstream signaling pathways. The released arachidonic acid that is not converted to prostaglandins by the COX enzymes is rapidly reincorporated into phospholipid membranes (31, 32). When the inhibitor dissociation rate, k_{off}, is slower that the rate of substrate disappearance, k_{-S}, then equilibrium will not be achieved.

This is illustrated in the following kinetic scheme, in which S is the substrate arachidonic acid, E is the COX enzyme, and I is the inhibitor:

$$EI \underset{k_{off}}{\overset{k_{on}}{\rightleftharpoons}} E + S \underset{k_{-s}}{\overset{k_2}{\rightleftharpoons}} ES \rightarrow PRODUCT$$

Consequently, less toxicity (and potency) should be observed with rapid dissociating, equilibrium COX1 inhibitors due to competition with substrate, while greater toxicity (and potency) should be observed with irreversible and slow dissociating, insurmountable COX1 inhibitors that cannot achieve equilibrium. The kinetic hypothesis is supported by COX1 specific cellular assays using different concentrations of arachidonic acid. In these assays the inhibition by the rapidly dissociating ibuprofen was reduced (surmountable) by increased arachidonic acid concentrations (33), whereas inhibition by the slow dissociating indomethacin was unaffected by higher concentrations of substrate (insurmountable) (Table 19.4) (34).

Table 19.4 Kinetic differentiation of the response to ibuprofen and indomethacin is dependent upon arachidonic acid concentration in COX1-expressing uninduced HFF 1491 cells.

Inhibitor	$t_{1/2}$ (s)	Low AA IC_{50}	High AA IC_{50}	Inhibition
Ibuprofen	7	2.5 μM	25 μM	Surmountable
Indomethacin	630	0.016 μM	0.023 μM	Insurmountable

See reference (33) for further details. Activity was measured as the amount of thromboxane B_2 formed as determined by enzyme immuno assays. (Reproduced with permission from Bentham Science Publishers Ltd (30), copyright 2006.)

Table 19.5   NSAID dependent GI toxicity correlates better with dissociation rate from COX1 than COX1 fractional occupancy.

Drug	Occupancy	Toxicity	k_{off}
Aspirin	**	*	*
Indomethacin	****	**	**
Ibuprofen	*	***	***
Celecoxib	***	****	****

Reproduced with permission from Bentham Science Publishers Ltd (30), copyright 2006.

The kinetic hypothesis for the GI toxicity correlates with the rank order of the dissociation rates (Table 19.5). The irreversible inhibitor, aspirin, and the non-equilibrium insurmountable inhibitor, indomethacin, have the greatest risk of GI toxicity, whereas the equilibrium inhibitors ibuprofen and celecoxib have the least risk. These observations are consistent with an inability of the non-equilibrium and irreversible inhibitors to effectively compete with the substrate during the time frame of its transient availability. The increasing concentration of substrate is unable to decrease the inhibition (insurmountable). In contrast, the substrate will effectively compete with rapidly reversible equilibrium inhibitors to reduce the inhibition (shift the dose–response curves to the right). The effectiveness of the rapid dissociating ibuprofen and celecoxib for COX1 will be determined by the laws of mass action competition and, as such, higher inhibitor concentrations will eventually result in effective inhibition. The inhibition at higher doses was observed clinically with ibuprofen. As noted above, the GI toxicity of ibuprofen increased with the dose of the drug until there was little differentiation from aspirin or indomethacin (23–25).

19.3.4 Slow Reversible Association Kinetics Associated with Conformational Change

The rate of ligand dependent interaction and stabilization of unique protein conformation states should be slower than the rate of diffusion controlled bimolecular reactions. Accordingly, slow reversible association rates can be associated with conformational changes, whereas the magnitude of the dissociation rate is the principle driver for the previously discussed kinetic mechanisms. A slower association rate can differentiate molecules by indicating the potential for different binding conformations. For many receptors systems, including G-protein coupled receptors (GPCRs) and nuclear receptors, unique conformations may result in the stabilization of specific receptor conformations that selectively interact with other proteins in the physiological system. This behavior is termed functional selectivity for GPCR agonists. In many of these cases changes in the binding kinetics and equilibrium constants associated with the bimolecular interaction between a series of structurally related molecules will not correlate with changes in function. This is because the pharmacological message is defined by the conformational structure, not the occupancy time. Conformational selectivity is most commonly observed with activation of receptor systems.

Conformational selectivity provides opportunities to minimize mechanism-based toxicity while retaining efficacy. Specific conformations may couple more effectively to desired pharmacological responses than undesirable responses. The prototype for this behavior is the selective estrogen receptors modulators (SERMs). Several classes of estrogen modulators have been discovered that have tissue-selective activity: beneficial effects of estrogen but do not promote growth of breast or uterine tissue. Tamoxifen and raloxifene are estrogen antagonists in breast, but have estrogenic effects in bone and the cardiovascular system. Raloxifene also did not stimulate growth of endometrial tissues. Raloxifene is differentiated from tamoxifen and estrogen by its ability to prevent post menopausal osteoporosis and heart disease without increasing the risk of breast or uterine cancer (35).

The tissue selective effects of the selective estrogen receptor modulators (SERMs) are mediated by binding to the ligand binding domain of the estrogen receptor. Binding to the receptor initiates a series of molecular events culminating in the activation or repression of target genes. The SERMs bind at the same site within the core of the ligand binding domain but demonstrate different binding modes, which translates to distinct conformations of the transactivation domain of the receptor. Transcriptional regulation of estrogen receptor is a complex process that involves the participation of coactivators and corepressors. The different conformations presumably change the affinity for the interacting proteins. The change in corepressor affinity alters the composition of the distinct cellular coregulatory complexes that modulate the transcriptional activity (36–38).

19.4 BINDING KINETICS DIFFERENTIATE PHYSIOLOGICAL RESPONSES

Physiology has evolved mechanisms that utilize binding kinetics and conformational changes as binding features to communicate the physiological message. Kinetic control has been suggested to provide physiology a mechanism for ensuring irreversibility in biological systems. In contrast, allostery or thermodynamic control allow for reversible regulation (39). Two examples that highlight the role of binding kinetics in differentiating physiological responses are briefly detailed below.

A linear type of proof reading has been associated with T-cell signaling. The key criteria for T-cell proofreading is the residence time of the antigen–MHC complex with the T-cell receptor. The ligands are molecular complexes between antigenic peptides and proteins of the MHC complex on the surfaces of antigen-presenting cells. Binding of ligand to receptor triggers a series of biochemical reactions in the T cell. If the ligand dissociates after these reactions are complete, the T cell receives a positive activation signal. However, dissociation of ligand after completion of the first reaction but prior to the generation of the final products result in partial T-cell activation, which acts to suppress a positive response (40). The interaction has to be of sufficient duration that a threshold is reached. Kinetic competition between the rate of debinding of a peptide–MHC complex and the rate at which the bound T-cell receptor (TCR) transitions to a signaling competent conformation differentiates the physiological responses.

Functional differentiation due to differential binding kinetics is also observed for antibody- mediated activation of the $Fc\gamma RI$ on mast cells. The long half-life of the complex of IgE bound to the $Fc\gamma RI$ on mast cells (approximately two weeks) as compared with only hours for a comparable IgG complex results in long term sensitization of mast cells and basophils toward activation by allergens and the type I immediate hypersensitivity reaction. The long dissociation rates associated with IgE binding provide the basis for the different immune response kinetics mediated by IgE versus those mediated by IgG (41).

19.5 UTILIZATION OF BINDING KINETICS IN DRUG DISCOVERY. HOW TO GET MAXIMUM VALUE OUT OF KINETIC ANALYSIS?

Effective utilization of binding kinetics and mechanism for drug discovery requires awareness that these features of drug action are important for the effective communication of the desired pharmacological response, and that the optimal kinetic mechanism will depend on the physiological context of the pharmacology. More value can be achieved in the target identification phase of drug discovery through early identification of the kinetic mechanism that enables efficient communication of the desired pharmacological response. Sometimes a very slow dissociation rate will be optimal, whereas in other cases a rapid reversible dissociation rate may be optimal, depending on the physiological context and potential for mechanism-based toxicity. Furthermore, the absolute magnitude of fast versus slow is context specific. Dissociation rates that are fast enough to allow equilibrium to be reached can be considered fast, whereas rates that result in a non-equilibrium response can be considered slow.

Identification of the kinetic mechanism should be a key component of target identification, or at least lead identification. The impact of the mechanism on therapeutic utility is clearly demonstrated by the medicines that bind to the same target but have different therapeutic uses as a result of differences in their kinetic mechanisms (Table 19.6) (4). The mechanistic revelation of the potential diversity of target specific pharmacological functions suggests that the current definition of a drug target is too limited and does not capture the value associated with

Table 19.6 Clinical differentiation of medicines based on binding kinetics and mechanism.

Medicines	Differentiated clinical end-point	Target	Biochemical differentiation
Candesartan/ losartan	Maximum efficacy	Angiotensin II receptor (GPCR)	Slow dissociation kinetics
Tiotropium/ ipratropium	Frequency of dosing	Muscarinic receptor (GPCR)	Slow dissociation kinetics, PD outlast PK
Memantine/ MK-801	Improved safety	NMDA receptor	Fast kinetics
Clozapine/ haloperidol	Improved safety	Dopamine receptor (GPCR)	Fast kinetics
Aspirin/ ibuprofen	High dose improved safety for ibuprofen Low dose therapeutic indication	COX enzymes	Irreversible vs. reversible kinetics
Verapamil/ dihydropyridines	Therapeutic indication	Ca^+ ion channel	Kinetics
Lidocaine/ flecainide	Therapeutic indication	Na^+ ion channels	Kinetics
Estrogen/ raloxifene	Safety	Estrogen receptor	Unique conformational states

discovering a strategy that is therapeutically effective. The definition of a drug target should be expanded to include the kinetic mechanism that communicates the desired functional response. The definition of a target would include (i) the macromolecular protein to which the drug binds and (ii) the kinetic mechanism that communicates a pharmacologically effective therapeutic response. For example, a tight-binding, mechanism-based inhibitor of a specific enzyme (42); a state dependent uncompetitive inhibitor of a specific channel (11); a drug induced conformational change leading to degradation of a specific nuclear receptor (37, 43), and so on. A mechanistic definition of a pharmaceutical target can work to increase focus on function as well as to capture the value created by the discovery of the optimal mechanism.

In practice, it is difficult to identify the optimal kinetic mechanism that communicates the desired response. The identification of an optimal mechanism generally requires physiology to direct the discovery. It is unrealistic in most cases to determine, a priori, the mechanism that will most effectively communicate the desired message. A balance must be maintained between the reductionist considerations required to optimize specific chemical interactions and the physiological considerations required to determine the optimal mechanism for communication. Additionally, the discovery must be driven by the idea and not the technology. Typically this balance will be shifted to the physiological, systems approach during the discovery phase and to the reductionist approach during the optimization phase (Figure 19.3). At no point should either approach be considered absolute, iterative checks between the chemistry of a specific interaction and its physiological consequences are required to identify the optimal mechanism.

Consistent with this opinion is an article by Ohlson on a role for transient binding drugs, which emphasized that we may have gone too far in our reductionist approach to drug discovery and are thus lacking in a proper understanding of the effects of new drugs on whole biological networks (44). He goes on to state that a major objective in the drug discovery process needs to be proper selection of target binding and Absorption, Distribution, Metabolism, Excretion, Toxicology (ADMET) properties as early as possible in the process in order to avoid late and costly failure for drug candidates that are inherently unsuitable. Ohlson draws attention to the potential of transient binding properties of drugs for providing maximum efficacy and at the same time reduced side effects.

The potential for serendipity is an aspect of the physiological approach for identification of the optimal kinetic mechanism that should

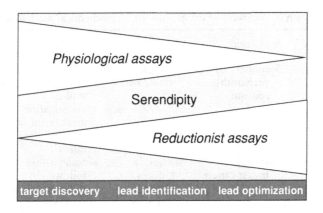

Figure 19.3 Identification and optimization of kinetic binding mechanisms requires physiological assays, reductionist assays, and serendipity. An appropriately balanced interplay between physiological assays to measure the response, reductionist assays to optimize the appropriate chemical interactions, and serendipity to account for physiological complexity is required to identify new medicines. Physiological assays will play a greater role in identification of the target and mechanism, while reductionist assays will have a more significant role in optimization of the chemical interactions that will initiate communication of the desired pharmacological message. Serendipity will be in the background at all stages of drug discovery.

also not be overlooked. There are numerous examples that highlight the importance of serendipity to innovation and drug discovery (Table 19.7). A classic example was the discovery of the H^+K^+ ATPase inhibitors, exemplified omeprazole. This class of highly successful drugs is irreversible inhibitors. They are delivered as prodrugs and are activated by the low pH of the acidic compartment of the parietal cell close to the proton pump. Initial screening using anesthetized dogs found this class of molecules to be active. The investigators originally thought that the pH was important for localizing the drug to the acidic compartment. It was much later that they learned the true nature of the pharmacological action (14).

19.6 CONCLUSION

An optimal binding mechanism will lead to an optimal therapeutic index, and thereby increase the utility of a medicine. Binding kinetics and conformational change are the features of binding through which the medicine interacts with physiology to communicate a safe, therapeutically useful response.

Table 19.7 Path to discovery of drugs with novel biochemical mechanisms.

Drug/Target	Indication	Mechanism	Discovery path	Ref.
Cinacalcet/ Calcium receptor	Secondary hyperparathyroidism	Allosteric modulator	Leads discovered serendipitously in studies investigating mechanism of extracellular Ca^{2+} influx	45, 46
Fulvestrant/ estrogen receptor	Metastatic breast cancer	Antagonist induces receptor degradation	Binding assays followed by functional assays, differentiating factors found serendipitously	47, 48
Memantine/ NMDA receptor	Alzheimer's Disease	uncompetitive blocker	Predecessor found serendipitously; subsequently found to have unique biochemical properties for differentiation	10
Pimecrolimus/ immunophilin	Atopic dermatitis	Indirect allosteric inhibitor	Class found originally in screen for antifungal activity; 20 years later anti-inflammatory activity identified	49
Azacitidine/ DNA methyltransferase	Myelodysplastic syndromes	Irreversible inhibitor	25 years after initial development, molecule's role as a hypomethylating agent discovered, leading to re-evaluation	50
Fuzeon/GP41	HIV infection	Allosteric inhibitor	Molecules discovered serendipitously as part of epitope mapping strategy.	51
Omeprazole/ H^+,K^+ ATPase	Duodenal ulcer; heart burn	Irreversible inhibitor	Optimization in animals leads to discovery of molecules that were activated to irreversible intermediates at the site of action	14

REFERENCES

1. P. Ehrlich, *Lancet* **182**, 445 (1915).
2. D. C. Swinney, *Curr. Top. Med. Chem.* **6**, 461 (2006).
3. D. C. Swinney, *Nature Rev Drug Disc* **3**, 801 (2004).
4. D. C. Swinney, *Pharm. Med.* **22**, 23 (2008).
5. D. C. Swinney, *Curr. Opin. Drug Discov. Dev.* **12**, 31 (2009).
6. R. A. Copeland, D. L. Pompliano, and T. D. Meek, *Nature Rev. Drug Discov.* **5**, 730 (2006).
7. P. J. Tummino and R. A. Copeland, *Biochemistry* **47**, 5481 (2008).
8. C.-H. Yun, K. E. Mengwasser, A. V. Toms *et al. Proc. Natl. Acad. Sci. USA* **105**, 2070 (2008).
9. S. Kapur and P. Seeman, *Am. J. Psychiatry* **158**, 360 (2001).
10. S. A. Lipton, *Nature Rev. Drug Disc.* **5**, 160 (2006).
11. S. A. Lipton, *Nature Rev. Neurosci.* **8**, 803 (2007).
12. P. Riederer, L. Lachenmayer, and G. Laux, *Curr. Med. Chem.* **11**, 2033 (2004).
13. J. Poirier, *Int. J. Clin. Pract. Suppl.* **127**, 6 (2002).
14. L. Olbe, E. Carlsson, and P. Lindberg, *Nature Rev. Drug Discov.* **2**, 132 (2003).
15. P. W. Majerus, G. J. Broze Jr., J. P. Miletich, and D. M. Tollefsen, in *Goodman & Gilman's The pharmacological basis of therapeutics* (eds J.G. Hardman and L.E. Limbird), McGraw-Hill, New York, NY, USA, 1353 (1996).
16. I. Van Liefde and G. Vauquelin, *Mol. Cell. Endo.*, **302**, 237–243 (2009).
17. F. Zannad and R. Fay, *Fund. Clin. Pharmacol.* **21**, 181 (2007).
18. M. Hudson, K. Humphries, J. V. Tu, *et al. Pharmacotherapy* **27**, 526 (2007).
19. G. A. Kidwell, A. J.Greenspon, R. M. Greenberg, and K. J. Volosin, *Circulation* **87**, 118 (1993).
20. D. M. Roden, in *Goodman & Gilman's The pharmacological basis of therapeutics* (eds J.G. Hardman and L.E. Limbird), McGraw-Hill, New York, NY, USA, 839 (1996).
21. E. A. Meade, W. L. Smith, and D. L. DeWitt, *J. Biol. Chem.* **268**, 6610 (1993).
22. C. Hawkey, N. J. Talley, N. D. Yeomans, *et al. Am. J. Gastroenterol* **100**, 1028 (2005).
23. D. Henry, L. L. Y. Lim, L. A. G. Rodriguez, *et al. Br. Med. J.* **312**, 1563 (1996).
24. F. L. Lanza, *Am. J. Med.* **77**, 19 (1984).
25. F. L. Lanza, G. L. Royer, R. S. Nelson, *et al. Am. J. Med.* **80**, 31 (1986).
26. L. S. Simon, F. L. Lanza, P. E. Lipsky, *et al. Arthritis Rheum.* **41**, 1591 (1998).
27. J. A. Mitchell, P. Akarasereenont, C. Thiemermann, *et al. Proc. Natl. Acad. Sci. USA* **90**, 11693 (1993).
28. T. D. Warner, F. Giulinao, I. Vojnovic, *et al. Proc. Natl. Acad. Sci. USA* **96**, 7563 (1999).
29. R. A. Copeland, J. M. Williams, J. Giannaras, *et al. Proc. Natl. Acad. Sci. USA* **91**, 11202 (1994).
30. D. C. Swinney, *Lett. Drug Des. Discov.* **3**, 569 (2006).
31. J. Balsinde and E. A. Dennis, *Eur. J. Biochem.* **235**, 480 (1996).
32. J. Balsinde, B. Fernandez, J. A. Solis-Herruzo, and E. Diez, *Biochim. Biophys. Acta* **1136**, 75 (1992).
33. D. C. Swinney, A. Y. Mak, J. Barnett, and C. S. Ramesha, *J. Biol. Chem.* **272**, 12393 (1997).

34. S. Kargman, E. Wong, G. M. Greig, *et al. Biochem. Pharmacol.* **52**, 1113 (1996).
35. P. D. Delmas, N. H. Bjarnason, B. H. Mitlak, *et al. N. Engl. J. Med.* **337**, 1641 (1997).
36. A. M. Brzozowski, A. C. W. Pike, Z. Dauter, *et al. Nature* **389**, 753 (1997).
37. H. Gronemeyer, J.-A. Gustafsson, and V. Laudet, *Nature Rev. Drug Discov.* **3**, 950 (2004).
38. B. W. O'Malley, *Mol. Endocrinol.* **21**, 1009 (2005).
39. D. Baker and D. Agard, *Biochemistry* **33**, 7505 (1994).
40. J. D. Rabinowitz, C. Beeson, D. L. Lyons, *et al. Proc. Natl. Acad. Sci. USA* **93**, 1401 (1996).
41. J. M. McDonnell, R. Calvert, R. L. Beavil, *et al. Nat. Struct. Biol.* **8**, 437 (2001).
42. G. Tian, J. D. Stuart, M. L. Moss, *et al. Biochemistry* **33**, 2291 (1994).
43. L. H. Long and K. P. Nephew, *J. Biol. Chem.* **281**, 9607 (2006).
44. S. Ohlson, *Drug Disc. Today* **13**, 433 (2008).
45. E. F. Nemeth, W. H. Heaton, M. Miller, *et al. J. Pharmacol. Exp. Ther.* **308**, 627 (2004).
46. R. Muff, E. F. Nemeth, S. Haller-Brem, and J. A. Fischer, *Arch. Biochem. Biophys.* **265**, 128 (1988).
47. V. C. Jordan, *J. Med. Chem.* **46**, 1081 (2003).
48. A. F. Wakeling, M. Dukes, and J. Bowler, *Cancer Res.* **51**, 3867 (1991).
49. C. Paul, M. Graeber, and A. Stuetz, *Exp. Opin. Investig. Drugs* **9**, 69 (2000).
50. J.-P. Issa and H. Kantarjian, *Nature Rev. Drug Disc.* **4**, S6 (2005).
51. T. Matthews, M. Salgo, M. Greenberg, *et al. Nature Rev. Drug Disc.* **3**, 215 (2004).
52. D. C. Swinney, *Expert Opin. Drug Discov.* **1**, 647 (2006).

20

ITC: More Than Just Binding Affinities

Ernesto Freire
Department of Biology, Johns Hopkins University, Baltimore, MD, USA

20.1 INTRODUCTION

Isothermal titration calorimetry (ITC) has developed into the gold standard for measuring binding affinities. It does so in solution, in a label free-format and without immobilization of any of the reactants. For that reason, it has become customary that any new binding technique is

Label-Free Technologies for Drug Discovery Edited by Matthew Cooper and Lorenz M. Mayr
© 2011 John Wiley & Sons, Ltd

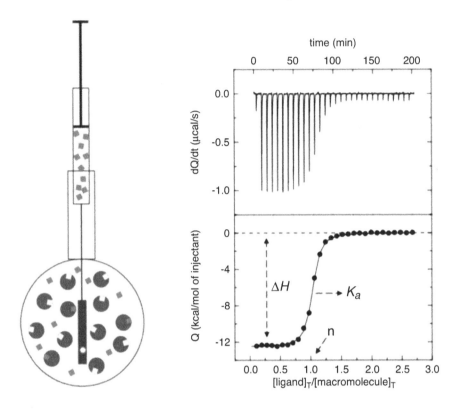

Figure 20.1 In a standard ITC experiment (left) the ligand is added in a step-wise fashion into the reaction cell containing macromolecule. After each ligand addition, the differential heat effects are measured (upper right panel). Integration of those peaks yields the characteristic ITC titration curve (lower right panel). Analysis of the titration curve provides the binding affinity, binding enthalpy, binding entropy and the stoichiometry of the reaction (see text for details).

validated by comparing its results with those of ITC. ITC measures the association between two or more molecules by directly determining the heat that is either absorbed (endothermic) or released (exothermic) when the binding reaction takes place. In modern ITC instruments (Figure 20.1) the binding reaction is triggered to occur in a reaction cell (200 μl in the current generation of instruments) where one of the reactants (usually the macromolecule) is placed.

In standard ITC titration experiments, the binding reaction is started by the injection of the second reactant into the reaction cell (~1.4 μl per injection) (1). Proper mixing is ensured by continuously stirring the solution. A complete titration is generated by the step-wise injection of the second reactant until saturation of the macromolecule is achieved. In the design of an ITC experiment, the concentration of reactants is cal-culated such that complete saturation occurs in fifteen injections or less. The heat associated with each injection is proportional to the amount of complex that is formed. As the macromolecule becomes saturated, the heat effects diminish in magnitude as fewer and fewer ligand molecules bind to the target. After saturation, additional injections produce small heat effects (due to dilution, mechanical or other effects) that must be subtracted from all the injection peaks before performing data analysis. Analysis of the ligand concentration dependence of the heat effect for each injection leads to the determination of the binding affinity (2–4).

Because the experimental observable in ITC is the heat of reaction, analysis of the data also yields the binding enthalpy and the binding entropy for the reaction. Having access to the enthalpy and entropy changes, in addition to the binding constant, provides a complete ther-modynamic description of the binding reaction: a knowledge of the forces involved in a particular binding process and a blueprint of the requirements to achieve extremely high affinity. All together, the infor-mation derived from ITC greatly accelerates the optimization of any lead candidate.

- ITC is the most accurate technique to measure binding affinities.
- In addition to binding affinities, ITC also measures the enthalpy and entropy of binding, thus providing a complete thermodynamic description of the binding reaction.
- ITC provides accurate guidelines for lead optimization.

20.2 WHY SHOULD WE CARE ABOUT ENTHALPY AND ENTROPY?

20.2.1 The Forces of Binding

Two types of forces determine the binding of a ligand to its target: (i) attractive forces between the ligand and the target molecule, like van der Waals interactions or hydrogen bonding; and (ii) repulsive forces between the solvent and ligand, like hydrophobicity, that drive the ligand away from the aqueous medium. It is apparent that maximal binding affinity will be achieved if both forces are maximized; that is, if the ligand is excluded vigorously from the solvent and simultaneously has great attraction to the target. When compounds are identified as potential drug leads by screening or some other methods, usually they exhibit binding affinities in the mid-micromolar range. This affinity level can be achieved without the need to synergistically combine both types of forces. Before they become viable drug candidates, the binding affinity of those compounds needs to be optimized by five orders of magnitude or more, in which case both types of forces need to be harnessed. Obviously, it would be of tremendous help in this optimization process if the balance of binding forces in the lead candidate was known and a strategy aimed at maximizing those forces that contribute marginally could be devised.

The binding affinity (K_a) or its inverse the dissociation constant $(K_D = 1/K_a)$, is determined by the Gibbs energy of binding (ΔG), which in turn is a function of the binding enthalpy (ΔH) and binding entropy (ΔS):

$$-RT \ln K_a = \Delta G = \Delta H - T\Delta S \qquad (20.1)$$

In Equation 20.1, all quantities can be measured by a single ITC experiment. Since different binding forces contribute differently to the enthalpy and entropy of binding, a single ITC experiment provides a clear picture of the binding mode of a compound in addition to its affinity for the target. Among the most important contributions to binding and their thermodynamic consequences, it was found:

- Favorable Enthalpy:
  - Strong Hydrogen Bonds
  - van der Waals Interactions (good shape complementarity)
- Unfavorable Enthalpy:
  - Burying polar groups without establishing strong hydrogen bonds
- Favorable Entropy:
  - Burying hydrophobic groups
- Unfavorable Entropy:
  - Lowering conformational degrees of freedom of compound and/or protein.

20.2.2 Thermodynamic Signature

A convenient way to represent the binding characteristics of a compound is by plotting the enthalpic and entropic contributions to the Gibbs energy in a format that has been called the thermodynamic signature (5–10), as shown in Figure 20.2 for three compounds with very different profiles.

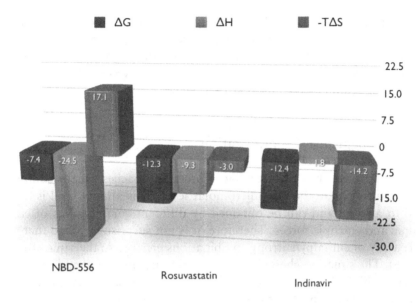

Figure 20.2 The thermodynamic signatures (in kcal/mol) of NBD-556 binding to HIV-1 gp120, rosuvastatin binding to HMG-CoA reductase, and indinavir binding to HIV-1 protease at 25°C. Different enthalpic and entropic contributions to the binding affinity reflect different types of interactions and processes as described in the text.

Figure 20.2 shows the thermodynamic signatures for: (i) rosuvastatin binding to HMG-CoA reductase (8); (ii) for the experimental HIV-1 entry inhibitor NBD-556 binding to gp120 (13); and (iii) Indinavir binding to the HIV-1 protease (9). Rosuvastatin, one of the most potent statins, binds to its target with an affinity of 0.9 nM in a process characterized by favorable enthalpy and entropy changes. The magnitude of the favorable enthalpy (-9.3 kcal/mol at 25 °C) is characteristic of small molecules that bind to proteins by establishing good hydrogen bonding and van der Waals interactions (11, 12). The also favorable entropy change is indicative that the binding is also coupled to the burial of hydrophobic groups. The thermodynamic signature of rosuvastatin should be contrasted with that of NBD-556. In this case, the inhibitor binds gp120 with a large favorable enthalpy and large unfavorable entropy. The large unfavorable entropy is indicative that the binding of NBD-556 is coupled to a large protein refolding event, as burial of hydrophobic groups is associated with a favorable entropy change (13, 14). Finally, the binding of indinavir to the HIV-1 protease is characterized by an unfavorable binding enthalpy and large favorable entropy. An unfavorable binding enthalpy is usually associated with the burial of a polar group that does not establish a hydrogen bond that is strong enough to overcome the unfavorable enthalpy of desolvation (15). The favorable binding entropy, on the other hand, reflects a significant burial of hydrophobic groups. These three examples illustrate the ability of the thermodynamic signature to capture the binding characteristics of a ligand.

20.2.3 Blueprint for Optimization

Compounds identified by screening or other approaches usually exhibit binding affinities in the mid-micromolar level. This affinity level is not hard to achieve and can be obtained by different combinations of enthalpic and entropic forces. Therefore, it is not surprising to find that a wide array of enthalpy/entropy combinations give rise to the same affinity (16). The situation changes as compounds are optimized and display extremely high affinity (e.g., picomolar level). In this case, both favorable enthalpic and entropic forces need to be combined (16).

From the affinity optimization point of view, the strategies will certainly be different if the binding of the lead candidate is either enthalpic or entropic. In the first case, better hydrophobic contributions will be required, whereas in the second case better hydrogen bonding interactions and/or the elimination of unsatisfied polar groups will be required. Experience has shown that entropic optimization by increasing the hydrophobicity of a compound can be easily accomplished, whereas enthalpic optimization of a compound is rather difficult. From this point of view, it is apparent that the optimization of a lead candidate that derives its binding affinity from enthalpic interactions will be easier to achieve; everything else being equal, the enthalpic compound should be preferred. In this respect, the ITC characterization of screening hits should provide important information for the selection of candidates for optimization.

The enthalpic optimization of a compound is difficult for two primary reasons. Firstly, there is a strong desolvation penalty for hydrogen bond donors and acceptors; if these groups do not participate in very strong hydrogen bonds with the target, the desolvation penalty will predominate resulting in enthalpic losses. Secondly, a favorable enthalpic contribution can be compensated by an entropic loss resulting in no affinity gain (11, 17). For those reasons, the development of a thermodynamic pharmacophore that identifies the best locations for enthalpic and entropic functionalities would be highly advantageous.

20.2.4 Thermodynamic Optimization Plot

The thermodynamic signature of a candidate for optimization, as measured by ITC, provides a representation of the contributions of enthalpic and entropic forces to its binding affinity. As such, it also outlines the type of interactions (enthalpic or entropic) that need to be optimized in order to achieve extremely high affinity. The main obstacle at the beginning of the optimization process is that chemical modifications of the compound cannot be made efficiently, since the structural locations for modification, addition or elimination of chemical groups that will have a favorable impact in the binding enthalpy or entropy are not known. The situation can be addressed by creating a Thermodynamic Optimization Plot (TOP) (17).

The thermodynamic optimization plot (Figure 20.3, left panel) is built by setting as ordinate the binding enthalpy (ΔH) and as abscissa the entropy contribution to affinity ($-T\Delta S$). A point corresponding to the experimental coordinates of the lead candidate is drawn $(-T\Delta S, \Delta H)_{lead\ candidate}$ and then a straight line (optimization line) between the experimental $(-T\Delta S, \Delta H)_{lead\ candidate}$ point and the point $(0, \Delta G)_{lead\ candidate}$ is drawn. The resulting optimization line has a slope of -1, and is built with a single experimental point corresponding to the binding thermodynamics of the lead candidate. The main characteristic of the optimization line is that all points that fall on the line have exactly the

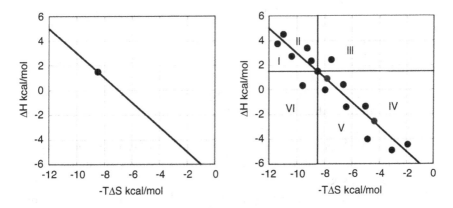

Figure 20.3 The thermodynamic optimization plot (built as described in the text) allows the medicinal chemist to map the impact of chemical modifications on the enthalpy and entropy changes and their impact on binding affinity.

same binding affinity (same ΔG), albeit with different enthalpy/entropy combinations. Likewise, all the points that fall above the line have a lower affinity (more positive ΔG) than the lead candidate and all the points that fall below the line have a higher affinity (more negative ΔG).

At the start of the optimization process, the lead candidate is chemically modified in different ways. The thermodynamic signatures of the resulting compounds are measured by ITC and plotted in the thermodynamic optimization plot (Figure 20.3, right panel). Some compounds will fall on the line and have the same affinity as the lead candidate. Some compounds will fall above the line and have lower affinity than the lead candidate; and some compounds will fall below the line and have better affinity than the lead candidate. By tracing vertical and horizontal lines across the coordinates of the lead candidate the plot can be divided into six different regions as indicated in the figure. Firstly, it should be noticed that all compounds which fall below the horizontal line have better binding enthalpy than the lead candidate and all that fall above, worse enthalpy. Similarly, all compounds that fall to the left of the vertical line have better binding entropy than the lead candidate and all that fall to the right, worse entropy. Together, the six regions indicate different impacts of chemical modifications on affinity, enthalpy and entropy and are used to develop a thermodynamic pharmacophore:

- Region I: More favorable binding entropy and less favorable binding enthalpy. A higher binding affinity because entropic gains are larger than enthalpic losses.
- Region II: More favorable binding entropy and less favorable binding enthalpy. A lower binding affinity because entropic gains are not sufficient to overcome enthalpic losses.
- Region III: Less favorable enthalpy and less favorable entropy. A lower binding affinity.
- Region IV: More favorable enthalpy and less favorable entropy. A lower binding affinity because the entropy losses are larger than the enthalpy gains.
- Region V: More favorable enthalpy and less favorable entropy. A higher binding affinity because the entropy losses are smaller than the enthalpy gains.
- Region VI: More favorable enthalpy and more favorable entropy. A higher binding affinity.

Regions I, V and VI identify modifications that result in improved binding affinities and can be additionally explored with similar functionalities in order to expand the gains. Regions II and IV are particularly important because they cause most bottlenecks in optimization; that is, chemical modifications show enthalpy or entropy gains that are overcompensated by opposite entropy or enthalpy losses. Different strategies to minimize and overcome enthalpy/entropy compensation and achieve higher binding affinity have been proposed (11, 12).

Since the structural locations of all chemical modifications in the lead candidate are known, the thermodynamic optimization plot allows the development of a thermodynamic pharmacophore and, consequently, a more efficient and faster optimization.

20.3 CONCLUSION

The ability of ITC to measure the binding enthalpy and the binding entropy in addition to the binding affinity provides a unique tool for the optimization of drug candidates. ITC allows identification of the forces that need optimization and the necessary requirements to achieve extremely high affinity. The thermodynamic optimization plot derived from ITC, maps structural regions of compounds in terms of their enthalpic and entropic potential, thus allowing the development of a thermodynamic pharmacophore.

ACKNOWLEDGEMENTS

This work was supported by grants from the National Institutes of Health (GM56550 and GM57144) and the National Science Foundation (MCB0641252).

REFERENCES

1. J. M. Brandts, R. K. Brown, R. O'Brien, and W. P. Peters, in *Label-Free Biosensors: Techniques and Applications* (ed. M. Cooper), Cambridge University Press, 2007.
2. T. Wiseman, S. Williston, J. F. Brandts, and L. N. Lin, *Anal. Biochem.* **179**, 131 (1989).
3. M. Straume and E. Freire, *Anal. Biochem.* **203**, 259 (1992).
4. A. Velazquez-Campoy and E. Freire, *Biophys Chem* **115**, 115 (2005).
5. H. Ohtaka, A. Velazquez-Campoy, D. Xie, and E. Freire, *Protein Sci* **11**, 1908 (2002).
6. H. Ohtaka and E. Freire, *Prog Biophys Mol Biol* **88**, 193 (2005).
7. E. Freire, *Drug Discovery Today* **1**, 295 (2005).

8. T. Carbonell and E. Freire, *Biochemistry* **44**, 11741 (2005).

9. E. Freire, *Drug Discov Today* **13**, 869 (2008).

10. J. E. Ladbury, G. Klebe, and E. Freire, *Nat Rev Drug Discov* **9**, 23 (2010).

11. V. Lafont, A. A. Armstrong, H. Ohtaka, *et al.*, *Chem Biol Drug Des* **69**, 413 (2007).

12. Y. Kawasaki, E. E. Chufan, V. Lafont, *et al.*, *Chemical Biology & Drug Design* **75**, 143 (2010).

13. A. Schön, N. Madani, J. C. Klein, *et al.*, *Biochemistry* **45**, 10973 (2006).

14. N. Madani, A. Schön, A. M. Princiotto, *et al.*, *Structure* **16**, 1689 (2008).

15. S. Cabani, P. Gianni, V. Mollica, and L. Lepori, *J. Solution Chem.* **10**, 563 (1981).

16. A. J. Ruben, Y. Kiso, and E. Freire, *Chemical Biology & Drug Design* **67**, 2 (2006).

17. E. Freire, *Chemical Biology & Drug Design* **74**, 468 (2009).

Index

Page numbers in **bold** refer to entries in tables. Page numbers in *italics* refer to entries in figures.